Mathematics for the Allied Health Professions

Mathematics for the Allied Health Professions

Michael P. Highers, M.A.
Associate Professor of Natural Science
Volunteer State Community College
Gallatin, Tennessee

Robert A. Forrester, M.A.
Aquinas Junior College
Nashville, Tennessee

APPLETON & LANGE
Norwalk, Connecticut/San Mateo, California

0-8385-6172-1

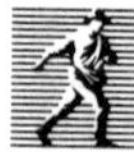

87 88 89 90 91 / 10 9 8 7 6 5 4 3 2 1

Prentice-Hall of Australia, Pty. Ltd., Sydney
Prentice-Hall Canada, Inc.
Prentice-Hall Hispanoamericana, S.A., Mexico
Prentice-Hall of India Private Limited, New Delhi
Prentice-Hall International (UK) Limited, London
Prentice-Hall of Japan, Inc., Tokyo
Prentice-Hall of Southeast Asia (Pte.) Ltd., Singapore
Whitehall Books Ltd., Wellington, New Zealand
Editora Prentice-Hall do Brasil Ltda., Rio de Janeiro

Library of Congress Cataloging-in-Publication Data

Highers, Michael P.
Mathematics for the allied health professions.

1. Medicine—Mathematics. I. Forrester, Robert A.
II. Title. [DNLM: 1. Allied Health Personnel.
2. Mathematics. QT 35 H634m]
R853.M3H54 1987 510'.2461 87-11437
ISBN 0-8385-6172-1

Production Editor: Jennifer L. Schwartz
Designer: M. Chandler Martylewski

PRINTED IN THE UNITED STATES OF AMERICA

To Our Parents
James and Virginia Highers
and
Howard and Wilene Forrester

Contents

Preface

This book is written to show the student how to use mathematics as a tool in the allied health professions. We have tried to present concepts that are applied in the various health fields. To that end, no topic is presented for its own sake.

Although the book assumes 1 year of high school algebra as a prerequisite, each topic is introduced gently, with straightforward language and various examples.

Some features that we feel noteworthy are:

1. A list of objectives at the beginning of each chapter that clarifies exactly what the student should be able to do upon completion of the chapter.
2. Examples, problems, and a chapter test to reinforce the ideas presented.
3. Examples that present not only the steps involved in the solution, but also a commentary that explains each step.
4. A simple "step" approach that makes conversions within the metric system easy to accomplish.
5. The dimensional analysis method of conversion, which can be universally applied to all unit conversions.
6. The division of each chapter into sections that are natural teaching units.

Both of the authors have had extensive teaching experience from junior high school through the university level. This book is written as a teacher would speak to a class. It is hoped that the student will find this style informative, easily comprehensible, and, if not absorbing, at least bearable as mathematics texts go.

The authors wish to thank the following reviewers for their helpful comments: Lawrence Dahl, M.S., Hawkeye Institute of Technology, Waterloo, Iowa; Leo Kling III, Ed.D., Auburn University, Pendleton, South Carolina; Alberta K. Metze, M.S., Trident Technical College, Charleston, South Carolina; and Charles J. Miller, Jr., Ph.D., Camden County College, Blackwood, New Jersey. We also acknowledge the assistance of Wilene Forrester and Bonnita Beasley in preparing the manuscript, and Janet Jones for explaining the profundities of the word processor to us. A tip of the hat goes to Steve Forrester for help in preparing many of the drawings in the text, and to the administration of Volunteer State Community College for its support, both moral and otherwise. Finally, a special thanks to Jennifer Schwartz, our editor, for her energy, thoroughness, and wit, which made finishing the text all the easier.

All mistakes are the sole responsibility of the authors and they would appreciate any suggestions that would make this a better book.

Michael P. Highers
Robert A. Forrester

January 23, 1987

Mathematics for the Allied Health Professions

chapter 1

Topics for Review

OBJECTIVES

After studying this chapter, the student should be able to:

1. Perform all operations involving signed numbers.
2. Simplify expressions involving basic exponential operations.
3. Simplify all expressions involving standard grouping symbols and more than one operation.

1.1 THE REAL NUMBER SYSTEM

Imagine that all numbers—positive, negative, and zero—are to be placed on a horizontal line. Pick a point and call it zero. Also pick a convenient distance that will equal one unit. Numbers to the right of zero will be considered positive. Numbers to the left of zero will be considered negative. Zero is neither positive nor negative. Every point will correspond to a unique number. Conversely, every number will correspond to a point on the line.

The following figure is a number line, with various numbers indicated on it.

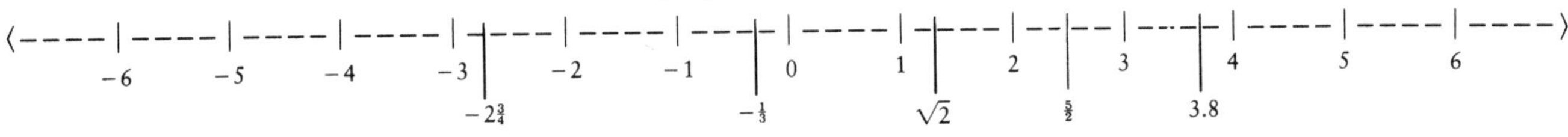

All numbers to the right of zero are positive and will be indicated with a plus sign (+) or no sign at all. All numbers to the left of zero are negative and will be indicated with a minus (−) sign.

Every number on the number line above is a **real number.** Real numbers can be subdivided into the following categories.

I. The **counting** or **natural numbers** are 1, 2, 3, 4 . . .

II. The **whole numbers** are 0, 1, 2, 3, 4, . . .

III. The **integers** are . . . −4, −3, −2, −1, 0, 1, 2, 3, 4 . . .

IV. The **rational numbers** are all numbers that can be expressed exactly as the ratio of two integers. For example, $-\frac{2}{3}$, $-\frac{17}{43}$, and $\frac{119}{2003}$ are rational numbers as well as all of the aforementioned numbers. For instance, 7 is a counting number, a whole number, an integer, and a rational number, since it can be expressed exactly as the ratio of two integers:

$$7 = \frac{7}{1} = \frac{14}{2} = \frac{21}{3}, \text{ etc.}$$

V. The **irrational numbers** are numbers that *cannot* be expressed exactly as the ratio of two integers. Such numbers as $\sqrt{11}$, $\sqrt{7}$, and π are irrational, since there are no integers whose ratios are exactly equal to these numbers. Referring back to the number line, every number indicated on the line is a real number. Moreover, each number is a special type of real number. For example, 2 is an integer, $-\frac{1}{2}$ is a rational number, and $\sqrt{2}$ is an irrational number. It should be emphasized, however, that all of these numbers are **real** numbers.

1.2 ABSOLUTE VALUE

The **absolute value** of a number is its distance from zero, regardless of direction. For example, the number 4 is 4 units to the right of zero and the number -4 is 4 units to the left of zero. Therefore, the absolute value of either 4 or -4 is equal to 4.

Absolute value is indicated by the symbol $|\ |$. The absolute value of 4 is indicated by $|4|$, and the absolute value of -4 is indicated by $|-4|$. Since 4 and -4 are the same distance from zero:

$$|4| = |-4| = 4.$$

The absolute value of any number is always positive since it represents a distance. You would not say that you live "minus" 4 miles from school.

EXAMPLE 1.2.1

Find the absolute value of: -3, -5, -15, $-\frac{2}{3}$.

Solution

$|-3| = 3$

$|5| = 5$

$|-15| = 15$

$$\left|-\frac{2}{3}\right| = \frac{2}{3}$$

1.3 ADDING SIGNED NUMBERS

Having defined the concept of absolute value, we can now proceed with the rules for adding signed numbers.

RULE 1

To add numbers *with the same sign,* add their absolute values and give this sum the common sign.

RULE 2

To add numbers *with different signs,* find the difference between their absolute values and give this difference the sign of the number with the larger absolute value. Always subtract the smaller absolute value from the larger.

EXAMPLE 1.3.1

Add $7 + 23$.

Solution

$|7| + |23| = 7 + 23 = 30$

Comments

Both numbers (or addends) are positive, so we add their absolute values and make the sum positive.

EXAMPLE 1.3.2

Add $-4 + (-32)$.

Solution

$|-4| + |-32| = 4 + 32$

$= -36$

Comments

Both numbers (or addends) are negative, so we add their absolute values. Since the numbers are both negative, we make the sum negative.

EXAMPLE 1.3.3

Add $-23.2 + 50.4$.

Solution

$$|50.4| - |-23.2| = 50.4 - 23.2 = 27.2$$

Comments

The numbers here have opposite signs. The absolute values of the addends are 50.4 and 23.2; their difference is 27.2. We leave this positive since the addend having the larger absolute value is positive in the original problem.

EXAMPLE 1.3.4

Add $7.03 + (-21.924)$.

Solution

$$|7.03| = 7.03$$
$$|-21.924| = 21.924 \text{ (larger absolute value)}$$
$$21.924 - 7.03 = 14.894$$
$$= -14.894$$

Comments

The numbers here have opposite signs. The absolute values of the addends are 7.03 and 21.924; their difference is 14.894.

We give this difference a minus sign since the addend with the larger absolute value is negative in the original problem.

1.4 SUBTRACTING SIGNED NUMBERS

There are two steps in subtracting signed numbers.

Step 1. Change the sign of the number being subtracted (this number is called the subtrahend).

Step 2. Add the numbers using the rules for addition.

RULE 3 $a - b = a + (-b)$; a **and** b **are rational numbers.**

EXAMPLE 1.4.1

Perform each of the following subtractions:

a. $-7 - 8$ **b.** $-\frac{2}{3} - \left(-\frac{1}{6}\right)$ **c.** $8.2 - (-0.85)$ **d.** $14\frac{1}{4} - 17\frac{1}{6}$

Solution

a. $-7 - 8 = -7 + (-8) = -15$

b. $-\frac{2}{3} - \left(-\frac{1}{6}\right) = -\frac{2}{3} + \frac{1}{6}$
$= -\frac{4}{6} + \frac{1}{6} = -\frac{3}{6} = -\frac{1}{2}$

c. $8.2 - (-0.85)$
$= 8.2 + 0.85 = 9.05$

Comments

a. When 8 is subtracted from -7, it is changed to -8 and added according to the rules of addition.

b. When $-\frac{1}{6}$ is subtracted from $-\frac{2}{3}$, it is changed to $+\frac{1}{6}$ and added to $-\frac{2}{3}$ according to the rules of addition.

c. When -0.85 is subtracted from 8.2, it is changed to $+0.85$ and added to 8.2 according to the rules of addition.

d. $14\frac{1}{4} - 17\frac{1}{6}$

$= \frac{57}{4} - \frac{103}{6}$

$= \frac{57}{4} + \left(-\frac{103}{6}\right)$

$= \frac{171 + (-206)}{12}$

$= -\frac{35}{12}$

d. Both mixed numbers are changed to improper fractions. The lowest common denominator is found and the numerators are combined using the rules for adding signed numbers.

1.5 MULTIPLYING OR DIVIDING SIGNED NUMBERS

RULE 4

The absolute value of the product or the quotient is obtained by multiplication or division of the absolute values of each number.

a. The sign of the result is positive if both numbers have the same sign.

b. The sign of the result is negative if the two numbers have different signs.

EXAMPLE 1.5.1

Perform each of the following operations:

a. $6\left(-\frac{1}{2}\right)$ b. $(-3)(-4)$ c. $(-0.25)(0.3)$ d. $\frac{2}{3} \div -\frac{1}{2}$

e. $-\frac{5}{2} \div \left(-\frac{3}{10}\right)$ f. $\left(-\frac{3}{2}\right)\left(\frac{7}{3}\right)\left(-\frac{6}{7}\right)$ g. $\frac{9}{4} \div \left(-\frac{2}{3}\right) \cdot \frac{44}{5}$

Solution

a. $6\left(-\frac{1}{2}\right) = -3$

b. $(-3)(-4) = 12$

c. $(-0.25)(0.3) = -0.075$

d. $\frac{2}{3} \div -\frac{1}{2} = \frac{2}{3} \cdot -\frac{2}{1} = -\frac{4}{3}$

e. $-\frac{5}{2} \div -\frac{3}{10} = -\frac{5}{2} \cdot \frac{10}{-3} = \frac{25}{3}$

f. $\left(-\frac{3}{2}\right)\left(\frac{7}{3}\right)\left(-\frac{6}{7}\right)$

$= -\frac{7}{2} \cdot -\frac{6}{7} = \frac{6}{2} = 3$

Comments

a. Each number has a different sign so the product is negative.

b. Both numbers have the same sign so the product is positive.

c. Each number has a different sign so the product is negative.

d. Each number has a different sign so the quotient is negative.

e. Both numbers have the same sign so the product is positive.

f. If there are more than two factors, work with two at a time, from left to right.

g. $\frac{9}{4} \div -\frac{2}{3} \cdot \frac{4}{5}$

$= \frac{9}{4} \cdot -\frac{3}{2} \cdot \frac{4}{5}$

$= -\frac{27}{{}^{2}\not{8}} \cdot \frac{{}^{1}\not{4}}{5} = -\frac{27}{10}$

$= -\frac{27}{10}$

g. Remember to invert only the fraction immediately behind the division sign. Then proceed as in example f.

PROBLEM SET 1

Perform each of the following operations and simplify your answers. Reduce all fractional answers to lowest terms.

1. $|-3|$
2. $|46|$
3. $|7 - 9|$
4. $8 + (-3)$
5. $-17.5 + (-18.2)$
6. $\frac{2}{5} + \frac{-1}{4}$
7. $-800.73 + 529.47$
8. $-18 - \left(-3\frac{1}{2}\right)$
9. $(-8.63) + (9.23)$
10. $\frac{100}{3} - \frac{205}{3}$
11. $1000 - (-2.5)$
12. $(600)(-40)$
13. $17 - (-1.48)$
14. $215\frac{2}{3} - 8\frac{5}{8}$
15. $(-20) - (-4)$
16. $(52)(4)$
17. $(692.55)(-3.5)$
18. $-768 - 3$
19. $450 + (-844.5)$
20. $\frac{92}{7} - 804$
21. $\frac{2}{3} + \left(-\frac{1}{2}\right) - \frac{6}{7}$
22. $(28)(-5)(3)$
23. $-(0.6) - 1.7 + (-2.5)$
24. $-8000 + (-80) - (-8)$
25. $-7 + (-3) + 5 - 8 + (-3)$
26. $|-(-2) + 3 - 40.6 + (-8.25)|$

(*Hint:* Simplify to a single value before taking absolute value.)

27. $|2 - 7 + (-3)|$
28. $|-8| - |6|$
29. $|2.6| - |-1.5|$
30. $-|-10|$
31. $|-(-2)|$
32. $|-6| - |8 - 12|$
33. $|-50| + |100| - |-25|$

Answers to odd-numbered problems appear on page 227.

1.6 BASIC EXPONENTIAL OPERATIONS

Sometimes it is necessary to multiply a number by itself repeatedly. Exponents allow us to conveniently express this occurrence.

For example, if we wish to use 2 as a factor in multiplication 5 times we would write $2 \cdot 2 \cdot 2 \cdot 2 \cdot 2$. However, this becomes cumbersome if 2 is to be used many times. If we wish 2 to be used as a factor 5 times, we write 2^5. The repeated number (the factor) is called the **base**. The number of times the base is used as a factor is called the **exponent**. The exponent is also called the **power** to which the base has been raised.

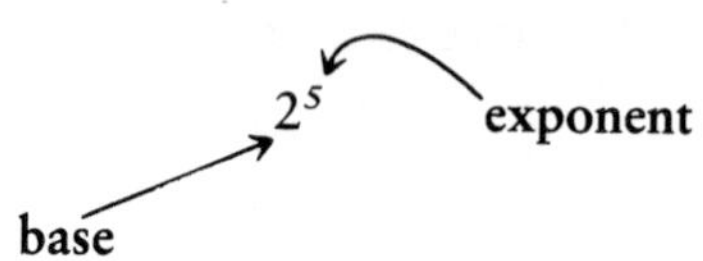

For the present we will make this definition.

RULE 5 $n^P = n \cdot n \cdot n \cdot n \ldots n$ P times, where P is a positive integer.

For this chapter, the exponents will be confined to the positive integers.

EXAMPLE 1.6.1

Evaluate each of the following:

a. 2^3 b. $\left(\frac{1}{2}\right)^4$ c. $(0.5)^3$ d. $(4^3)(2^4)$ e. $3^1 \cdot 2^3$ f. $(3x^2)^3$

Solution	**Comments**
a. $2^3 = 2 \cdot 2 \cdot 2 = 8$	a. Two is used as a factor 3 times.
b. $\left(\frac{1}{2}\right)^4 = \frac{1}{2} \cdot \frac{1}{2} \cdot \frac{1}{2} \cdot \frac{1}{2} = \frac{1}{16}$	b. One half is used as a factor 4 times.
c. $(0.5)^3 = (0.5) \cdot (0.5) \cdot (0.5) = 0.125$	c. The base (0.5) is used as a factor 3 times.
d. $(4^3)(2^4) = 4 \cdot 4 \cdot 4 \cdot 2 \cdot 2 \cdot 2 \cdot 2 = 1024$	d. Four is used as a factor 3 times, and 2 is used 4 times. Then all factors are multiplied together.
e. $3^1 \cdot 2^3 = 3 \cdot 2 \cdot 2 \cdot 2 = 24$	e. Three is used as a factor once. Two is used as a factor 3 times. (If a number has no exponent, its exponent is understood to be 1.)
f. $(3 \cdot 2)^3 = 6^3 = 216$	f. Note how the placement of the parenthesis alters the quantity expressed.

The elevated dot "·" represents multiplication, while the lowered dot represents a decimal point.

PROBLEM SET 2

Evaluate each of the following:

1. $(3)^3$
2. $(4)^2 \cdot (5)^3$
3. $(3)(4^2)$
4. $(2^3) \cdot (4^2)$
5. $(7.2)^2$
6. $\left(-\frac{1}{2}\right)^2$
7. $(-2.5)^2$
8. $(-80)^2$
9. $5 \cdot \left(\frac{1}{5}\right)^4$
10. $(10)^8$
11. $(-2)^4(3)^2$
12. $\left(\frac{1}{2}\right)^3$
13. $(-3.2)(4)^2$
14. $(10)^3(0.375)$
15. $8^2 \cdot 3^2$

16. $\left(-\frac{3}{4}\right)^3$

17. $-\left(\frac{1}{2}\right)^2$

18. $(-0.125)(10)^4$

19. $2^3 \cdot (-3)^2$

20. $(3)^3(2)(-1)^5$

Answers to odd-numbered problems appear on page 227.

1.7 ORDER OF OPERATIONS

It is necessary that we be able to handle correctly a formula or expression that involves a series of different operations. Consider the expression

$$2 + 5 \cdot 3.$$

There are two operations to be performed here, but which one do we do first? If we add 2 + 5 and then multiply by 3, the answer is 21. If we multiply 5 times 3 and then add 2, our answer is 17. The need for a set of rules that tell us the correct **order of operations** is obvious.

The order in which operations are carried out are as follows:

1. Remove *Parentheses* by performing all operations inside them.
2. Remove all *Exponents* by raising all exponential terms to the indicated powers.
3. Do all *Multiplications* and *Divisions* as indicated, from left to right.
4. Do all *Additions* and *Subtractions* as indicated, from left to right.

If we focus on the words in italics and look at their first letters, we get the acronym P-E-M-D-A-S. These letters are also the first letters in the sentence "Please Examine My Dear Aunt Sarah." This may seem an eccentric reminder, but it may also help us to remember the correct order of operations.

A brief note here about parentheses. Symbols, such as a parenthesis, which group numbers or other quantities together are called **grouping symbols**. Examples are:

( ) parenthesis

[ ] brackets

{ } braces

| | absolute value

We will use the first two of these extensively throughout the book. The parenthesis and the brackets serve the same purpose. If, however, a parenthesis is nested inside a bracket, always simplify inside the parenthesis first. In other words, always evaluate grouping symbols from the inside out.

EXAMPLE 1.7.1

Simplify $2^2 - (3 \cdot 2) + 9$.

Solution	**Comments**
$2^2 - (3 \cdot 2) + 9$	Remove parenthesis.
$= 2^2 - 6 + 9$	Evaluate exponent.
$= 4 - 6 + 9$ $= -2 + 9$ $= 7$	There are no indicated multiplications or divisions, so move on to the additions and subtractions as they occur from left to right.

EXAMPLE 1.7.2

Simplify $2 \cdot 3 \div 2 - 6 \cdot 3$.

Solution	**Comments**
$2 \cdot 3 \div 2 - 6 \cdot 3$ $= 6 \div 2 - 6 \cdot 3$	Do multiplications and divisions first as they occur from left to right.
$= 3 - 18$ $= -15$	Do subtraction.

EXAMPLE 1.7.3

Simplify $3 - (2 + 5)^2 - 8 \div 4 \cdot \frac{1}{2}$.

Solution

$3 - (2 + 5)^2 - 8 \div 4 \cdot \frac{1}{2}$

$= 3 - 7^2 - 8 \div 4 \cdot \frac{1}{2}$

$= 3 - 49 - 1$
$= -46 - 1 = -47$

Comments

Remove parenthesis.

Evaluate exponents, do multiplications and divisions as they occur from left to right.

Do subtractions as they occur from left to right.

EXAMPLE 1.7.4

Simplify $4^2 \cdot 3\left(2 - \frac{1}{3}\right) - 5^2$.

Solution

$4^2 \cdot 3\left(2 - \frac{1}{3}\right) - 5^2$

$= 16 \cdot 3\left(\frac{5}{3}\right) - 25$

$= \frac{240}{3} - 25$

$= 80 - 25$
$= 55$

Comments

Simplify inside parenthesis; evaluate exponents.

Do multiplications and division.

Do subtraction.

EXAMPLE 1.7.5

Simplify $-2\left[\frac{1}{2} + \frac{1}{4} + (-8)\right] - 2^3 \cdot 3^2$.

Solution

$-2\left[\frac{1}{2} + \frac{1}{4} + (-8)\right] - 2^3 \cdot 3^2$

$= -2\left[-\frac{29}{4}\right] - 2^3 \cdot 3^2$

$= -2\left[-\frac{29}{4}\right] - 8 \cdot 9$

$= \frac{29}{2} - \frac{72}{1}$

$= -\frac{115}{2}$

Comments

Remove bracket (add fractions).

Evaluate exponents.

Do multiplications.

Do subtraction.

EXAMPLE 1.7.6

Simplify $\frac{(2 - 3)(4 + 2)^2}{(7 - 2)(1 + 3)}$.

Solution

Numerator: $(2 - 3)(4 + 2)^2$
$= (-1)(36)$
$= -36$

Comments

Simplify the numerator and denominator separately using the order of operations and then divide.

Denominator: $(7 - 2)(1 + 3)$
$= (5)(4)$
$= 20$

Note that the division line separates the problem into two parts that are simplified separately before division takes place.

$-\frac{36}{20} = -\frac{9}{5}$

PROBLEM SET 3

Simplify each of the following:

1. $(3 - 2)^2 + 4 \cdot 5$
2. $4 - (2 + 5)^2$
3. $7^2 - (2 + 1) \div 3 \cdot 4$
4. $81 + 4^2 - (2 \cdot 6) \div 3$
5. $(3 + 2)^2 - 9^2 \cdot 3^2 \div 27$
6. $9 \cdot 3 - 9 \cdot 2^2 - (4 + 5)^2$
7. $(2 \cdot 3)^2 - (5 \cdot 4)^2 \div (2 \cdot 4)$
8. $39 \div 13 \cdot 3 - 2 + 5$
9. $(10 + 2)^2 + (5 - 2)^3 - 4^2 \cdot 3$
10. $6 + (5 - 2)^3 \cdot 4 \div 2 \cdot (3 \cdot 2)^4$
11. $6 + 3 \cdot (-2)3 - 8[1 - 20 \div 10) \cdot 2^2]$
12. $7^2 + 3(-2)^3 - 2(1 - 11)$
13. $(60 - 2^2) \div (-2) + 2[2 - 6(1 - 3)]$
14. $(6 - 2)^3 \div (-4)^2$
15. $-5 - (3 - 5) + 4(2 - 8)^2$
16. $(8 \cdot 2)^2 \div (-2)^3 - (2 - 3)^2$
17. $-45 \div -\frac{5}{3} \cdot (-2) - (-100)$
18. $[14 - 2^2 \div (-2)]^2$
19. $(2 \cdot 3)^2 - [6 - 2(3^2 - 1)]$
20. $(4 \cdot 5)^2 \div 2 - 50 \cdot \frac{1}{2}$

Answers to odd-numbered problems appear on page 227.

CHAPTER REVIEW

(1.1)

Characterize each number by one or more of the following descriptions: real, rational, natural, integer, whole, irrational.

1. -37
2. $\frac{5}{3}$
3. $\sqrt{9}$
4. $-\frac{400}{7}$
5. $\sqrt{3}$

(1.2; 1.3; 1.4)

Perform the following operations and simplify.

6. $|-8|$
7. $-|7|$
8. $|-3| - |-4|$
9. $|200 - 3| + |-100|$
10. $|-50| - |200|$
11. $|8.6 - (-1.2)| - |0.05|$
12. $6 + 3$
13. $9 + (-3)$
14. $100 - 52$
15. $-32 + (-6)$
16. $-(-4) + 8$
17. $-15 - 1.5$

(1.5)

18. $(-3.5)(-1.2)$
19. $(-3) - (-1.5)(2)$

(1.6)

20. 3^4

21. $(-2)^5$

22. $(1 - 2)^5$

23. $\left(-\frac{2}{3}\right)^3$

(1.2–1.7)

24. $\frac{13}{2} + \left(-\frac{1}{2}\right) - \left(-\frac{4}{39}\right)$

25. $(6 - 2)^2 - (2 \cdot 5) - 3^2$

26. $20 - (2 \cdot 5) \div 2 + 4^2$

27. $8 \cdot 2^2 \div 4 \cdot 2^4$

28. $38 \cdot 2 + 5 - (-8)^2$

29. $1000 \div 10^2 \cdot 4 \div 2 - (-4)^3$

30. Given the formula $(a - b)(a + 3)^2 - b^2 = K$, find K when $a = -4$ and $b = \frac{1}{2}$.

(*Hint*: Substitute -4 for a and $\frac{1}{2}$ for b, and then use the order of operations.)

Answers to odd-numbered problems appear on page 228.

chapter **2**

Algebra Review—Exponents and Radicals

OBJECTIVES

After studying this chapter, the student should be able to:

1. Understand the concepts of exponents and successfully solve problems that involve their manipulation.
2. Understand the concepts of radicals and square roots and solve problems involving them.
3. Extend the rules of exponents to apply to zero and rational exponents.
4. Write radical expressions in terms of exponents and exponential expressions in terms of radicals.
5. Simplify the combination of exponential terms using the concept of like terms.

2.1 DEFINITION OF EXPONENT

As discussed in Section 1.6, it is sometimes necessary to use the same quantity repeatedly as a factor. To indicate this, we use the exponent.

Suppose the number 2 is to be used as a factor five times. This is indicated by writing $2 \cdot 2 \cdot 2 \cdot 2 \cdot 2$.

We make use of the exponent to express this same quantity as follows:

$$2 \cdot 2 \cdot 2 \cdot 2 \cdot 2 = 2^5 = 32$$

The "5" is the exponent, since it indicates how many times 2 is to be used as a factor; 2 is called the base. We can generalize to give the following definition:

An **exponent** is a number that indicates how many times another quantity, the **base**, is used as a factor in multiplication.

An exponent may also be referred to as the **power** of a base. For example, we can say that 32 is 2 raised to the fifth power. Consider the following example.

EXAMPLE 2.1.1

Evaluate each of the following:
a. 4^4 **b.** 7^3 **c.** 20^2 **d.** $(1.6)^5$

Solution	**Comments**
a. $4^4 = 4 \cdot 4 \cdot 4 \cdot 4 = 256$	a. 4 is the base as well as the exponent; 256 is 4 raised to the fourth power.
b. $7^3 = 7 \cdot 7 \cdot 7 = 343$	b. 7 is the base; 3 is the exponent; 343 is the third power of 7.
c. $20^2 = 20 \cdot 20 = 400$	c. 20 is the base; 2 is the exponent; 400 is 20 to the second power or 20 squared.
d. $(1.6)^5 = (1.6) \cdot (1.6) \cdot (1.6) \cdot (1.6) \cdot (1.6) = 10.5$	d. 1.6 is the base; 5 is the exponent; 10.5 is the fifth power of 1.6 (to the nearest tenth).

Note that when a quantity is raised to the second power, it is said to be **squared.** When a quantity is raised to the third power it is said to be **cubed.** A base with no exponent shown is understood to have an exponent of 1; for example, $2 = 2^1$.

We may use exponents to evaluate specific quantities expressed by certain formulas.

EXAMPLE 2.1.2

Using the formula $k = vt^2$, find k (the symbol used to represent a constant) when $v = 10$ ft/sec and $t = 2$ sec.

Solution	**Comments**
$k = 10 \dfrac{\text{ft}}{\text{sec}} (2 \text{ sec})^2$	Replace variables with values given for those quantities.
$k = 10 \dfrac{\text{ft}}{\cancel{\text{sec}}} \cdot 4 \text{ sec}^{\cancel{2}\,1}$	Perform the calculations using order of operations. Be careful with the units.
40 ft sec	Notice that constants also have units.

EXAMPLE 2.1.3

Using the formula $k = (vt)^2$, find k when $v = 10$ ft/sec and $t = 2$ sec.

Solution	**Comments**
$k = \left(10 \dfrac{\text{ft}}{\text{sec}} \cdot 2 \text{ sec}\right)^2$	Replace variables with values given for these quantities.
$k = \left(\dfrac{20 \text{ ft} \cancel{\text{sec}}}{\cancel{\text{sec}}}\right)^2 = 400 \text{ ft}^2$	Perform the calculations using order of operations. Be careful with the units.

Notice that in the preceding examples, the presence or absence of the parenthesis made a difference in the outcome.

The quantity vt^2, without the parenthesis, indicates that only the t is squared. However, the quantity $(vt)^2$, with the parenthesis, indicates that the product of v and t is found first, then the product is squared.

Another example further illustrates the importance of the parenthesis.

EXAMPLE 2.1.4

Evaluate $-x^2$ when $x = 3$.

Solution	**Comments**
$-x^2 = -3^2 = -(3 \cdot 3) = -9$	Replace x with 3 and perform the calculation. Notice that, without the parenthesis, only the 3 is squared and the answer is negative.

EXAMPLE 2.1.5

Evaluate $(-x)^2$ when $x = 3$.

Solution

$(-x)^2 = (-3)^2 = (-3)(-3) = 9$

Comments

Replace x with 3 and perform the calculation. Notice that the parenthesis encloses the minus sign and the product is positive.

EXAMPLE 2.1.6

Evaluate $Q = 3t^2 - t + 3$ when $t = -1$.

Solution

$$Q = 3(-1)^2 - (-1) + 3$$
$$= 3(1) + 1 + 3$$
$$= 3 + 1 + 3 = 7$$

Comments

Let $t = -1$ and evaluate Q using order of operations.

EXAMPLE 2.1.7

Evaluate $E = 0.5MV^2$ when $M = 9.11$ g and $V = 3.0$ m/sec.

Solution

$$E = 0.5(9.11\text{ g})(3.0\text{ m/sec})^2$$

$$= 0.5(9.11\text{ g})(3.0\text{ m/sec})(3.0\text{ m/sec})$$

$$= 40.995\,\frac{\text{g}\cdot\text{m}^2}{\text{sec}^2}$$

$$= 41\,\frac{\text{g}\cdot\text{m}^2}{\text{sec}^2}$$

Comments

Let $M = 9.11$ g and $V = 3.0$ m/sec.

Perform the calculations using the order of operations.

Obtain the proper units.

PROBLEM SET 1

1. Evaluate: (Remember to use the order of operations.)
   a. 7^4
   b. $(-3)^3$
   c. 2^4
   d. $\frac{6^3}{2}$
   e. $(1.5)^2$
   f. $9^2 \cdot 3^2$
   g. $\frac{8^3 \cdot 2^2}{4^2}$
   h. $(-2)^3(-1)^4(3)^2$
   i. $\frac{8(-2)^3}{2^2}$
   j. $-(-3)^3$
2. Given $E = mc^2$, find E when $m = 2$ g and $c = 3$ m/sec.
3. Given $S = 2\pi r^2 + 2\pi rh$, find S when $r = 2$ m and $h = 10$ m. ($\pi = 3.14$.)
4. Given $V = \frac{1}{3}\pi r^3 h$, find V when $r = 4$ ft and $h = 12$ ft. ($\pi = 3.14$.)
5. Given $P = -x^2 + 5x - 3$, find P when $x = -2$.
6. Given $s = gt^2 + vt$, find s when $g = 32$, $t = 4$, and $v = 80$.
7. Given $v = \frac{1}{3}\pi r^2 h$, find v when $r = 0.5$ inches and $h = 10$ inches. ($\pi = 3.14$.)
8. Given $A = 4\pi r^2 h$, find A when $r = \frac{1}{4}$ yard and $h = 2.5$ yards.
9. Given $v = \pi r^2 h$, find v when $r = 3.2$ m and $h = 1.0$ m.
10. Given $v = \frac{4}{3}\pi r^3$, find v when $r = 0.3$ feet.

Answers to odd-numbered problems appear on page 228.

2.2 RULES FOR EXPONENTS

It is important that the student undertstand and apply the following rules regarding exponents. Until now all exponents have been positive integers (i.e., 1, 2, 3, 4, . . .). We shall see, however, that this set of rules can be extended to fractional exponents, but first, let us review the basic rules governing exponents.

RULE 1

$$b^m \cdot b^n = b^{m+n}$$

When exponential terms, with the same base, are multiplied, the exponents are added.

EXAMPLE 2.2.1

Simplify each of the following:
a. $2^3 \cdot 2^4$ b. $x^5 \cdot x^7$ c. $(2x)^3(2x)^1$

Solution

a. $2^3 \cdot 2^4 = \underbrace{2 \cdot 2 \cdot 2}_{2^3} \cdot \underbrace{2 \cdot 2 \cdot 2 \cdot 2}_{2^4} = 2^7 = 2^{4+3}$

b. $x^5 \cdot x^7 = \underbrace{x \cdot x \cdot x \cdot x \cdot x}_{x^5} \cdot \underbrace{x \cdot x \cdot x \cdot x \cdot x \cdot x \cdot x}_{x^7} = x^{12} = x^{5+7}$

c. $(2x)^3 \cdot (2x)^1 = 2x \cdot 2x \cdot 2x \cdot 2x = (2x)^4$
$(2x)^3 \cdot 2x^1 = (2x)^{3+1}$

Comments

a. Definitions of exponent $b = 2, m = 3, n = 4.$

b. Definition of exponent $b = x, m = 5, n = 7.$

c. Definition of exponent $b = 2x, m = 3, n = 1.$
Note that when the exponent is equal to one, it is not usually written explicitly.

RULE 2

$$\frac{b^m}{b^n} = \begin{cases} b^{m-n} \text{ if } m > n \\ \dfrac{1}{b^{n-m}} = \text{ if } m < n \\ 1 \text{ if } m = n \end{cases}$$

When exponential terms with the same base are divided, their exponents are subtracted. The symbol ">" means "greater than" and the symbol "<" means "less than." Notice that when Rule 2 is followed, the exponent will always be positive. Later, we will see that exponents do not always have to be positive.

EXAMPLE 2.2.2

Simplify: a. $\frac{2^4}{2^3}$ b. $\frac{x^7}{x^5}$ c. $\frac{(2x)^3}{(2x)}$ d. $\frac{2^3}{2^4}$ e. $\frac{(2x)^1}{(2x)^3}$ f. $\frac{2^3}{2^3}$ g. $\frac{(5y)^7}{(5y)^7}$

Solution

a. $\frac{2^4}{2^3} = \frac{2 \cdot 2 \cdot 2 \cdot 2}{2 \cdot 2 \cdot 2} = 2^{1=4-3}$

b. $\frac{x^7}{x^5} = \frac{x \cdot x \cdot x \cdot x \cdot x \cdot x \cdot x}{x \cdot x \cdot x \cdot x \cdot x} = x^{2=7-5}$

Comments

a. Definition of exponent, and canceling like factors.

b. Definition of exponent, and canceling like factors.

c. $\frac{(2x)^3}{(2x)^1} = (2x)^{3-1} = (2x)^2$

c. This time, use Rule 2, as it is much faster.

d. $\frac{2^3}{2^4} = \frac{1}{2^{4-3}} = \frac{1}{2^1} = \frac{1}{2}$

d. Use Rule 2, $m < n$.

e. $\frac{(2x)^1}{(2x)^3} = \frac{1}{(2x)^{3-1}} = \frac{1}{(2x)^2}$

e. Use Rule 2, $m < n$.

f. $\frac{2^3}{2^3} = \frac{2 \cdot 2 \cdot 2}{2 \cdot 2 \cdot 2} = 1$

f. Use Rule 2, $m = n$.

g. $\frac{(5y)^7}{(5y)^7} = \frac{5y \cdot 5y \cdot 5y \cdot 5y \cdot 5y \cdot 5y \cdot 5y}{5y \cdot 5y \cdot 5y \cdot 5y \cdot 5y \cdot 5y \cdot 5y} = 1$

g. Use Rule 2, $m = n$.

RULE 3

$$(b^m)^n = b^{mn}$$

When an exponential term is raised to a power, the exponents are multiplied. This property is sometimes called the "power to a power property."

EXAMPLE 2.2.3

Simplify: a. $(2^4)^3$ b. $(x^7)^5$ c. $[(2x)^6]^2$

Solution

a. $(2^4)^3 = 2^4 \cdot 2^4 \cdot 2^4 = 2^{4+4+4} = 2^{12}$

b. $(x^7)^5 = x^{7 \cdot 5} = x^{35}$

c. $[(2x)^6]^2 = (2x)^{6 \cdot 2} = (2x)^{12}$

Comments

a. We may solve this using the definition of exponents, and Rule 1.

b. It is easier to use Rule 3, which follows from the definition of exponents and Rule 1, where $b = x$, $m = 7$, and $n = 5$.

c. Use Rule 3, where $b = 2x$, $m = 6$, and $n = 2$.

RULE 4

$$(bc)^m = b^m c^m$$

A product of bases raised to a power is equal to the product of the bases each raised individually to that power. This property is sometimes called the "distributive property of exponents over multiplication."

EXAMPLE 2.2.4

Simplify: a. $(2 \cdot 3)^3$ b. $(xy)^4$ c. $(2pq)^2$ d. $(3^2a^3b^4)^3$

Solution

a. $(2 \cdot 3)^3 = (2 \cdot 3)(2 \cdot 3)(2 \cdot 3)$
$= 2 \cdot 3 \cdot 2 \cdot 3 \cdot 2 \cdot 3$
$= 2 \cdot 2 \cdot 2 \cdot 3 \cdot 3 \cdot 3$
$= 2^3 \cdot 3^3$

b. $(xy)^4 = (x^1)^4 \cdot (y^1)^4 = x^4y^4$

c. $(2pq)^2 = (2^1)^2 \cdot (p^1)^2 \cdot (q^1)^2$
$= 2^2p^2q^2 = 4p^2q^2$

Comments

a. Definition of exponent; Associative property; Commutative property. Definition of exponent.

b. Use Rule 4 to distribute the exponent; then multiply the exponents together (Rule 3).

c. Use Rule 4 to distribute the exponent; then use Rule 3.

d. $(3^2a^3b^4)^3 = (3^2)^3 \cdot (a^3)^3 \cdot (b^4)^3 = 3^6a^9b^{12} = 729a^9b^{12}$

d. Distribute exponent; then multiply exponents together.

RULE 5

$$\left(\frac{b}{c}\right)^m = \frac{b^m}{c^m}$$

A fraction raised to a power is equal to numerator raised to that power divided by the denominator raised to that power. This property is sometimes called the "distributive property of exponents over division."

EXAMPLE 2.2.5

Simplify: a. $\left(\frac{2}{3}\right)^3$ b. $\left(\frac{x}{y}\right)^4$ c. $\left(\frac{2p}{q}\right)^2$ d. $\left(\frac{4m^2}{n^3}\right)^4$

Solution

a. $\left(\frac{2}{3}\right)^3 = \frac{2}{3} \cdot \frac{2}{3} \cdot \frac{2}{3} = \frac{2^3}{3^3} = \frac{8}{27}$

b. $\left(\frac{x}{y}\right)^4 = \frac{x^{1\cdot 4}}{y^{1\cdot 4}} = \frac{x^4}{y^4}$

c. $\left(\frac{2p}{q}\right)^2 = \frac{2^{1\cdot 2}p^{1\cdot 2}}{q^{1\cdot 2}} = \frac{2^2p^2}{q^2} = \frac{4p^2}{q^2}$

d. $\left(\frac{4m^2}{n^3}\right)^4 = \frac{4^{1\cdot 4}m^{2\cdot 4}}{n^{3\cdot 4}} = \frac{4^4m^8}{n^{12}} = \frac{256m^8}{n^{12}}$

Comments

a. We can use the definition of the exponents; Rule 1.

b. Use Rule 5 and distribute the exponent to each base; then multiply the exponents of the bases together.

c. Use Rule 5 and distribute exponent to each base; multiply exponents together.

d. Use Rule 5 and distribute exponent to each base; multiply exponents together.

We often make use of more than one rule to simplify an exponential expression.

EXAMPLE 2.2.6

Simplify $(3x^2y)^2 \cdot \left(\frac{2xy}{z}\right)^4$

Solution

$$(3x^2y)^2 \cdot \left(\frac{2xy}{z}\right)^4 = 3^2x^4y^2 \cdot \frac{2^4x^4y^4}{z^4}$$

$$= \frac{9 \cdot 16x^8y^6}{z^4} = \frac{144x^8y^6}{z^4}$$

Comments

Use distributive property and power to a power property (Rules 3–5).

Combine like bases (Rule 1); then subtract exponents of like bases (Rule 2).

2.3 ZERO AND NEGATIVE EXPONENTS

Consider the fraction $\frac{2^2}{2^2}$. We know this is equal to 1 because

$$\frac{2^2}{2^2} = \frac{4}{4} = 1.$$

However, we wish our rules to cover *all* situations where one exponential term is divided by another with the same base. Therefore, according to Rule 2,

$$\frac{4}{4} = \frac{2^2}{2^2} = 2^{2-2} = 2^0 = 1.$$

We generalize this to say

RULE 6

$b^0 = 1$, where $b \neq 0$.

That is, any nonzero number raised to the zero power is equal to 1. We emphasize that raising a number to the zero power is *not* the same thing as multiplying it by zero. In the latter case zero is a factor; in the former it is an exponent.

For example, $b \cdot 0 = 0$, whereas $b^0 = 1$.

In the first case b can be zero; in the second case it cannot. 0^0 is a meaningless expression.

EXAMPLE 2.3.1

Simplify: **a.** $3x^0$ **b.** $(5x^2y^0)^2$ **c.** $(3x^3y^4)^0$ (Assume no variable is equal to zero.)

Solution	**Comments**
a. $3x^0 = 3 \cdot 1 = 3$	**a.** Definition of zero exponent.
b. $(5x^2y^0)^2 = (5x^2)^2 = 5^2x^4 = 25x^4$	**b.** Definition of zero exponent. Rules 3 and 4.
c. $(3x^3y^4)^0 = 1$	**c.** Definition of zero exponent when $3x^3y^4 \neq 0$.

Examine the following product:

$$b^2 \cdot b^{-2} = b^{2+(-2)} = b^0 = 1 \ (b \neq 0)$$

According to Rule 1, we add the exponents 2 and -2 to get zero. Then $b^0 = 1$. Now examine another product:

$$b^2 \cdot \frac{1}{b^2} = 1; \ (b \neq 0)$$

We say that $1/b^2$ is the multiplicative inverse (or reciprocal) of b^2 because their product is equal to 1. This is also true of b^{-2}. Since we obtain 1 when we multiply b^2 by either $\frac{1}{b^2}$ or b^{-2}, we can say that

$$b^2 \cdot b^{-2} = b^2 \cdot \frac{1}{b^2} \qquad (b \neq 0)$$

If we divide both sides of this equation by b^2 we obtain

$$b^{-2} = \frac{1}{b^2}$$

We can generalize this to say

RULE 7

$$b^{-m} = \frac{1}{b^m} \qquad (b \neq 0).$$

That is, a quantity raised to a negative power is equal to the reciprocal of that quantity raised to the same numerical positive power.

That is,

$$b^{-2} = \left(\frac{b}{1}\right)^{-2} = \left(\frac{1}{b}\right)^2 = \frac{1}{b^2}.$$

What about an expression such as $\frac{1}{b^{-2}}$? We can convert the negative exponent into a positive one by the following method:

$$\frac{1}{b^{-2}} = \frac{1}{\frac{1}{b^2}}$$ Rule 7

$$= 1 \div \frac{1}{b^2}$$ Divide numerator of fraction by denominator

$$= 1 \cdot \frac{b^2}{1}$$ Invert and multiply

$$= b^2.$$

We can generalize this outcome by stating:

RULE 8

$$\frac{1}{b^{-m}} = b^m.$$

Rules 7 and 8 may be combined to give the following steps to write any fraction with only positive exponents:

Step 1. Any factor in the numerator containing a negative exponent may be moved to the denominator, and be rewritten with a positive exponent.

Step 2. Any factor in the denominator containing a negative exponent may be moved to the numerator and rewritten with a positive exponent.

Using the rules for negative exponents, and these steps, study the following examples.

EXAMPLE 2.3.2

Write each of the following *without* negative exponents.

a. 2^{-3} b. $\left(\frac{1}{2}\right)^{-4}$ c. $\left(\frac{x}{y}\right)^{-1}$ d. $(4)^{-2}$ e. $\frac{2xy^{-4}}{3^{-1}}$ f. $\frac{(2x^2y^{-3})^2}{x^{-3}}$

g. $\left(\frac{2x^2y^{-2}}{y^4}\right)$

Solution

a. $2^{-3} = \frac{1}{2^3} = \frac{1}{8}$

b. $\left(\frac{1}{2}\right)^{-4} = \frac{1^{-4}}{2^{-4}} = \frac{2^4}{1^4} = 16$

c. $\left(\frac{x}{y}\right)^{-1} = \frac{x^{-1}}{y^{-1}} = \frac{y^1}{x^1} = \frac{y}{x}$

d. $4^{-2} = \frac{1}{4^2} = \frac{1}{16}$

e. $\frac{2xy^{-4}}{3^{-1}} = \frac{3^1 2x}{y^4} = \frac{6x}{y^4}$

f. $\frac{(2x^2y^{-3})^2}{x^{-3}} = \frac{4x^4y^{-6}}{x^{-3}}$

$= \frac{4x^4x^3}{y^6}$

$= \frac{4x^7}{y^6}$

Comments

a. Definition of negative exponent (Rule 7).

b. Distributive property (Rules 7 and 8).

c. Distributive property (Rules 7 and 8).

d. Definition of negative exponent (Rule 7).

e. Rules 7 and 8; leave factors with positive exponents alone.

f. Use the distributive property of exponents; Rules 7 and 8.

Combine like bases.

g. $\left(\dfrac{2x^2y}{y^4}\right)^{-2} = \dfrac{2^{-2}x^{-4}y^{-2}}{y^{-8}}$

$= \dfrac{y^8}{2^2x^4y^2}$

$= \dfrac{y^{8-2}}{4x^4}$

$= \dfrac{y^6}{4x^4}$

g. Distribute exponent. Move all three factors in the numerator with negative exponents to denominator. Move factor with negative exponent in denominator to numerator.

Divide like bases by subtracting exponents.

PROBLEM SET 2

Simplify, and evaluate if possible. Leave answers with positive exponents.

1. $2^3 \cdot 2^6$
2. $3^2 \cdot 3^4 \cdot 3^{-2}$
3. $\dfrac{2^8}{2^2}$
4. $\dfrac{4^7 \cdot 4^{-3}}{4^4}$
5. $(x^4)^3$
6. $(y^3)^{-2}$
7. $(xy)^5$
8. $(a^2b)^{-1}$
9. $(2x)^3(xy)^4$
10. $x^5(2x)^4$
11. $\left(\dfrac{x^2}{2y}\right)^4$
12. $(5xy^{-1})^3$
13. $\left(\dfrac{2x}{y^{-1}}\right)^3\left(\dfrac{4x^2y}{x^4}\right)^{-2}$
14. $\left(\dfrac{3x^0}{y^4}\right)^{-1}$
15. $\left(\dfrac{10x^2}{y^{-1}}\right)^0$
16. $\left[x^0\left(\dfrac{1}{y^{-3}}\right)\right]^{-2}$
17. $\left(\dfrac{2x^{-1}y^{-3}}{y^{-4}z^{-2}}\right)^{-1}$
18. $\left(\dfrac{3x^2y^{-4}}{x^0}\right)^2 \cdot \left(\dfrac{5x^{-1}y}{z^{-2}}\right)^{-3}$

Answers to odd-numbered problems appear on page 228.

2.4 RADICALS AND FRACTIONAL EXPONENTS

A **radical** is indicated by the symbol $\sqrt{}$. The quantity under the radical is called the **radicand.** The **index** of the radical indicates what root of the radicand we are taking. It is always a positive integer, and is placed in the slot of the radical unless we have the square root, which has an index number of 2. In this case the index is understood. In all other cases, it is explicitly stated. For example, the square root of 7 is indicated as follows:

$$\sqrt{7}$$

where 7 is the radicand and 2 is understood to be the index.

The cube root of 7 is indicated as follows:

$$\sqrt[3]{7}$$

where 7 is the radicand and 3 is the index.

The fourth root of 7 would be written as $\sqrt[4]{7}$, where 7 is the radicand and 4 is the index.

The nth root of 7 would be written as $\sqrt[n]{7}$, where 7 is the radicand and n is the index.

The nth root of a number is defined as follows:

RULE 9 $\sqrt[n]{b} = r$ if and only if $r^n = b$.

For example, $\sqrt{4} = 2$, since $2^2 = 4$, or 2 is one of the two equal factors of 4; $\sqrt[3]{8} = 2$, since $2^3 = 8$, or 2 is one of the three equal factors of 8; and $\sqrt[5]{243} = 3$, since $3^5 = 243$.

When the index is an even integer, the root indicated is always positive: $\sqrt{4}$ could also be -2, since $(-2)^2 = 4$; but, to avoid confusion, roots indicated by radicals with an even index are always considered positive and are called **principal roots.** Therefore, $\sqrt{4}$ always means $+2$, $\sqrt{9} = +3$, $\sqrt[4]{81} = +3$, and $\sqrt[6]{64} = +2$.

When the index is an odd integer, the **principal root** may be positive or negative. If the radicand is negative the principal root will be negative. For example,

$$\sqrt[3]{-27} = -3, \text{ since } (-3)^3 = -27$$

and

$$\sqrt[5]{-32} = -2, \text{ since } (-2)^5 = -32.$$

If the radicand is positive, the principal root will be positive. For example,

$$\sqrt[3]{64} = 4, \text{ since } 4^3 = 64$$

and

$$\sqrt[5]{243} = 3, \text{ since } 3^5 = 243.$$

Most calculators have **square root** keys on them. They are indicated as follows:

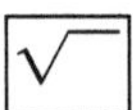

To find the square root of a number, say 52 to the nearest tenth, enter 52 and press the square root button, and round off.

Enter 52

Press [$\sqrt{\ }$]

$\rightarrow 7.2111025 = 7.2$

EXAMPLE 2.4.1 Find each of the following to the nearest tenth.

a. $\sqrt{100}$ b. $\sqrt[3]{1000}$ c. $-\sqrt[3]{27}$ d. $-\sqrt[4]{256}$ e. $\sqrt{105}$ f. $\sqrt{17}$ g. $\sqrt[3]{-1000}$ h. $\sqrt[3]{-64}$

Solution	**Comments**
a. $\sqrt{100} = 10$	a. $10^2 = 100$
b. $\sqrt[3]{1000} = 10$	b. $10^3 = 1000$
c. $-\sqrt[3]{27} = -3$	c. $3^3 = 27$. Be sure to put the $(-)$ sign before the 3.
d. $-\sqrt[4]{256} = -4$	d. $4^4 = 256$
e. $\sqrt{105} = 10.2$	e. Use [$\sqrt{\ }$] on calculator.
f. $\sqrt{17} = 4.1$	f. Use [$\sqrt{\ }$] on calculator.

g. $\sqrt[3]{-1000} = -10$ g. $(-10)^3 = -1000$

h. $\sqrt[3]{-64} = -4$ h. $(-4)^3 = -64$

EXAMPLE 2.4.2

Given $T = \sqrt{l/g}$, find T to the nearest tenth when $l = 9$ ft, and $g = 32$ ft/sec^2.

Solution

$$T = \sqrt{\frac{9 \text{ ft}}{\frac{32 \text{ ft}}{\text{sec}^2}}} = \sqrt{\frac{9 \cancel{\text{ft}} \cdot \text{sec}^2}{32 \cancel{\text{ft}}}}$$

$$= \sqrt{0.28125 \text{ sec}^2} = 0.5 \text{ sec.}$$

Comments

Obtain proper units and use a calculator.

Consider the following equation:

$$(\sqrt{4})^2 = 2^2 = 4$$

This is true because of the definition of a radical. We can generalize this to say

$$(\sqrt{b})^2 = b.$$

We can extend this to any index. For example $(\sqrt[3]{b})^3 = b$, and $(\sqrt[4]{b})^4 = b$. As a general rule, it is true that

RULE 10 $(\sqrt[n]{b})^n = b.$

Now consider another equation

$$(b^{1/2})^2 = b.$$

This is true because of Rule 3. Since $(\sqrt{b})^2 = b$ because of Rule 10 and $(b^{1/2})^2 = b$, we can say

$$(\sqrt{b})^2 = (b^{1/2})^2$$

Therefore, $\sqrt{b} = b^{1/2}$.

We can generalize this to say

RULE 11 $\sqrt[n]{b} = b^{1/n}.$

In the case where the index is even, the radicand "b" is assumed to be zero or positive. A discussion of a negative radicand with an even index, such as $\sqrt{-4}$ or $\sqrt[4]{-81}$, is beyond the scope of this text.

We now have a connection between radicals and fractional exponents with a numerator of 1. For example, $\sqrt[3]{2} = 2^{1/3}$, $\sqrt[5]{xz^4} = (xz^4)^{1/5}$, $\sqrt[4]{xy} = (xy)^{1/4}$, $\sqrt{2y} = (2y)^{1/2}$.

Let us consider the connection between radicals and fractional exponents where the numerator is something other than 1.

Consider $8^{2/3}$. We can also write this as $(8^{1/3})^2$ since $\frac{1}{3} \cdot 2 = \frac{2}{3}$. But $8^{1/3} = \sqrt[3]{8}$, so $8^{2/3} = (\sqrt[3]{8})^2 = 2^2 = 4$.

We can also write $8^{2/3}$ as $(8^2)^{1/3}$, since $2 \cdot \frac{1}{3} = \frac{2}{3}$. But $(8^2)^{1/3} = \sqrt[3]{8^2} = \sqrt[3]{64} = 4$.

So $8^{2/3} = (\sqrt[3]{8})^2 = \sqrt[3]{8^2}$. Notice that the denominator of the fraction, 3, becomes the index of the radical. The numerator becomes the exponent either on the 8 or on $\sqrt[3]{8}$.

RULE 12 $b^{m/n} = (\sqrt[n]{b})^m = \sqrt[n]{b^m}$.

EXAMPLE 2.4.3

Rewrite without radicals.
a. $\sqrt{2x}$ b. $\sqrt[3]{3x^2y}$ c. $\sqrt[4]{4xy^5}$ d. $\sqrt[5]{32zq^3}$

Solution	Comments
a. $\sqrt{2x} = (2x)^{1/2}$	a. Definition of fractional exponent.
b. $\sqrt[3]{3x^2y} = (3x^2y)^{1/3} = 3^{1/3}x^{2/3}y^{1/3}$	b. Definition of fractional exponent.
c. $\sqrt[4]{4xy^5} = (4xy^5)^{1/4} = 4^{1/4}x^{1/4}y^{5/4}$	c. Definition of fractional exponent.
d. $\sqrt[5]{32zq^3} = (32zq^3)^{1/5}$	d. Definition of fractional exponent.
$= 32^{1/5}z^{1/5}q^{3/5} = 2z^{1/5}q^{3/5}$	$2^5 = 32$.

EXAMPLE 2.4.4

Rewrite with radicals.
a. $2xy^{1/3}$ b. $(2xy)^{1/3}$ c. $2^{1/3}x^{1/3}y^{4/3}$ d. $5x^{1/2}y^{1/4}$

Solution	Comments
a. $2xy^{1/3} = 2x\sqrt[3]{y}$ b. $(2xy)^{1/3} = \sqrt[3]{2xy}$	a. Note the placement of the parenthesis and how it affects the outcome of **b** compared to problem **a**.
c. $2^{1/3}x^{1/3}y^{4/3} = \sqrt[3]{2xy^4}$	c. The denominator becomes the index. The numerator becomes the exponent.
d. $5x^{1/2}y^{1/4} = 5x^{2/4}y^{1/4}$ $= 5\sqrt[4]{x^2y}$	d. There must be a common denominator that determines the index of the radical.

PROBLEM SET 3

Evaluate to the nearest tenth. Use a calculator when necessary.

1. $\sqrt{18}$
2. $\sqrt{196}$
3. $\sqrt{25x^2}$
4. $\sqrt[3]{125y^3}$
5. Given $r = \sqrt[3]{vt}$, find r to the nearest tenth in feet if $V = 100$ ft/sec and $t = 4$ sec.

Evaluate.

6. $9^{1/2}$
7. $27^{2/3}$
8. $64^{3/2}$
9. $125^{-1/3}$
10. $81^{-3/4}$

Rewrite without radicals.

11. $\sqrt{2x^2y^3}$
12. $2x\sqrt{y^3}$
13. $\sqrt[3]{64yz^4}$
14. $\sqrt[4]{81q^3}$
15. $\sqrt[5]{32y^4z^2}$

Rewrite using radicals. Note carefully the placement of parentheses.

16. $(144x^2y)^{1/2}$
17. $144x^2y^{1/2}$
18. $25^{1/3}x^{2/3}y^{4/3}$
19. $(2x^2y)^{1/4}$
20. $(100x^4y^2z^3)^{1/5}$
21. $(3x^{2/3}y^{1/4})^{4/5}$

Answers to odd-numbered problems appear on page 228.

2.5 SIMPLIFYING EXPRESSIONS BY COMBINING LIKE TERMS

Examine the exponential terms "$3x^2y$" and "$7x^2y$." These terms are said to be **like terms** because they have the same variables and associated exponents. The numbers (3 and 7) multiplied by the variable factors are called **numerical coefficients**, or simply **coefficients.**

Exponential terms may only be added or subtracted if they are like terms. This is done by combining their coefficients using the rules for signed numbers. For example,

$$3x^2y + 7x^2y = (7 + 3)x^2y = 10x^2y.$$
$$12ab^3 - 4ab^3 = (12 - 4)ab^3 = 8ab^3.$$

The terms "$3x^2y$" and "$7xy^2$" are not like terms because the variables do not have the same exponents. They cannot be added or subtracted into a single term.

To summarize:

1. Like terms may differ only in their coefficients.
2. They may be added and subtracted by combining coefficients using the rules for signed numbers.

EXAMPLE 2.5.1

Underline the pair of like terms in each group.

a. $3yz^3, 7y^2z, 8yz^3, -6yz^3q$ **b.** $-10x, 5xy, -9xyz, 6xy$

Solution	**Comments**
a. $\underline{3yz^3}, 7y^2z, \underline{8yz^3}, -6yz^3q$	**a.** These two terms differ only in their coefficients.
b. $-10x, \underline{5xy}, -9xyz, \underline{6xy}$	**b.** These two terms differ only in their coefficients.

EXAMPLE 2.5.2

Simplify each of the following expressions by combining like terms.

a. $7xy - 6x^2y^3 + 4x^2y^2 + 4x^2y^3 + 9xy$
b. $3x^2 - 7x^2y + 100xy^2 - 14x^2y - 10x$
c. $\frac{1}{2}x - \frac{3}{4}y + \frac{2}{3}x + \frac{1}{5}y$

Solution **Comments**

a. $7xy - 6x^2y^3 + 4x^2y^2 + 4x^2y^3 + 9xy$
$= (7 + 9)xy + (-6 + 4)x^2y^3 + 4x^2y^2$
$= 16xy - 2x^2y^3 + 4x^2y^2$

b. $3x^2 - 7x^2y + 100x^2y^2 - 14x^2y - 10x^2y^2$
$= 3x^2 + (-7 - 14)x^2y + (100 - 10)x^2y^2$
$= 3x^2 - 21x^2y + 90x^2y^2$

Combine coefficients only for terms which are identical except for coefficients.

You may use the commutative rule for addition to rearrange terms.

c. $\frac{1}{2}x - \frac{3}{4}y + \frac{2}{3}x + \frac{1}{5}y$

$= \left(\frac{1}{2} + \frac{2}{3}\right)x + \left(\frac{-3}{4} + \frac{1}{5}\right)y$

$= \frac{7}{6}x - \frac{11}{20}y$

PROBLEM SET 4

Determine if each of the following pairs of terms are like terms.

1. $4x^2y, 3xy$
2. $-\frac{2}{3}xzq, \frac{1}{2}xzq$
3. $-\frac{8}{5}xr^2, \frac{9}{2}x^2r$
4. $\frac{1}{4}xyz^2, -7xy^2z$
5. $21xpt^2, -\frac{14}{5}xt^2p$

Simplify each of the following expressions by combining like terms.

6. $6x + 4x$
7. $5y - 3y + 7y$
8. $11x + 3y - 4x + 8y - 2x$
9. $33xy - 22yz + 6xz - 4xy$
10. $8x - 2yz + 9x - 7yz^2 + 9yz + 15x$
11. $7prs^2 - 15pr^2s + 16p^2rs - 4pr^2s - 6prs^2$
12. $-3a^2b^3c^4 - 5a^2b^3c^3 + 12a^2b^3c^4$
13. $9qz^2 + 6qzt - 4qzt^2 + 8qzt$
14. $8ab - 4ab^2 + 7a^2b + 5b^2a$
15. $18ab^3 - 91a^3b - 6a^3b^3 + 17ab - 4(ba)^3$

Answers to odd-numbered problems appear on page 229.

CHAPTER REVIEW

(2.1)

1. Write each of the following as an exponential term.
   a. $3 \cdot 3 \cdot 3 \cdot 3$
   b. $x \cdot x \cdot x \cdot x \cdot x$
   c. $2y \cdot 2y \cdot 2y$

(2.1) 2. Given the formula $S = at^2$, find S when $a = 32$ ft/sec^2 and $t = 3$ sec.

(2.1) 3. Given the formula $S = 4\pi r^2$, find S when $r = 1.2$ ft. ($\pi = 3.14$.)

(2.2) 4. Simplify:

a. $(2x^2)^3$

b. $5y \cdot (3y^2)$

c. $\left(\frac{2z^3}{y}\right)^4$

d. $(3x^2yz)^4(2yz^4)^2$

e. $\left(\frac{x^2}{y}\right)(2xy^4)^3$

(2.3) 5. Simplify. Do not leave negative exponents in your answer. Note carefully the placement of parentheses.

a. $5y^0$

b. $(5y)^0$

c. $(6y^{-2})^3(2y)^{-1}$

d. $(3x^0)^4$

e. $(2x^{-1}y^{-2})^4(3y^{-1})^{-2}$

f. $\left(\frac{4y^{-1}}{2y^2}\right)^{-1}$

g. $\left(\frac{8y^2z^{-1}}{qr^3}\right)^0$

h. $\frac{3x^{-1}y^{-2}z^3}{zy^2z^{-1}}$

i. $\left(\frac{x^{-1}y^{-1}}{3}\right)^{-1}$

j. $\left(\frac{3xy^2z^{-4}}{9y^{-1}}\right)^2\left(\frac{2y^{-1}z^{-2}}{y^4}\right)^{-3}$

(2.4) 6. Evaluate to the nearest tenth.

a. $\sqrt{109}$

b. $\sqrt{3140}$

c. $\sqrt{2.93}$

d. $-\sqrt{81}$

(2.4) 7. Given the formula $d = \sqrt{a^2 + b^2}$, find d to the nearest tenth when $a = 7$ and $b = 6$.

(2.4) 8. Rewrite using radicals. Note carefully the placement of parentheses.

a. $3x^{1/3}$

b. $(3x)^{1/3}$

c. $2^{2/5}y^{3/5}z^{1/5}$

d. $4x^{2/3}y^{1/3}$

e. $\dfrac{7y^{3/4}}{z^{-1/4}}$

(2.4) 9. Rewrite without radicals.

a. $\sqrt[4]{2xy^3}$

b. $\sqrt{\dfrac{l}{g}}$

c. $3\sqrt{x^2y}$

d. $\sqrt[3]{5x^2y^4}$

e. $\sqrt[3]{\dfrac{3}{4}v^2}$

(2.4) 10. Evaluate.

a. $64^{2/3}$

b. $121^{3/2}$

c. $36^{3/2}$

d. $81^{-1/2}$

e. $27^{-4/3}$

(2.5) 11. Simplify by combining like terms.

a. $0.5x^2 - 5x^2y + 25x^2 - 2.5xy^2$

b. $12x^2yz - 3x^2yz - 4xyz^2 - 100\,xy^2z$

c. $\dfrac{1}{2}pr^2 - \dfrac{3}{4}pr^2 + \dfrac{5}{6}p^2r + \dfrac{1}{3}p^2r^2 - \dfrac{1}{8}p^2r$

d. $4y^2z - 6zy^2 - 6.5yz^2 - 3yz$

e. $-x^2z^2q - 9xz^2q^2 + 20x^2zq^2 - 5x^2qz^2$

Answers to odd-numbered problems appear on page 229.

chapter **3**

Significant Digits and Scientific Notation

OBJECTIVES

After studying this chapter, the student should be able to:

1. Determine the number of significant digits in a given measurement.
2. Round off the result after performing the operations of addition, subtraction, multiplication, or division on measured values.
3. Write any number or measurement in exponential or scientific notation.
4. Perform the operations of addition, subtraction, multiplication, and division with measurements written in exponential or scientific notation.

3.1 UNCERTAINTY IN MEASUREMENT

No measurement, however carefully made, can ever be exact, with the exception of a counting of items. The uncertainty of the measurement will be due either to the nature of the measuring device or the limitations of the person making the measurement.

When we make a measurement, we are allowed to report all of the digits we can measure plus one guessed digit—this becomes our **uncertain digit**. In a few cases are we allowed to guess at two digits (if guessing $\frac{1}{4}$ of a unit, this would equal 0.25 unit). Most reported measurements are assumed to be accurate to ± 1 in the smallest place value reported. For example, if a metal object has a mass of 27.21 g, the mass may be as much as 27.22 g or as low as 27.20 g. This uncertainty may be shown as

27.21 g $\pm$ 1 in the hundredth place, or 27.21 $\pm$ 0.01 g.

Other measurements may have a greater or lesser uncertainty, but it will usually be indicated, such as:

15.2 $\pm$ 0.5 mL

which means the volume could be as high as 15.7 mL or as low as 14.7 mL. This uncertainty is largely determined by the measuring device used.

3.2 ACCURACY AND PRECISION

The terms **accuracy** and **precision** are sometimes used interchangeably. In laboratory situations, we want accuracy and precision to have the same meanings, but often they do not.

Accuracy may be defined as closeness of a measurement to a standard or to a true value. **Precision** is reflected in the smallest place value measured. A measurement may be precise and not accurate if the measuring device is not properly calibrated or is not used properly.

To illustrate the difference between accuracy and precision, consider three time measuring devices below: a clock, a wrist watch, and a digital stopwatch.

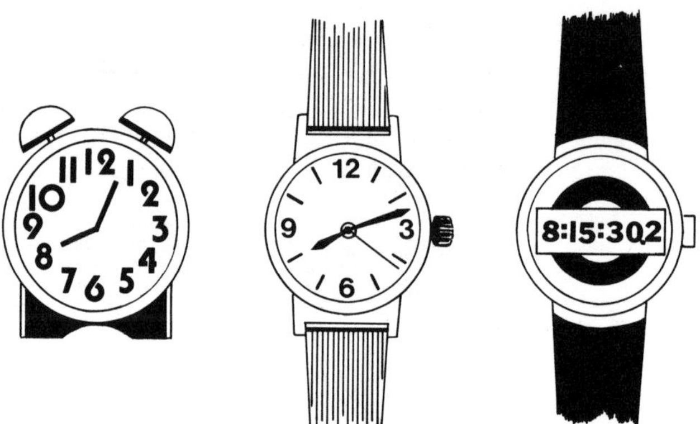

(Adapted from Malone, L., *Basic concepts of chemistry* (2nd ed.). New York: John Wiley & Sons, Inc., 1985.)

The clock can be read only to the nearest minute, and shows a time of 8:03. The wrist watch can be read to the nearest second, and shows a time of 8:12:22. The digital stopwatch indicates a time to the nearest tenth of a second, 8:15:30.2. It is the most precise measurement of time of the three. If, however, the actual time as determined from a reliable source is found to be 8:05:15.2, then the clock is the most accurate of the three.

Remember that in laboratory situations we want accuracy and precision to mean the same thing; we must be sure, however, that our instruments are properly used and calibrated to a standard that assures accuracy.

Numbers that result from a measurement are called **significant digits.** These significant digits are really "measured" digits. The number of significant digits in a measurement determine how many digits will be used in a result obtained when the measurement is used in a computation. The significant digits also determine the precision of the measurement. For example, the measurement

14.20 g

shows an uncertainty of ± 0.01 g, whereas the measurement

14.2 g

shows an uncertainty of ± 0.1 g. The first measurement is more precise, because the nearest *hundredth* of a gram was measured. Let us look at the rules for determining how many significant digits are in a reported measurement.

3.3 RULES FOR DETERMINING THE NUMBER OF SIGNIFICANT DIGITS

RULE 1 All nonzero digits (1–9) are significant.

RULE 2 Zeroes between two other significant digits are significant.

RULE 3 Zeroes that are both to the right of the decimal point and also to the right of any other nonzero digit are significant.

RULE 4 Zeroes to the left of all other nonzero digits are not significant.

RULE 5 Terminal zeroes in a whole number (no decimal point indicated) are not significant unless indicated with a bar placed over the last significant zero in the measurement. Many zeroes of this type are the result of rounding off, and therefore are not significant.

Explanation of the Rules

It is easier to understand the need for the rules if we consider the car odometer, which is used to measure the amount of miles the car has been driven. If we begin a journey in a brand new car, our odometer (assume this one records the nearest *hundredth* of a mile) reads

0 0 0 . 0 0

There is no measurement made, and therefore no significant digits. We travel a short distance, and the odometer reads

0 0 0 . 0 4

Now there is one significant digit (Rule 4). Notice that the dials with the zeros have not budged, so have not measured anything. We travel further. The odometer now reads

0 0 0 . 1 0

There are now two significant digits (Rule 3). The zero on the far right is significant because it is the result of a measurement: the dial has made one complete revolution. The zeroes to the left have not moved yet. We begin moving again. The odometer reads

0 0 1 . 0 1

There are now three significant digits (Rule 2). Our final measurement on the odometer is

1 0 0 . 0 0

There are now five significant digits (Rules 2 and 3). All of the zeroes in this last measurement are the result of having been measured, since all of the dials have turned over at least once.

Consider the measurements in the following example, and study the application of the rules for determining significant digits in a measurement.

EXAMPLE 3.3.1

Determine the number of significant digits in each measurement: **a.** 2.80 mL **b.** 0.02 cg **c.** 30.09 inches **d.** 100.0 kL **e.** 99.987 g **f.** 93,000,000 miles; and **g.** 10,000 miles.

Solution	**Comments**
a. 2.80 mL	**a.** Three significant digits (Rules 1 and 3)
b. 0.02 cg	**b.** One significant digit (Rules 1 and 4)

c. 30.09 inches — c. Four significant digits (Rules 1 and 2)

d. 100.0 kL — d. Four significant digits (Rules 1, 2, 3)

e. 99.987 g — e. Five significant digits (Rule 1)

f. 93,000,000 miles — f. Two significant digits (Rules 1 and 5)

g. $10,\bar{0}00$ miles — g. Three significant digits (Rules 1, 2, and 5)

Did you notice the bar over the third zero in the last measurement in the example? It indicated that that zero is significant, but that the two zeroes farther to the right are not. The last two zeroes are important, however, because they maintain the place value of the 1, which is in the ten-thousands place.

One Last Comment

If any value is exact, such as a pure number or a number of objects, or is defined, such as

12 inches = 1 ft

then these values have an infinite number of significant digits, because exactly 12 inches equals exactly 1 ft. Other examples of exact or defined values are given in example 3.3.2.

EXAMPLE 3.3.2

1000 M = 1 km
5280 ft = 1 mile
10 dm = 1 m
4 qt = 1 gal
1 mile = 1.609 km

exact (1 mile); four significant figures (1.609) (it is an approximation)

PROBLEM SET 1

Determine the number of significant digits in each measurement.

1. 4.93 cm
2. 11.10 g
3. 0.07 ft
4. 100.0 miles
5. 99.01 mL
6. 240,000 miles
7. 200 kg
8. 15.998 a.m.u.
9. 9.010 mg
10. 1,000,001 cm
11. exactly 20 people
12. about 20 people
13. 3.00 kL
14. 9.99 dL
15. 70.40 qt
16. 430 m
17. 3000 nm
18. 0.0008 g
19. 1.0008 g
20. 1.010 cg

Answers to odd-numbered problems appear on page 229.

3.4 ROUNDING OFF MEASUREMENTS

If a calculation contains more digits than can be justified based on the data from which it came, you will be forced to round the measurement off to the proper number of significant digits. This happens often when a calculator is used to make computations. The rules for rounding off are given below.

Rules for Rounding Off Measurements

RULE 6 If the first digit to be dropped from the measurement is greater than 5, or is 5 followed by any nonzero digit, drop those digits, and add 1 to the first digit on the left (the last one to be kept).

RULE 7 When the first digit to be dropped is less than 5, drop it and all others that follow. Leave the rest of the measurement as it is.

RULE 8 If the first digit to be dropped is exactly 5, or 5 followed only by zeroes, round the first digit to the left to an even number.

EXAMPLE 3.4.1 Round 3.87 to the nearest tenth.

Solution	**Comments**
$3.\underline{8}7$	Eight is in the tenths place. Keep it.
$3.\overset{1}{8}7$	The first digit to be dropped is 7, which is greater than 5, so drop it, and add 1 to the 8 (Rule 6).
3.9	This is the rounded-off figure.

EXAMPLE 3.4.2 Round 14.501 to the nearest whole number.

Solution	**Comments**
$1\underline{4}.501$	Keep the 4.
$1\overset{\cancel{1}}{4}.\cancel{5}\cancel{0}\cancel{1}$	The first digit to be dropped is 5, and it is followed by a 0 and a 1. Drop the 5, 0, and 1, and add 1 to the first digit on the left (Rule 6).
15	This is our rounded-off measurement.

EXAMPLE 3.4.3 Round off 0.0374 to the nearest thousandth.

Solution	**Comments**
$0.03\underline{7}4$	Locate the thousandths place.
$0.03\underline{7}\cancel{4}$	The first digit to be dropped is less than 5, so drop it (Rule 7).
0.37	Leave the rest of the measurement as it is.

EXAMPLE 3.4.4 Round 3.0524 to three significant digits.

Solution	**Comments**
$3.0\underline{5}24$ g	Count over three significant digits from the left.
$3.0\underline{5}\cancel{2}\cancel{4}$ g	The first digit to be dropped is less than 5, so drop it, and all others (Rule 7).
3.05 g	Leave the rest of the measurement as it is.

EXAMPLE 3.4.5

Round 3850 to two significant digits.

Solution	Comments
$3\underline{8}50$	Count from the left two digits. The last digit we keep is the 8.
$3\underline{8}50$	The first digit to be dropped is 5, followed by nothing but a zero; therefore, drop the 5 and 0. Since the 8 is already even, leave it as it is (Rule 8).
3800	You must place two zeroes at the end of the number to keep the 3 and 8 in their proper place values. These zeroes, however, are not significant (measured), but are important.

PROBLEM SET 2

Round off each measurement to *two* significant digits.

1. 39.49 cm
2. 9.38 ft
3. 7.726 m
4. 0.0211 nm
5. 100.7 mL
6. 4,976,285 people
7. 0.368 cg
8. 1102 kg
9. 5.05 g
10. 4350 cL
11. 1.94 mm
12. 0.2508 g

Using a periodic table, find the atomic weights of the following elements, and round each weight to the nearest tenth.

13. H
14. O
15. C
16. Na
17. K
18. U
19. Mg
20. Cl
21. N
22. Fe
23. Cu
24. Au

Answers to odd-numbered problems appear on page 230.

3.5 OPERATIONS WITH SIGNIFICANT DIGITS

Multiplication and Division

When multiplying and dividing measurements, the result of these computations must be rounded off to reflect the precision of the measurements. We may paraphrase the old adage "A chain is no stronger than its weakest link." This old saying is true when applied to the result of a multiplication and division process.

RULE 9

The result of multiplication and division processes may contain no more significant digits than the least precise measurement, that is, the measurement with the fewest significant digits.

EXAMPLE 3.5.1

Multiply (3.83 ft)(4.2 ft) and round off your measurement.

Solution	**Comments**
(3.83 ft)(4.2 ft) $= 16.086\ ft^2$	Multiply measurements and units.
$= 1\underline{6}.086\ ft^2$	Since 4.2 ft contains only two significant digits, round off your answer to two significant digits.
$= 16\ ft^2$	

EXAMPLE 3.5.2

The density of an object is given by the formula

$$\text{Density} = \frac{\text{Mass}}{\text{Volume}}.$$

Find the density of aluminum if a 3.620-g piece of aluminum has a volume of 1.34 cc.

Solution	**Comments**
$d = \frac{m}{v}$	Write the formula for density.
$d = \frac{3.620\ g}{1.34\ cc}$	In the formula, substitute 3.620 g for mass and 1.34 cc for volume.
$d = 2.7\underline{0}14925$ g/cc	This is the result after division. Since the volume measurement has only three significant digits, the answer must be rounded off to three significant digits.
$d = 2.70$ g/cc	This is the rounded-off answer.

EXAMPLE 3.5.3

Find P_2 if $P_2 = \frac{(54\bar{0}\ \text{torr})(2.4\ \text{L})}{(4.82\ \text{L})}$.

Solution	**Comments**
$P_2 = \frac{(540\ \text{torr})(2.4\ \text{L})}{(4.82\ \text{L})}$	Multiply the factors in the numerator. Notice that "liters" divides out.
$P_2 = \frac{1296\ (\text{torr})(\cancel{\text{L}})}{4.82\ \cancel{\text{L}}}$	Divide.
$P_2 = 2\underline{6}8.8796$ torr	The least precise of all measurements in the problem is 2.4 L, which has two significant digits. Round the answer to two significant digits.
$P_2 = 270$ torr	Notice that the terminal zero here is not significant.

Addition and Subtraction

When adding and subtracting measurements, we are not interested in the total number of significant digits, but only in the precision of the measurements.

RULE 10

When adding or subtracting measurements, the answer must be rounded to the smallest place value (precision) that all measurements have in common.

EXAMPLE 3.5.4

The weights of three gold nuggets are 2.11 g, 4.2g, and 11.4081 g. What is the total weight of the gold nuggets?

Solution	Comments
2.11 g 4.2 g +11.4081 g 17.7181 g	Add the weights. Be sure to line up decimal points. The smallest place value all measurements have in common is the tenths place.
= 17.7~~181~~ g	The first digit to be dropped is less than 5, so drop it.
= 17.7 g	This answer reflects the precision of all the measurements.

Note in the foregoing example of addition and subtraction, we do not consider the total number of significant digits, but only the level of precision, or the smallest place value all measurements have in common.

EXAMPLE 3.5.5

A graduated cylinder contains 9.2 mL of water. A solid object is dropped into the cylinder, and the water level rises to 17.2 mL. What is the volume of the object?

Solution	Comments
17.2 mL − 9.2 mL	Subtract the original volume from the final volume.
8.0 mL	Both measurements are precise to the nearest tenth, and we keep the tenths place.
8.0 mL, **not** 8 mL	A common mistake students make is to leave off the zero. The zero must be written to indicate the level of precision is to the nearest ±0.1 mL.

PROBLEM SET 3

Carry out the following computations, and round off your answers. Assume all numbers are measurements.

1. (8.43)(2.00)
2. (91.27)(0.0201)
3. (1.277)(0.38)(100)
4. (1000)(92,000)(0.0010)
5. (0.0040)(0.0300)(0.5280)
6. $\dfrac{8.43}{2.1}$
7. $\dfrac{19.76}{0.03121}$
8. $\dfrac{(5240)(3.81)}{4.6}$
9. $\dfrac{(11{,}277)(0.730)}{(40)(0.09)}$
10. $\begin{array}{r} 13.73 \\ 2.818 \\ +\ 6.60 \\ \hline \end{array}$
11. $\begin{array}{r} 0.0217 \\ 5.022 \\ +17.19 \\ \hline \end{array}$
12. $\begin{array}{r} 47.87 \\ -17.67 \\ \hline \end{array}$
13. $\begin{array}{r} 483 \\ 2.96 \\ +\ 14.234 \\ \hline \end{array}$

14. $(6.81)(2.25) + 14.1$

15. $(0.935)(18.74) - 16$

16. $\frac{11.12}{10.4} + 13.7 + 8.880$

17. $\frac{(516.0)(.436)}{(1.000)} - (58.16)$

18. $(3200)(8400) + 14{,}000$

Answers to odd-numbered problems appear on page 230.

3.6 SCIENTIFIC NOTATION

Basic Rules

When a factor is multiplied by itself, such as

$$5 \cdot 5 \cdot 5 = 125$$

it can be written in a shorthand notation:

$$5^3 = 5 \cdot 5 \cdot 5 = 125.$$

Other examples are

$$2^4 = 2 \cdot 2 \cdot 2 \cdot 2 = 16$$
$$3^2 = 3 \cdot 3 = 9$$
$$4^5 = 4 \cdot 4 \cdot 4 \cdot 4 \cdot 4 = 1024$$

exponential number (4^5) — decimal number (base 10) (1024)

We can write large numbers as a **base** (X) to a **power** (m).

RULE 11 $X^m = X \cdot X \cdot X \cdot X \ldots m$ factors of X.

In this section, we will deal with the base ten, since our number system is based on the number "10."

EXAMPLE 3.6.1 Write 10^6, 10^3, 10^2, 10^1, and 10^0 as decimal numbers.

Solution	Comments
$10^6 = 10 \cdot 10 \cdot 10 \cdot 10 \cdot 10 \cdot 10 = 1{,}000{,}000$	10^6 is 1 with 6 zeroes
$10^3 = 10 \cdot 10 \cdot 10 = 1000$	10^3 is 1 with 3 zeroes
$10^2 = 10 \cdot 10 = 100$	10^2 is 1 with 2 zeroes
$10^1 = 10$	10^1 is 1 with 1 zero
$10^0 = 1$	10^0 is 1 with no zeroes

RULE 12 $X^0 = 1$, assuming $X \neq 0$.

Any number (X) to the zero power is equal to 1, but 0^0 is undefined.

Very large or very small measurements are often written in exponential notation in order to make computations with these measurements easier. It is also easier to comprehend the magnitude of a measurement when it is written in this manner. For example, the distance from the earth to the sun is roughly 93,000,000 miles. This may be written as follows:

$$\begin{aligned} 93{,}000{,}000 &= 93 \cdot 10^6 \ (93 \cdot 1{,}000{,}000) \\ &= 930 \cdot 10^5 \ (930 \cdot 100{,}000) \\ &= 9.3 \cdot 10^7 \ (9.3 \cdot 10{,}000{,}000) \end{aligned}$$

All of the above equal to 93,000,000. An important pattern emerges as we look at these values. Notice as the numbers written to the left of the power of ten increases, the exponent decreases, and as the number to the left of the exponent decreases, the exponent increases:

$$93 \cdot 10^6 = 930 \cdot 10^5$$
$$93 \cdot 10^6 = 9.3 \cdot 10^7$$

EXAMPLE 3.6.2

Determine the exponent needed when $17 \cdot 10^5$ is rewritten as $1.7 \cdot 10^X$.

Solution	**Comments**
$17 \cdot 10^5 = 1.7 \cdot 10^X$	Rewrite 17 as 1.7 If 17 decreases to 1.7, then the exponent "5" should increase to "6."
$1.7 \cdot 10^6$	This is the same number as $17 \cdot 10^5$.

Very small numbers can also be written in exponential notation. The following rule governs numbers less than one.

RULE 13

$$X^{-m} = \frac{1}{X^m}, \ X \neq 0.$$

EXAMPLE 3.6.3

Write 10^{-6}, 10^{-3}, 10^{-2}, and 10^{-1} as decimal numbers.

Solution	**Comments**
$10^{-6} = \frac{1}{10^6} = \frac{1}{1{,}000{,}000} = 0.000001$	Note: 10^{-6} can be written as a fraction or a decimal.
$10^{-3} = \frac{1}{10^3} = \frac{1}{1000} = 0.001$	
$10^{-2} = \frac{1}{10^2} = \frac{1}{100} = 0.01$	
$10^{-1} = \frac{1}{10^1} = \frac{1}{10} = 0.1$	X^{-m} is the *reciprocal* of X^m.

Any number or measurement written as the product of a number and a power of 10 is said to be in **exponential notation.** If the number before the power of 10 is between 1 and 10, we say that it is written in **scientific notation.**

Definition of Scientific Notation

$N \cdot 10^P$ is in scientific notation if the measurement, (N), is equal to or greater than 1 and less than 10. The exponent (or power) (P) may be any integer.

Writing a Measurement in Scientific Notation

To write any measurement in scientific notation, follow these steps:

Step 1. Write down all significant digits.
Step 2. Place a decimal point after the first digit on the left. This is known as the **standard position.**

Step 3. Multiply by a power of 10. Next, we need to find the correct exponent (P).

Step 4. Count the number of places the decimal point must be moved to obtain the original measurement. This gives the absolute value of the power.

Step 5. If the decimal in step 4 was moved to the **right** to obtain the original measurement, the exponent is **positive**.
If the decimal in step 4 was moved to the **left**, the exponent is **negative**.

Now, consider the following example.

EXAMPLE 3.6.4

Write 6024 km in scientific notation.

Solution	Comments
6024	Write down all significant digits.
6.024	Now, place a decimal point after the first digit on the left. This is known as the **standard position.**
$6.024 \cdot 10^P$	Multiply by a power of 10. Next, we need to find the correct exponent (P).
$6\,.\,0\,2\,4\,\cdot 10^3$ (moves 1 2 3)	Count the number of places the decimal point must be moved to obtain the original measurement. This gives you the value of the power.
$6.024 \cdot 10^{+3}$ km	Since the decimal in the previous step was moved to the **right** to obtain the original measurement, the exponent is **positive.** (If the decimal in the previous step had been moved to the **left**, the exponent would have been **negative.**)

In example 3.6.4, the decimal was moved to the right, and the exponent was positive. The positive sign associated with any exponent may be omitted, but a negative exponent must be preceded by a negative sign. Observe that $6024 = 6.024 \cdot 10^3$. The number value before the power of 10 is between 1 and 10. This number may be referred to as the **significant digit portion** of the measurement.

EXAMPLE 3.6.5

Write 0.00201 cg in scientific notation.

Solution	Comments
201	Write down all significant digits.
2.01	This is standard position.
$2.01 \cdot 10^P$	Multiply by 10.
$0\,.\,0\,0\,2\,0\,1$ = 3 decimal places (moves 3 2 1)	Count decimal places to obtain original measurement.
$2.01 \cdot 10^{-3}$ cg	The decimal point was moved to the left to obtain original measurement; therefore the exponent is negative.

EXAMPLE 3.6.6

Write 12.60 g in scientific notation.

Solution	Comments
1260	Significant digits.
1.260	Standard position.

$1.260 \cdot 10^P$	Multiply by 10 to a power P.
1. 2 6 0 = 1 decimal place (1)	Count decimal places necessary to obtain original measurement.
$1.260 \cdot 10^1$ g	The decimal was moved to the right to obtain the original position; therefore the exponent is positive.

Any number greater than one, when written in scientific notation, will have a zero or positive power of ten, and any number less than one will have a negative exponent.

3.7 MULTIPLICATION BY SCIENTIFIC NOTATION

When multiplying like bases, what happens to the exponents? From algebra, we have the following definition:

RULE 14 $x^m \cdot x^n = x^{m+n}$, **where** m **and** n **are integers.**

In other words, when multiplying like bases, add the exponents:

$10^4 \cdot 10^3 = 10^7$
$4^3 \cdot 4^2 = 4^5$
$3^{-2} \cdot 3^6 = 3^4$
$3^2 \cdot 2^3 = ?$ (*Note*: You cannot add exponents where the bases are different.)

If there are measurements or numbers before the powers, multiply them as usual.

EXAMPLE 3.7.1

Multiply $(2.34 \cdot 10^6)(1.22 \cdot 10^4)$.

Solution	**Comments**
$(2.34 \cdot 10^6)(1.22 \cdot 10^4)$	Multiply significant digit portion.
$= 2.8548 \cdot 10^6 \cdot 10^4$	Add the exponents on the powers of 10.
$= 2.8548 \cdot 10^{10}$	Round off to the proper number of significant digits.
$= 2.85 \cdot 10^{10}$	It is already in standard form.

EXAMPLE 3.7.2

Multiply $(6.88 \cdot 10^{-3})(4.1 \cdot 10^8)(0.077 \cdot 10^4)$.

Solution	**Comments**
$(6.88 \cdot 10^{-3})(4.1 \cdot 10^8)(0.077 \cdot 10^4)$	Multiply the significant digit portions.
$= 2.172016 \cdot 10^{-3} \cdot 10^8 \cdot 10^4$	Add the powers of 10. $-3 + 8 + 4 = 9$
$= 2.172016 \cdot 10^9$	Round off your answer to two significant digits.
$= 2.2 \cdot 10^9$	The answer is already in standard form.

EXAMPLE 3.7.3

Multiply $(8.24 \cdot 10^{-3})(5.2 \cdot 10^{2})$.

Solution	Comments
$(8.24 \cdot 10^{-3})(5.2 \cdot 10^{6})$	Multiply the significant digit portion.
$= 42.848 \cdot 10^{-3} \cdot 10^{6}$	Add exponents.
$= 42.848 \cdot 10^{+3}$	Round off your answer to two significant digits.
$= 43 \cdot 10^{3}$ $= 4.3 \cdot 10^{4}$	Rewrite this answer in standard form. Move the decimal point one place to the left and increase the exponent by 1; thus, 43 becomes 4.3 and the power of 10 becomes 4.

3.8 DIVISION BY SCIENTIFIC NOTATION

When multiplying, we add the exponents of like bases. When dividing, we subtract them.

RULE 15 $\dfrac{X^m}{X^n} = X^{m-n}$, when m and n are integers.

$$\frac{4^3}{4^4} = 4^{3-4} = 4^{-1} \text{ or } \frac{1}{4}$$

$$\frac{8^3}{8^{-2}} = 8^{3-(-2)} = 8^{3+2} = 8^5$$

$$\frac{10^{17}}{10^{13}} = 10^{17-13} = 10^4$$

To divide like bases, subtract the exponent in the denominator from the exponent in the numerator.

EXAMPLE 3.7.4

Divide $\dfrac{8.11 \cdot 10^{6}}{2.000 \cdot 10^{-4}}$.

Solution	Comments
$\dfrac{8.11 \cdot 10^{6}}{2.000 \cdot 10^{-4}}$	Divide significant digit portion.
$= 4.06 \cdot \dfrac{10^{6}}{10^{-4}}$	Subtract the exponents.
$= 4.06 \cdot 10^{6-(-4)}$	
$= 4.06 \cdot 10^{6+4}$	
$= 4.06 \cdot 10^{10}$	The answer should contain three significant digits and it is already in standard form.

EXAMPLE 3.7.5

Simplify $\dfrac{(9.11 \cdot 10^3)(2.111 \cdot 10^{-5})}{(6.27 \cdot 10^4)}$.

Solution

$$\frac{(9.11 \cdot 10^3)(2.111 \cdot 10^{-5})}{(6.27 \cdot 10^4)}$$

$$= \frac{19.23 \cdot 10^3 \cdot 10^{-5}}{6.27 \cdot 10^4}$$

$$= \frac{19.23 \cdot 10^{-2}}{6.27 \cdot 10^4}$$

$$= 3.07 \cdot 10^{-2-4}$$
$$= 3.07 \cdot 10^{-6}$$

Comments

Multiply the significant digit portion of the numerator. For convenience, you may round off the product to one more significant digit than your least precise measurement.

Add exponents in the numerator.

Divide significant digits, and subtract exponents.

The result is in standard form, with the proper number of significant digits.

EXAMPLE 3.7.6

Simplify $\dfrac{(0.42 \cdot 10^4)(0.277 \cdot 10^{-3})}{(16.4)(7.001 \cdot 10^{-5})}$.

Solution

$$\frac{(0.42 \cdot 10^4)(0.277 \cdot 10^{-3})}{(16.4)(7.001 \cdot 10^{-5})}$$

$$= \frac{0.116 \cdot 10^4 \cdot 10^{-3}}{114.8 \cdot 10^{-5}}$$

$$= \frac{0.116 \cdot 10^1}{114.8 \cdot 10^{-5}}$$

$$= \frac{0.0010 \cdot 10^1}{10^{-5}}$$

$$= 0.0010 \cdot 10^{1-(-5)}$$
$$= 0.0010 \cdot 10^{1+5}$$
$$= 0.0010 \cdot 10^6$$
$$= 1.0 \cdot 10^3$$

Comments

Multiply significant digits in numerator and denominator. Keep one extra significant digit for convenience, but remember, the final answer must be rounded off to *two* significant digits.

Add exponents in numerator and denominator. *Note:* 16.4 is the same as $16.4 \cdot 10^0$.

Divide significant digits, and round off.

Subtract exponents. Be careful with the signs.

Write in standard form.

3.9 ADDITION AND SUBTRACTION USING EXPONENTIAL OR SCIENTIFIC NOTATION

Consider the following problem:

$$\begin{array}{r} 3.17 \cdot 10^3 \\ \underline{+2.41 \cdot 10^2} \end{array}$$

What is the sum of the two values? Can we add the significant digit portions as the problem is written? Look at the decimal form of both numbers.

$$\begin{array}{rcr} 3.17 \cdot 10^3 & = & 3170 \\ \underline{+2.41 \cdot 10^2} & = & \underline{+ \quad 241} \end{array}$$

The digits do not have the same place values when written in decimal form. Never add or subtract the significant digit portion of numbers if they do not have the same power of ten. Always use the following rule when adding and subtracting numbers or measurements written in exponential notation. We will complete the above problem as Example 3.9.1.

RULE 16

To add numbers written in exponential notation, the powers of ten *must* be the same. Only after all exponents have the same integral value may the significant digit portions be added or subtracted.

EXAMPLE 3.9.1

Add $\begin{array}{r} 3.17 \cdot 10^3 \\ \underline{+2.41 \cdot 10^2} \end{array}$

Solution

$\begin{array}{r} 3.17 \cdot 10^3 \\ \underline{+0.241 \cdot 10^3} \end{array}$

Comments

Rewrite $2.41 \cdot 10^2$ to have an exponent of 10^3. As a rule of thumb, *make the smaller exponent like the larger one.*

$\begin{array}{r} 3.17 \cdot 10^3 \\ \underline{+0.241 \cdot 10^3} \\ 3.411 \cdot 10^3 \end{array}$

Add the significant digit portions. Leave power of 10 as it is.

$= 3.41 \cdot 10^3$

Round off the sum to the nearest hundredth (why?).

EXAMPLE 3.9.2

Subtract $\begin{array}{r} 14.83 \cdot 10^{-3} \\ \underline{-\ 7.07 \cdot 10^{-5}} \end{array}$

Solution

$\begin{array}{r} 14.83 \cdot 10^{-3} \\ \underline{-\ 0.0707 \cdot 10^{-3}} \end{array}$

Comments

Rewrite 10^{-5} as 10^{-3}. As the exponent of the 10 increases from -5 to -3, the significant digit portion decreases from 7.07 to 0.0707.

$\begin{array}{r} 14.83 \cdot 10^{-3} \\ \underline{-\ 0.0707 \cdot 10^{-3}} \\ 14.7593 \cdot 10^{-3} \end{array}$

Subtract the significant digit portion, and round off. Leave the exponent of 10 as is.

$= 14.76 \cdot 10^{-3}$
$= 1.476 \cdot 10^{-2}$

Write the answer in scientific notation with the decimal point in standard position.

PROBLEM SET 4

Perform the indicated operations, and round off your answers. Assume all values are measurements. Leave answers in scientific notation.

1. $(7.3 \cdot 10^4)(6.9 \cdot 10^2)$
2. $(8.37 \cdot 10^6)(2.9 \cdot 10^2)$
3. $(1.977 \cdot 10^5)(1.977 \cdot 10^5)$
4. $(9.9 \cdot 10^{-3})(1.000 \cdot 10^{-3})$
5. $(5.33 \cdot 10^{-7})(8.6 \cdot 10^7)$
6. $(38.2 \cdot 10^{-1})(47.7 \cdot 10^{-2})$
7. $(1.22 \cdot 10^6)(8.34 \cdot 10^3)(5.00 \cdot 10^{-1})$
8. (0.001(0.001)(0.100)
9. $(10^6)(10^2)(10^0)$
10. $\dfrac{15.4 \cdot 10^7}{4 \cdot 10^3}$
11. $\dfrac{1.227 \cdot 10^{-3}}{4.6 \cdot 10^3}$
12. $\dfrac{8.88 \cdot 10^3}{4.0 \cdot 10^{-3}}$
13. $\dfrac{482 \cdot 10^3}{24 \cdot 10^3}$

14. $\dfrac{0.732 \cdot 10^{-1}}{1.65 \cdot 10^{-4}}$

15. $\dfrac{3.14 \cdot 10^{0}}{9.02 \cdot 10^{-5}}$

16. $\dfrac{(16.43 \cdot 10^{4})(2.00 \cdot 10^{3})}{4.00 \cdot 10^{2}}$

17. $\dfrac{(0.001)(100.0)(0.002)}{0.00001}$

18. $\dfrac{(10^{7})(10^{5})(10^{3})}{10^{-3}}$

19. $\dfrac{7.06 \cdot 10^{4}}{10^{-3}}$

20. $\dfrac{40.08}{10^{-5}}$

21. $\begin{array}{r} 1.23 \cdot 10^{5} \\ +7.11 \cdot 10^{5} \\ \hline \end{array}$

22. $\begin{array}{r} 48.6 \cdot 10^{7} \\ +31.5 \cdot 10^{7} \\ \hline \end{array}$

23. $\begin{array}{r} 16.2 \cdot 10^{-3} \\ -14.1 \cdot 10^{-3} \\ \hline \end{array}$

24. $\begin{array}{r} 19.7 \cdot 10^{6} \\ +21.3 \cdot 10^{5} \\ \hline \end{array}$

25. $\begin{array}{r} 3.26 \cdot 10^{-2} \\ -1.77 \cdot 10^{-3} \\ \hline \end{array}$

26. $\begin{array}{r} 1.83 \cdot 10^{5} \\ 7.01 \cdot 10^{4} \\ +8.33 \cdot 10^{3} \\ \hline \end{array}$

27. $(79.28 \cdot 10^{3} + 14.6 \cdot 10^{2}) - 1.52 \cdot 10^{3}$

28. The diameter of a hydrogen atom is about $1 \cdot 10^{-10}$ m. How long would a string of 1,000,000 of these atoms extend if placed side by side?

29. A computer can complete an addition problem in $1 \cdot 10^{-7}$ seconds. How many problems can the computer complete in $6 \cdot 10^{1}$ seconds?

30. A patient is prescribed $2.5 \cdot 10^{5}$ units of penicillin. How many doses of the penicillin can the patient receive from a bottle containing $1.0 \cdot 10^{6}$ units?

31. The speed of light is $3.00 \cdot 10^{8}$ m/sec. How far can a beam of light travel in exactly 60 seconds?

32. One mole of carbon contains about $6.02 \cdot 10^{23}$ atoms of carbon. How many atoms are there in $1.0 \cdot 10^{2}$ moles of carbon?

33. A patient's blood albumin level measured $4.3 \cdot 10^{3}$ mg/dL. How many milligrams are present in a 2.4-dL sample?

Answers to odd-numbered problems appear on page 230.

CHAPTER REVIEW

(3.1–3.3)

Determine the number of significant digits in each measurement:

1. 3.82 cm
2. 230 L
3. 14.70 kg
4. $9.80 \cdot 10^{3}$ mm
5. 0.301 mL
6. 0.002 g

(3.4)

Round off each measurement to *three* significant digits.

7. 4.841 cL
8. 864.50 m
9. 2.0097 dg
10. 1,292,611 miles
11. $9.997 \cdot 10^{4}$ hm
12. 15.9994 amu

(3.5)

Perform the following computations and round off your answers. Assume all numbers result from measurements.

13. $(1.32)(2.008)$

14. $\dfrac{(8.53)(12)}{0.0032}$

15. $\begin{array}{r} 85.21 \\ 16 \\ +39.176 \\ \hline \end{array}$

16. $\dfrac{16}{4.99} - 2.186$

(3.6–3.9)

Write in scientific notation.

17. 320.14 mm

18. 0.801 g

19. $18.21 \cdot 10^{7}$ nm

20. $0.0222 \cdot 10^{-2}$ m

Perform the indicated operations. Round off your answers, and leave in scientific notation.

21. $(4.11 \cdot 10^{2})(1.12 \cdot 10^{3})$

22. $(49.6 \cdot 10^{-3})(6.02 \cdot 10^{23})$

23. $\dfrac{(10)(10^{3})(10^{2})}{10^{6}}$

24. $\begin{array}{r} 14.7 \cdot 10^{5} \\ -12.1 \cdot 10^{4} \\ \hline \end{array}$

25. $\dfrac{(1500)(2.1 \cdot 10^{-1})}{14.7 \cdot 10^{4}}$

26. The wavelength (λ) of a typical x-ray beam may be determined by using the formula $c = \lambda\nu$, where c is the speed of light and ν is the frequency. Find the wavelength of the x-ray beam if $c = 3.00 \cdot 10^{8}$ m/sec and $\nu = 3.45 \cdot 10^{17}$ sec^{-1}. Leave your answer in scientific notation.

Answers to all problems appear on page **xx.**

chapter 4

The Metric System and Dimensional Analysis

OBJECTIVES

After studying this chapter, the student should be able to:

1. Define the prefixes commonly used in the metric system.
2. Convert from one metric unit to another.
3. Convert a measurement from one system of measurement to any other by using dimensional analysis.
4. Define and use the interrelationships among metric units of length, volume, and mass.

4.1 THE METRIC SYSTEM

In the laboratory and other scientific work, measurements are made using the metric system. The metric system was devised by the French during the latter part of the 18th century.

The metric system is the official system of measurement in many countries throughout the world, and is used chiefly in laboratory and in scientific work in the United States. It is slowly being adopted by the industrial community, and is already a legal system of measurement for anyone wishing to use it.

For each of the quantities of length, volume, and mass, there is defined a base unit. The metric system is a **decimal system**, that is, every prefix in the system is a multiple of 10 of the base unit. The key to understanding the metric system is to know the prefixes used with each base unit. You must memorize these prefixes and their abbreviations.

Prefix	Means	Abbreviation	Notes
kilo	1000 ×	k	A "kilodollar" is 1000 dollars
hecto	100 ×	h	A "hectogram" is 100 grams
deka	10 ×	da	A "decade" is 10 years
deci	$\frac{1}{10}$ ×	d	A "decidollar" is $\frac{1}{10}$ of a dollar or a dime
centi	$\frac{1}{100}$ ×	c	A "centidollar" is one cent

Prefix	Means	Abbreviation	Notes
milli	$\frac{1}{1000}\times$	m	
micro	$\frac{1}{1{,}000{,}000}\times$	μ or mc	Used to make very small measurements (such as those on the cell, molecular, or atomic level)
nano	$\frac{1}{1{,}000{,}000{,}000}\times$	n	

Let us examine the three base units used for length, volume, and mass in more detail.

4.2 MEASURING LENGTH

The base unit for length in the metric system is the **meter**, abbreviated m. Originally, the meter was defined as one ten-millionth of the distance from the equator to the North Pole along a meridian through Paris, France. Although that definition was changed somewhat in 1960, the meter is still basically the same length as before, which is approximately 3 inches longer than the English yard.

Notice how the prefixes given above are used to define the multiples of the meter:

1 kilometer (km) = 1000 m	1 decimeter (dm) = $\frac{1}{10}$ m
1 hectometer (hm) = 100 m	1 centimeter (cm) = $\frac{1}{100}$ m
1 dekameter (dam) = 10 m	1 millimeter (mm) = $\frac{1}{1000}$ m

In laboratory work, the prefixes "hecto" and "deka" are seldom used, but they may be considered when making conversions from one metric unit to another. The relationship between the centimeter and the inch is shown below:

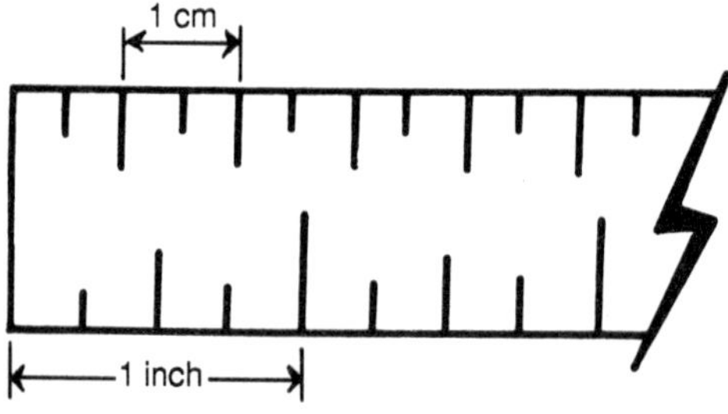

EXAMPLE 4.2.1

If 2 mm are $2 \cdot \frac{1}{1000}$ m or $\frac{2}{2000}$ m, then 4 km are how many meters?

Solution	Comments
kilo = 1000	Recall that the prefix kilo means 1000.
4 km = $4 \cdot 1000$ m	
= 4000 m	

EXAMPLE 4.2.2

Write $\frac{3}{10}$ m as decimeters.

Solution	Comments
$\frac{3}{10}$ m = $3 \cdot \frac{1}{10}$ m	Recall that $\frac{1}{10}$ m = 1 dm.
$\frac{1}{10}$ m = 1 dm	Substitute 1 dm for $\frac{1}{10}$ m.
$3 \cdot 1$ dm = 3 dm	
$\frac{3}{10}$ m = 3 dm	

4.3 MEASURING VOLUME

The official version of the metric system is called the Système Internationale (SI). In this version, the **cubic meter** (m^3) is the basic unit of volume. In health-related occupations, however, the **liter** (L) is accepted as the base unit for volume. A liter is only slightly larger than the English quart:

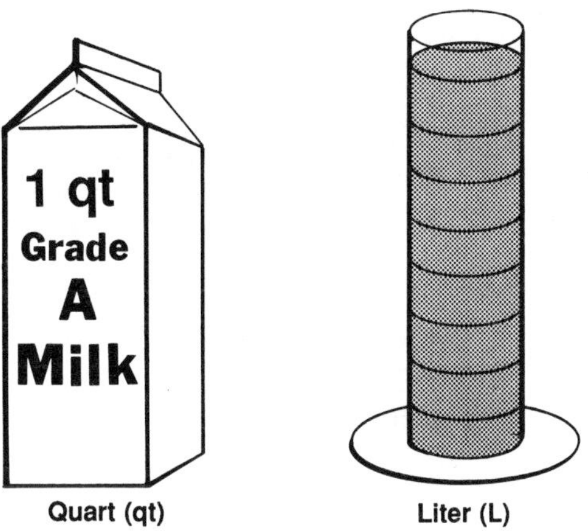

Quart (qt) Liter (L)

We use the metric system prefixes to obtain the multiples of the liter in the same way we obtained the multiples of the meter:

1 kiloliter (kL)	= 1000 L	1 deciliter (dL)	= $\frac{1}{10}$ L
1 hectoliter (hL)	= 100L	1 centiliter (cL)	= $\frac{1}{100}$ L
1 dekaliter (daL)	= 10 L	1 milliliter (mL)	= $\frac{1}{1000}$ L

A milliliter is a small volume; roughly 15–20 drops of water are equal to 1 mL.

EXAMPLE 4.3.1

How many centiliters is $\frac{4}{100}$ of a liter?

Solution	**Comments**
$\frac{4}{100}\text{ L} = 4 \cdot \frac{1}{100}\text{ L}$	Recall that centi $= \frac{1}{100}$.
$= 4 \cdot 1\text{ cL}$	Substitute $1\text{ cL} = \frac{1}{100}\text{ L}$.
$= 4\text{ cL}$	

EXAMPLE 4.3.2

How many liters is 5 hL?

Solution	**Comments**
$5\text{ hL} = 5 \cdot 100\text{ L}$ $= 500\text{ L}$	Recall that hecto = 100 times the base unit. Substitute 100 L for 1 hL.

4.4 MEASURING MASS

Mass is the amount of matter an object contains. Weight is the result of gravity pulling on a mass. Since for all practical purposes, gravity exerts the same pull all over the earth, and since it pulls on equal masses with the same force, equal masses have equal weights. Often, we speak of the weight of an object when we are really referring to the mass of the object.

The fundamental unit of mass in the SI system is the kilogram, but in health-related occupations, we may consider the **gram** (g) to be the basic unit of mass. Two small paper clips have a mass of approximately 1 gr:

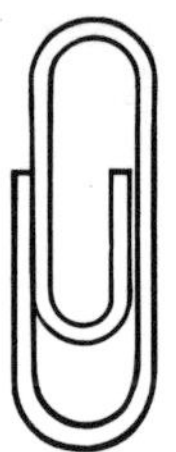

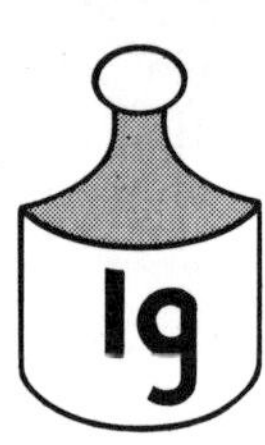

1 kilogram (kg)	= 1000 g	1 decigram (dg)	$= \frac{1}{10}$ g
1 hectogram (hg)	= 100 g	1 centigram (cg)	$= \frac{1}{100}$ g
1 dekagram (dag)	= 10 g	1 milligram (mg)	$= \frac{1}{1000}$ g

EXAMPLE 4.4.1

If $1 \text{ dg} = \frac{1}{10}$ g, how many grams are in 10 dg?

Solution	**Comments**
$1 \text{ dg} = \frac{1}{10} \text{ g}$	Defined.
$10 \cdot 1 \text{ dg} = 10 \cdot \frac{1}{10} \text{ g}$	Multiply both sides of the definition by 10.
$10 \text{ dg} = 1 \text{ g}$	This is the solution. It is another version of the original definition of the decigram that appears in the first step.

EXAMPLE 4.4.2

How many milligrams are in 1 g?

Solution	**Comments**
$1 \text{ mg} = \frac{1}{1000} \text{ g}$	Defined.
$1000 \cdot 1 \text{ mg} = 1000 \cdot \frac{1}{1000} \text{ g}$	Multiply both sides of the definition by 1000.
$1000 \text{ mg} = 1 \text{ g}$	This is the solution.

4.5 THE STAIRSTEP METHOD TO METRIC CONVERSIONS

An easy mental way to make metric conversions from one metric unit to another is to think of each metric prefix as occupying a stairstep, as shown in the following figure:

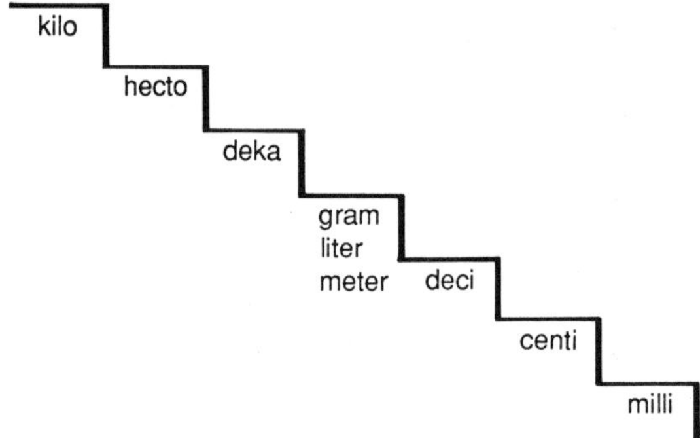

As you climb the stairs, you go from right to left, and as you descend the stairs, you go from left to right. Also notice that the value of the prefixes increase by a factor of 10 as you climb, and decrease by a factor of 10 as you descend. The base units occupy the center step.

EXAMPLE 4.5.1

Change 15.2 kg to grams.

Solution

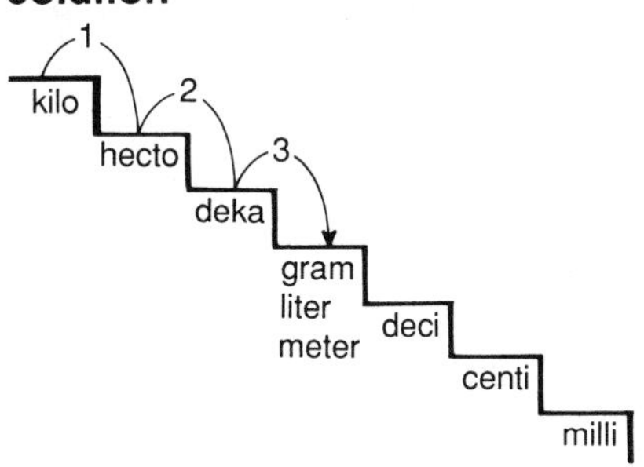

Comments

You are converting from kilograms to grams. Begin on the prefix "kilo" and then descend to the gram step. You have moved three steps to the right.

15.2 kg = 1 5 . 2 0 0 . = 15,200 g

15.2 kg = 15,200 g

Now, move the decimal point three places to the right in the given measurement.

EXAMPLE 4.5.2

Change 1.022 cm to meters.

Solution

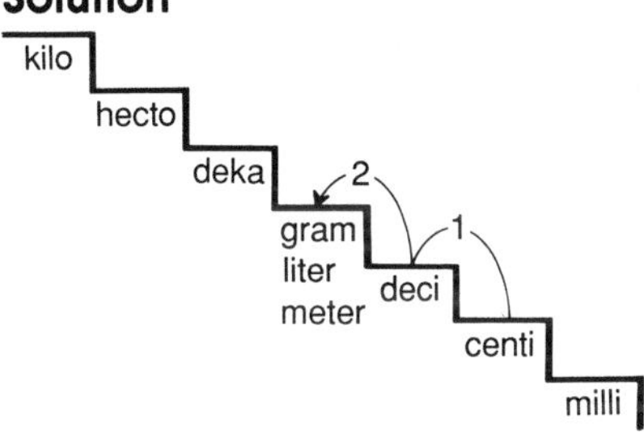

Comments

You are changing from centimeters to meters.

Begin on the "centi" step and move up two steps to the meter step.

1.022 cm = 0 . 0 1 . 0 2 2 m
= 0.01022 m

Notice that you moved up to the left two steps. Move the decimal point in your original measurement to the left two places.

EXAMPLE 4.5.3

Change 4733 mL to kiloliters.

Solution

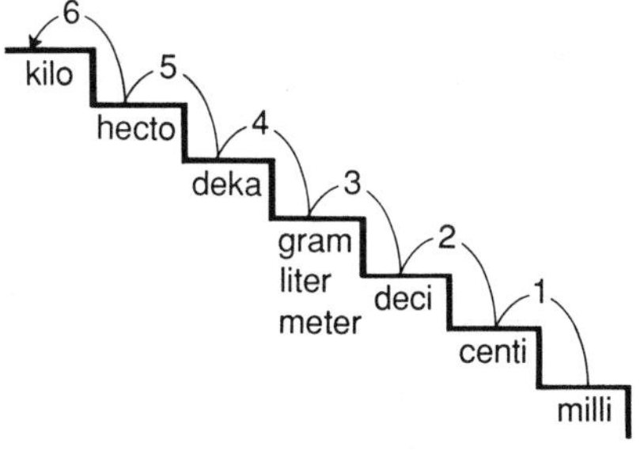

Comments

Start on the "milli" step. Move up left to the "kilo" step.

4733 mL = 0 . 0 0 4 7 3 3 kL = 0.004733 kL

You moved six steps to the left, so move the decimal point six places to the left.

4.6 A PATTERN TO REMEMBER

If the above examples are studied carefully, an important pattern emerges. When converting from one metric unit to another, the sequence of given numbers in the measurement never changes; only the position of the decimal point changes.

EXAMPLE 4.6.1

Study the pattern in these metric equivalences.

$$\begin{aligned} 43 \text{ mL} &= 0.043 \text{ L} \\ 2.03 \text{ kL} &= 2030 \text{ L} \\ 0.042 \text{ cg} &= 0.0042 \text{ dg} \end{aligned}$$

Along with the moving of the decimal point right or left, you may see that as we go from a larger unit to a smaller unit, the number associated with the measurement increases. Also, as we convert from a smaller unit to a larger unit, the numerical value of the measurement decreases. This kind of relationship is called an **inverse relationship**. As one quantity increases, the other quantity decreases, and vice versa.

EXAMPLE 4.6.2

Study the inverse relationship between the unit and the associated measurement.

Large unit to smaller unit:

$$\begin{aligned} 22 \text{ g} &= 220 \text{ dg} \\ 220 \text{ dg} &= 2200 \text{ cg} \end{aligned}$$

Small unit to larger unit:

$$\begin{aligned} 19.3 \text{ g} &= 1.93 \text{ dag} \\ 1.93 \text{ dag} &= 0.193 \text{ hg} \end{aligned}$$

PROBLEM SET 1

Convert from the given metric unit to the indicated metric unit using the definition of the prefixes or by using the stairstep method.

1. 2.6 g = _____ mg
2. 8.01 kg = _____ hg
3. 0.004 daL = _____ L
4. 18.3 L = _____ cL
5. 100 m = _____ mm
6. 10 cm = _____ dm
7. 0.002 kL = _____ dL
8. 1 200 cg = _____ dag
9. 43.3 hm = _____ mm
10. 0.0101 hg = _____ kg
11. 8.4 mg = _____ g
12. 20.00 mm = _____ cm
13. 0.2999 cm = _____ dm
14. 0.2999 dm = _____ m
15. 1000 kL = _____ hL
16. 10,000 hL = _____ daL
17. 100,000 daL = _____ L
18. 1 dg = _____ g
19. 10 dg = _____ g
20. 1000 mg = _____ g
21. 0.207 dam = _____ mm

Two other smaller metric prefixes often encountered in laboratory work are "micro" (μ) and "nano" (n). The relationship of "micro" and "nano" to the other metric prefixes in the following figure:

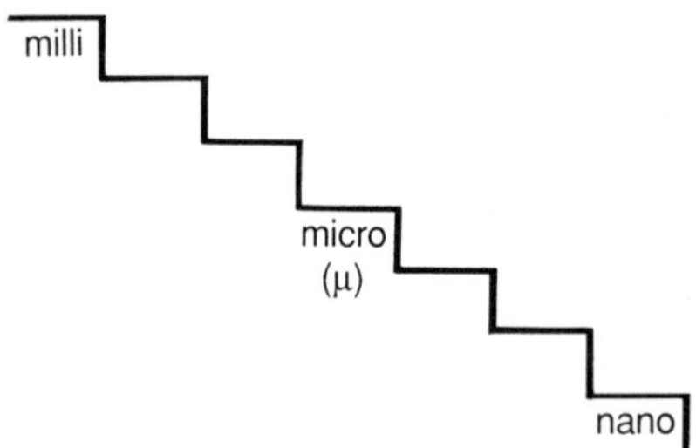

Using the "stairstep" method, make these conversions.

22. 9.97 μL = _____ mL

23. 2384 ng = ______ cg
24. 0.423 μg = ______ g
25. 1000 μL = ______ nL
26. 0.101 mm = ______ nm
27. 3267 μg = ______ g
28. 25.2 kg = ______ hg = ______ dag = ______ g = ______ dg = ______ cg = ______ mg

Answers to odd-numbered problems appear on page 231.

4.7 RELATIONSHIPS AMONG THE METRIC UNITS

Using the centimeter, we can derive a metric unit of volume. Consider a cube 1 cm on an edge:

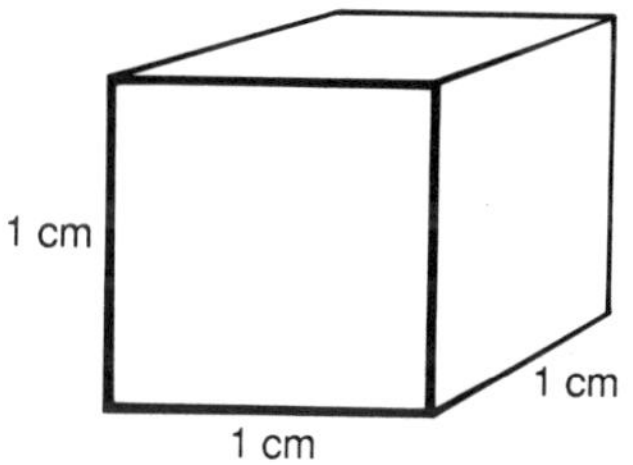

The volume of the cube is given by the formula

$$V = l \cdot w \cdot h.$$

Therefore

$$\begin{aligned} V &= (1\text{ cm}) \cdot (1\text{ cm}) \cdot (1\text{ cm}) \\ &= 1\text{ cm}^3, \text{ or 1 } \underline{c}\text{ubic } \underline{c}\text{entimeter } (= 1\text{ cc}) \end{aligned}$$

By definition,

$$\begin{aligned} 1\text{ cc} &= 1\text{ mL} \\ 1000\text{ cc} &= 1000\text{ mL} \\ 1000\text{ cc} &= 1\text{ L, etc.} \end{aligned}$$

EXAMPLE 4.7.1

Study the following cubic centimeter–milliliter equivalences.

$$\begin{aligned} 100\text{ cc} &= 100\text{ mL} \\ 15.4\text{ cc} &= 15.4\text{ mL} \\ 10\text{ cc} &= 10\text{ mL} = 1\text{ dL} \\ 15{,}667\text{ cc} &= 15{,}667\text{ mL} = 15.667\text{ L} \end{aligned}$$

If we could fill a cube like that pictured above with pure water at a temperature of 4.5°C (slightly above the freezing point), then the mass of the water is defined to equal exactly 1 g:

$$1\text{ cc of } H_2O = 1\text{ mL of } H_2O \text{ and is equivalent to } 1\text{ g (at } 4.5°\text{C)}$$

What about temperatures nearer those encountered in most laboratory environments? At temperatures near 20°–22°C, the mass of 1 cc of water is still close to 1 g:

$$1\text{ cc of } H_2O = 1\text{ mL } H_2O \approx 1\text{ g}$$

The symbol "≈" means "approximately equal to." We will make greater use of these relationships when we discuss the properties of solutions in a later chapter.

PROBLEM SET 2

1. 14.7 cc = ______ mL
2. 0.025 L = ______ cc
3. 0.12 kL = ______ cc
4. A beaker containing 45.0 cc of has a mass of approximately how many grams?
5. A chemist asks an assistant to quickly obtain approximately 520 g of distilled water. What is the fastest method for the assistant to measure the required amount?
6. How much mass does 9.5 kL of water have
   a. in grams?
   b. in kilograms?
7. A cube that is 2.0 cm long, 7.0 cm wide, and 5.0 cm deep is completely filled with distilled water. What is the approximate mass of the water?
8. A 250-mL beaker contains 182 g of water. How much more water can be added to the beaker to fill it to its capacity?

Answers to odd-numbered problems appear on page 231.

4.8 DIMENSIONAL ANALYSIS: ANOTHER METHOD OF PROBLEM SOLVING

When solving problems, students sometimes become confused because they overlook the units associated with the measured values. In this section, we use the units (or dimensions) to help set up the problems, such as those involving conversions from one unit to another. This method of problem solving is called **dimensional analysis.** It is also called the "factor unit method," since it involves multiplication by a fraction equal to "1." Examples of such fractions are

$$\frac{1 \text{ kL}}{1000 \text{ L}} = 1; \quad \frac{1000 \text{ g}}{1 \text{ kg}} = 1; \quad \frac{1 \text{ mL}}{1 \text{ cc}} = 1; \quad \frac{1 \text{ kL}}{1000 \text{ L}} = 1; \quad \frac{12 \text{ inches}}{1 \text{ ft}} = 1$$

These fractions are equal to "1" because the numerator of each is divided by a value equal to itself.

There are occasions when two different items may be written in the fractional form as above, even though they are not "equal" to each other. We say such items are "equivalent" to each other. For example, suppose the price of gasoline is $1.05 per gallon:

$$\$1.05 \simeq 1 \text{ gal which, in fraction form, becomes } \frac{\$1.05}{1 \text{ gal}} \text{ or } \frac{1 \text{ gal}}{\$1.05}.$$

The symbol "$\simeq$" means "equivalent to." We may still think of this fraction as equal to "1."

Examine the examples that follow to learn the steps involved in dimensional analysis. In these problems, we will be changing from one unit to another; in some instances, the given unit will be from one system, for example, the metric system, while the desired unit is from another, for example, the English system.

EXAMPLE 4.8.1

Change 8 ft to inches.

Solution	**Comments**
Given: 8 ft To find: ? inches	8 ft is given. You are trying to find inches.
8 ft · ______ (12 inches = 1 ft)	Always multiply by a fraction that will contain the conversion factor.

$8\ \cancel{ft} \cdot \frac{12\ \text{inches}}{1\ \cancel{ft}}$

The numerator of the conversion factor will contain the unit you are trying to find, and the denominator will contain the unit you are given. The given unit will divide or "cancel" out, and the unit you are trying to find will be left in the numerator.

$= \frac{8 \cdot 12\ \text{inches}}{1} = 96\ \text{inches}$

Carry out the computation. Leave "inches" in the answer.

Note that if the conversion factor in example 4.8.1 had been inserted upside down, the given unit would not have canceled out, and some undesired units would be left in the answer:

$$8\ \text{ft} \times \frac{1\ \text{ft}}{12\ \text{inches}} = \frac{8\ \text{ft}^2}{12\ \text{inches}} = \frac{2\ \text{ft}^2}{3\ \text{inches}}$$

This answer, of course, is not the one we want.

EXAMPLE 4.8.2

Change 2.3 L (of water) to drops

Solution

Liters → milliliters → drops

Comments

Plan a strategy based on the given unit and the unit you are trying to find.

$2.3\ \text{L} \cdot \frac{1000\ \text{mL}}{1\ \text{L}} \cdot \frac{15\ \text{drops}}{1\ \text{mL}}$

$2.3\ \cancel{L} \cdot \frac{1000\ \cancel{mL}}{1\ \cancel{L}} \cdot \frac{15\ \text{drops}}{1\ \cancel{mL}}$

$(2.3) \cdot (1000) \cdot (15)$ drops

There are 1000 mL in 1 L, and approximately 15 drops in 1 mL. Write down the given measurement, and multiply by the conversion factors. You can place several together. Cancel out the units to check the setup. Finish the computation. The unit "drops" should be the only unit left in the answer.

= 34,500 drops
= 34,000 drops

Round off your answer to two significant digits.

Notice that in example 4.8.2 we can place the conversion factors together and proceed to our solution according to the strategy we planned. If we had inserted one or both of the conversion factors into the setup incorrectly, the units would not have canceled out in the desired manner.

There may be an occasion where we want to convert from a measurement in the English system to one in the metric system. We can use the conversion table below for many of these problems.

Length	Volume	Mass
1 mile = 1. 609 km	1 L = 1.06 qt	1 kg = 2.2 lb
1 inch = 2.54 cm		1 lb = 453.6 g

EXAMPLE 4.8.3

Convert 180 lb to grams.

Solution

pounds → kilograms → grams

Comments

Plan a strategy.

$180\ \cancel{lb} \cdot \frac{1\ \cancel{kg}}{2.2\ \cancel{lb}} \cdot \frac{1000\ \text{g}}{1\ \cancel{kg}}$

Set up the conversion factors so that the desired unit is left in the answer.

$$\frac{(180) \cdot (1000)}{2.2} \text{ g} = 81{,}818 \text{ g}$$

Finish the computation.

$$= 82{,}000 \text{ g}$$

Round to two significant digits.

EXAMPLE 4.8.4

Change 7 ft, 4 inches to centimeters.

Solution / **Comments**

$$7 \cancel{\text{ft}} \cdot \frac{12 \text{ in}}{1 \cancel{\text{ft}}} = 84 \text{ inches}$$

$$84 \text{ inches} + 4 \text{ inches} = 88 \text{ inches}$$

First, change either feet to inches, or inches to feet. To make use of the conversion factor 1 inch = 2.54 cm, we will change feet to inches.

$$88 \cancel{\text{inches}} \cdot \frac{2.54 \text{ cm}}{1 \cancel{\text{inch}}} = 223.52 \text{ cm}$$

$$= 220 \text{ cm}$$

Change inches to centimeters. Inches should divide out, with centimeters left in the numerator. Round your answer.

EXAMPLE 4.8.5

The distance from the earth to the moon is approximately $3.86 \cdot 10^8$ m. What is this distance in miles?

Solution / **Comments**

meters → kilometers → miles

Plan a strategy.

$$3.86 \cdot 10^8 \cancel{\text{m}} \cdot \frac{1 \text{ km}}{10^3 \cancel{\text{m}}}$$

Change meters to kilometers. Do not do the arithmetic yet.

$$3.86 \cdot 10^8 \cancel{\text{m}} \cdot \frac{1 \cancel{\text{km}}}{10^3 \cancel{\text{m}}} \cdot \frac{1 \text{ mile}}{1.609 \cancel{\text{km}}}$$

Add a second conversion factor to change kilometers to miles: 1 mile = 1.609 km.

$$= \frac{3.86 \cdot 10^8}{1.609 \cdot 10^3} \text{ miles}$$

$$= 2.40 \cdot 10^5 \text{ miles}$$

Finish the computation. Notice that miles is left in the numerator. Round off your answer.

We can use dimensional analysis to convert from a measurement with two units (like miles/hour) to some other set of units (such as feet/second). Study the following example.

EXAMPLE 4.8.6

The density of an object was found to be 4.2 kg/L. What is the density of the object in grams per deciliter?

Solution / **Comments**

From kilograms → grams, and from liters → deciliters.

Note that there are two conversions to make. We can make both of these conversions using one setup.

$$\frac{4.2 \text{ kg}}{1 \text{ L}} \cdot \frac{1000 \text{ g}}{1 \text{ kg}} \cdot ?$$

First, change kg to g.

$$\frac{4.2 \text{ kg}}{1 \text{ L}} \cdot \frac{1000 \text{ g}}{1 \text{ kg}} \cdot \frac{1 \text{ L}}{10 \text{ dL}}$$

Second, change liters to deciliters.

$$\frac{4.2 \cancel{\text{kg}}}{1 \cancel{\text{L}}} \cdot \frac{1000 \text{ g}}{1 \cancel{\text{kg}}} \cdot \frac{1 \cancel{\text{L}}}{10 \text{ dL}}$$

The only units left are grams per deciliter.

$$\frac{(4.2) \cdot (1000) \cdot (1) \text{ g}}{10 \text{ dL}}$$

$$= \frac{420 \text{ g}}{\text{dL}}$$

Finish the computation.

Dimensional analysis may be used for any problem where conversions are required. You will encounter this method again, especially when the mole concept is introduced in Chapter 6.

PROBLEM SET 3

Make all conversions using dimensional analysis.

1. 75.2 kg to lb
2. 10.41 gal to liters
3. 7 lb 1 oz to kilograms
4. 35 mm to inches
5. $10\bar{0}$ yd to meters
6. 12.0 oz to milliliters
7. 6 ft 2 inches to centimeters
8. 50.0 miles/hour to feet per hour ("per" means "divided by")
9. 88.0 ft/sec to miles per hour
10. 3.5 qt to milliliters
11. Change your age, in years, to seconds using dimensional analysis.
12. How far can you drive an ambulance on $15.00 worth of gas if gas cost $1.09 per gallon, and the ambulance gets 22 miles per gallon of gas?
13. An IV set delivers 32 drops/min into a patient's vein. How much IV solution in milliliters can be delivered in 1 hour if there are 16 drops of the IV fluid in 1 mL?
14. The muzzle velocity of a certain rifle cartridge is 2200 ft/sec (The bullet is travelling this fast as it exits the rifle barrel.) What is the speed of the bullet in miles per hour?
15. A laboratory floor has a length of 25.0 ft and a width of 12.4 ft. What is the area of the floor in square meters?

    $$\left[\textit{Hint: } \left(\frac{12 \text{ inches}}{1 \text{ ft}}\right)^2 = \frac{144 \text{ inches}^2}{1 \text{ ft}^2}\right]$$

16. A typical IV bag holds $100\bar{0}$ cc of fluid. How many pints of fluid is this?
17. The average adult male has 13 pints of blood in his body. Convert this to milliliters.
18. A Pasteur pipette used in a chemistry laboratory was calibrated and found to deliver 20 drops of water per milliliter. A procedure calls for 2.5 mL reagent to be delivered dropwise. How many drops of the reagent should be delivered?
19. An automobile engine has a cubic inch displacement of 350 inches^3. (This is the volume of all of the cylinders of the car's engine.) What is the displacement in liters? [*Hint*: If 2.54 cm = 1 inch, then $(2.54 \text{ cm})^3 = (1 \text{ inch})^3$]
20. A certain laboratory chemical costs 15 cents per 150 mL of solution. At this price, how much would exactly 1 gallon of the chemical cost?
21. A 20% solution of sodium hydroxide contains 1.0 g of sodium hydroxide per 5 mL of solution. How much sodium hydroxide is dissolved in 4000 mL of a 20% solution?
22. The earth rotates once in 24 hours. If the circumference of the earth at the equator is 25,000 miles, how far will a point on the equator move in 120 minutes?

Answers to odd-numbered problems appear on page 231.

CHAPTER REVIEW

(4.1–4.6)

Make the following metric conversions:

1. 2.35 cm = _____ mm
2. 19.2 kg = _____ g
3. 0.39 cL = _____ dL
4. 20,000 mg = _____ dag
5. 2.1 cc = _____ mL
6. 80.3 kL = _____ dL
7. 14.2 g = _____ mg
8. 2.4 nL = _____ L
9. 7.8 dag = _____ dg
10. 9630 cm = _____ km

(4.7)

11. A box 4.8 cm × 2.1 cm × 5.0 cm is completely filled with distilled water. Approximately how much mass does the distilled water have?
12. A chemist pours 25.2 mL of distilled water into a beaker resting on a balance. Approximately how much does the mass recorded by the balance increase?

(4.7–4.8)

13. A swimming pool $3\overline{0}$ ft long, 15 ft wide, and 6.0 ft deep is completely filled with water. What is the approximate mass of the water in kilograms?

(4.8)

14. Change 77 kg to pounds.
15. A baby weighs 8 lb 12 oz at birth. What is the mass of the baby in kilograms?
16. A laboratory chemical costs $2.00 per $20\overline{0}$ mL. How many milliliters of the chemical can be bought for $25.00?
17. Last year, Dr. Med I. Care gave 5.0 pints of blood to the local bloodmobile. How many liters of blood is this?
18. A student must deliver 15.0 mL of acid into a reaction beaker. The pipette delivers 18 drops of acid per milliliter. How many drops will the student add to the beaker?
19. If the normal level of glucose in the bloodstream is 65 mg/dL, how much glucose is present in the bloodstream of a person whose blood capacity is exactly 7 L?

Answers to odd-numbered problems appear on page 231.

chapter **5**

Algebra as a Tool

OBJECTIVES

After studying this chapter, the student should be able to:

1. Solve equations with one unknown.
2. Express a formula (or literal equation) in terms of any of its parts.
3. Solve problems dealing with the application of ratio and proportion.
4. Solve problems dealing with the application of direct, inverse, and joint variation.

5.1 INTRODUCTION

Algebra has been called the "arithmetic of symbols." The purpose of this chapter is to explain how to solve equations and correctly manipulate formulas with more than one unknown part. It attempts to provide enough background to handle the algebra involved in the various allied health fields.

5.2 DEFINITION OF EQUATION

An **equation** is the statement that two quantities are equal. An equation may contain an unknown quantity that we will want to isolate on one side of the "equals" sign. When this is done, we have solved the equation.

The following section outlines rules and procedures that make possible the solution of equations and formulas encountered in the allied health professions.

5.3 SOME USEFUL RULES OF ALGEBRA

To describe the following rules of algebra, we review the concept of variable. A **variable** is a symbol, usually a letter of the alphabet, which may represent more than one value. A **constant**, on the other hand, is a symbol that always represents the same value. For example, the product of $2 \cdot x$ contains the variable x and the constant 2.

Let us assume that you work for an hourly wage of \$4.00. Your weekly salary would then be equal to \$4.00 times the number of hours that you work. Suppose that your schedule varies and you work a different number of hours each week. We can now employ variables and write an equation that will calculate your salary every week regardless of your schedule, provided your hourly wage does not change. Let W represent your weekly salary and H represent the number of hours that you work. Then

$$\mathrm{W} = 4.00 \cdot H$$

W and H are variables since they may represent different values during different weeks and 4.00 is a constant. W is called the **left side** of the equation because it comprises all that is to the left of the equals sign; similarly, $4.00 \cdot \mathrm{H}$ is called the **right side** of the equation. Each part of the equation connected by a plus or minus sign is called a **term**.

Generally the numerical part of each term is called a **coefficient.** For example, in the term 4.00 H, 4.00 is the coefficient of H in that particular term.

Let us look at another example of an equation to review our nomenclature. In the equation

$$x - 5(x - 3) = 7x - 2$$

$x - 5(x - 3)$ is the **left side** of the equation

$7x - 2$ is the **right side** of the equation

x, $-5(x - 3)$, $7x$, and -2 are each **terms** of the equation

1 is the **coefficient** of x in the x term

-5 is the **coefficient** of $(x - 3)$ in the $-5(x - 3)$ **term**

7 is the **coefficient** of x in the $7x$ **term**

-2 is simply called a **constant term** since it contains no variable

Now that we understand what variables and constants are, we can look at some important rules that provide essential background for solving equations.

RULE 1

The Commutative Rule

In Algebra

$x + y = y + x$

and

$xy = yx$, where x and y represent any real numbers.

In Words

Addition and *multiplication* when carried out in any order will produce the same result. This rule also applies to any situation where more than two values are either *added* or *multiplied.* This rule applies *only* to the operations of *addition* and *multiplication.*

Examples

$3 + 2 = 2 + 3 = 5$

$3 \cdot 2 = 2 \cdot 3 = 6$

$7 + x = x + 7$

$xyf = yfx$

$x + 2y + 5y + 7r = 7r + 5y + x + 2y$

$(6f)(12q)r = r(6f)(12q)$

$(x + 2)(y - 5) = (y - 5)(x + 2)$

RULE 2

The Associative Rule

In Algebra

$(x + y) + z = x + (y + z)$

and

$(xy)z = x(yz)$, where x, y, and z are any real numbers.

In Words

When more than two values are *added* or *multiplied* they may be grouped or associated in any manner (by means of parentheses and brackets) without changing the result. This rule applies *only* to the operations of *addition* and *multiplication.*

Examples

$(2 + 3) + 5 = 2 + (3 + 5) = 10$

$(2 \cdot 3) \cdot 5 = 2 \cdot (3 \cdot 5) = 30$

$(x + 3) + q = x + (3 + q)$

$(2x)z = 2(xz)$

$(2x + y) + 3z = 2x + (y + 3z)$

$(9y)(zq) = 9yzq$*

* Observe that this rule allows us to remove or put in grouping symbols as well as rearrange them.

RULE 3

The Identity Rule for Addition

In Algebra	In Words	Examples
$x + 0 = 0 + x = x$, where x is any real number.	Any value remains unchanged when it is added to zero or zero is added to it.	$6 + 0 = 6$ $0 + \frac{19}{3} = \frac{19}{3}$ $x + 0 = x$ $0 + 5x = 5x$ $-\frac{2fq}{y} + 0 = -\frac{2fq}{y}$ $0 - 3f = -3f$ $\frac{3y}{4} = 0 + \frac{3y}{4}$

RULE 4

The Identity Rule for Multiplication

In Algebra	In Words	Examples
$x \cdot 1 = 1 \cdot x = x$, where x is any real number.	Any value remains unchanged when it is multiplied by 1 or 1 is multiplied by it.	$1 \cdot 3 = 3 \cdot 1 = 3$ $\frac{401}{2} \cdot 1 = \frac{401}{2}$ $-\frac{3}{2} \cdot 1 = -\frac{3}{2}$ $3x \cdot 1 = 3x$ $\frac{x}{y} \cdot 1 = \frac{x}{y}$ $-\frac{2x}{f} \cdot 1 = -\frac{2x}{f}$

RULE 5

The Inverse Rule for Addition

In Algebra	In Words	Examples
For every real number x, there exists a real number, $-x$, such that $x + (-x) = (-x) + x = 0$ x and $-x$ are said to be opposites or *additive inverses* of each other.	Every real number has its opposite, which is the same numerical value with only the sign changed. These two values when added together always equal zero.	$-3 + 3 = 0$ $5 + (-5) = 0$ $\frac{6}{7} - \frac{6}{7} = 0$ $3x - 3x = 0$ $\frac{2y}{3} + \left(-\frac{2y}{3}\right) = 0$ $-8ab + 8ab = 0$

RULE 6

The Inverse Rule for Multiplication

In Algebra

For every real number x except 0, there exists a number $\frac{1}{x}$ such that

$$x \cdot \frac{1}{x} = \frac{1}{x} \cdot x = 1$$

x and $\frac{1}{x}$ are called *multiplicative inverses* of each other. They are also said to be *reciprocals* of each other.

In Words

If any real number is inverted (turned upside down), its reciprocal or multiplicative inverse is obtained. The product of a number and its reciprocal is always equal to 1.

Examples

$3 \cdot \frac{1}{3} = 1$

$\frac{4}{3} \cdot \frac{3}{4} = 1$

$\frac{x}{2} \cdot \frac{2}{x} = 1$

$\frac{pq}{r} \cdot \frac{r}{pq} = 1$

$-\frac{1}{8x} \cdot -\frac{8x}{1} = 1$

$-\frac{x}{2} \cdot -\frac{2}{x} = 1$

$-\frac{5y}{4} \cdot -\frac{4}{5y} = 1$

RULE 7

The Distributive Property of Multiplication over Addition or Subtraction

In Algebra

$x(y + z) = xy + xz$

or

$(y + z)x = yx + zx$, where x, y, and z are real numbers.

In Words

If a sum or difference of terms is multiplied by another term, then each part of that sum or difference can be multiplied separately by that term and the products added or subtracted. This rule also applies to the case where more than two terms are combined inside the parenthesis or brackets.

Examples

$3(z + q) = 3z + 3q$

$4r(t - p) = 4rt - 4rp$

$9(x + 3) = 9x + 27$

$7(2x - 5y - z) = 14x - 35y - 7z$

$(z + q)R = zR + qR$

$(1 - q)7 = 7 - 7q$

$x(y - z + 1) = xy - xz + x$

$5(2x - 3y + 7r - 5) = 10x - 15y + 35r - 25$

$-(pq - tv + 1) = -1(pq - tv + 1) = -pq + tv - 1$

In examples of the distributive property, observe that the grouping symbol containing the sum or difference may appear on the left *or* right of the other term without changing the result. This is true because multiplication follows the commutative rule. Here is another example:

$$f(r + t) = fr + ft = rf + tf = (r + t)f$$

PROBLEM SET 1

Indicate which rule (or rules) justifies each of the following statements. Be careful! More than one rule may be needed to justify some of these statements.

1. $3x \cdot 1 = 3x$
2. $5xyf = 5yfx$
3. $7q + (-7q) = 0$
4. $\frac{2x}{3y} \cdot \frac{3y}{2x} = 1$
5. $2x + 3y + f = 2x + (3y + f)$
6. $(sx)(2y)(cx) = (sy)(2x)(xc)$
7. $-\frac{1}{3}r + 0 = -\frac{1}{3}r$
8. $-\frac{2}{3} \cdot -\frac{3}{2} = 1$
9. $-3q(r - 3 + pt) = -3qr + 9q - 3qpt$
10. $-(x - 2y + 5t - 8) = -x + (2y - 5t + 8)$

Answers to odd-numbered problems appear on page 231.

5.4 SOLVING EQUATIONS

An equation is the statement that two quantities are equal. For example, the statements

$$2x = 3$$
$$9x - 2 = 5$$
$$3(y - 2) + 5(y - 3) = 7y$$
$$f = \frac{pq}{r}$$

are all equations.

To solve an equation is to find, by proper means, a value that, when substituted for the variable, will make the statement true. For example, the equation $2x + 5 = 11$ is called an **open sentence.** That is, before we substitute a known value for x the statement is neither true nor false. However, once we substitute 3 for x, the equation becomes a true statement. Thus the equation is solved. Notice,

$$2x + 5 = 11$$
$$2(3) + 5 = 11$$
$$6 + 5 = 11$$
$$11 = 11$$

The following equations involve more than one variable, that is, they relate more than one unknown quantity:

$$D = rt$$
$$F = \frac{9}{5}C + 32$$
$$E = IR$$

We will do more with these kinds of equations in another section. We begin by solving equations containing one unknown quantity. To do this we need two more rules that deal specifically with solving equations.

RULE 8

Keep the Equation Balanced: Whatever operation is applied to one side of an equation must be applied to the other side. Think of the equation as two weights balanced on either side of the equal sign. If the weight is increased or diminished on one side, the weight on the other side must be increased or diminished by the same amount.

This keeps the equation balanced. For example, in the equation

$$2x - 3 = 7,$$

if we add 3 to the left side, we must add 3 to the right side as well:

$$\begin{array}{rcr} 2x - 3 & = & 7 \\ +\ 3 & = & +\ 3 \\ \hline 2x \quad & = & 10 \end{array}$$

Now, to solve for x, divide $2x$ by 2. However, if we divide the left side of our resulting equation ($2x = 10$) by 2, we must do the same to the right side.

$$2x = 10$$

$$\frac{2x}{2} = \frac{10}{2}$$

$$x = 5$$

The equation is now solved properly because throughout the solution process we kept the equation balanced.

RULE 9

Use Inverse Operations Correctly

Any operation in mathematics can be undone by means of an inverse operation. We saw examples of this in the previous section. Addition and subtraction are **inverse operations** because they undo each other. If we have x and add 4 to it, we can undo that operation by simply subtracting 4. This brings us back to x.

x	
$x + 4$	Add 4.
$-\ 4$	Subtract 4.
$x + 0 = x$	Back to our starting point

If we have x and multiply it by 4, we can undo that operation with division by 4. This brings us back to x.

$4x$	Multiply by 4
$\frac{4x}{4}$	Divide by 4
x	Back to x

The important thing to remember is that you must use the correct operation to undo what has been done. For example, in the equation $3x + 7 = 19$, we can find x by undoing the operations that have been performed on x. We can undo the addition of 7 *only* by the *subtraction* of 7. In keeping with Rule 8 we must subtract 7 from the other side as well.

$$\begin{array}{rcr} 3x + 7 & = & 19 \\ -\ 7 & = & -\ 7 \\ \hline 3x \quad & = & 12 \end{array} \qquad \text{Subtract 7 from both sides.}$$

To isolate x, we must next undo the multiplication by 3. This is done with division by 3. Once again, we must also divide the other side by 3 to keep the equation balanced.

$$3x = 12$$

$$\frac{\cancel{3}x}{\cancel{3}} = \frac{12}{3} \qquad \text{Divide both sides by 3.}$$

$$x = 4$$

Now the equation is solved because we have used the correct inverse operations in the correct order. The variable x is multiplied by 3 and then 7 is added to that product.

To reverse this process, we undo the addition first and then divide by 3 to recover x.

Do not try to undo multiplication with subtraction. Multiplication can only be undone with division and vice versa. Addition can only be undone with subtraction and vice versa.

Incorrect	*Correct*
$7x = 15$	$7x = 15$
$7x = 15$	$\frac{7x}{7} = \frac{15}{7}$
$-7 = -7$	$x = \frac{15}{7}$
$x = 8$	

We now proceed with some examples of solving equations with one unknown quantity.

EXAMPLE 5.4.1

Solve $x + 5 = 23$.

Solution

$$\begin{aligned} x + 5 &= 23 \\ -5 &= -5 \\ \hline x &= 18 \end{aligned}$$

Comments

Subtract 5 from both sides of the equation to undo addition of 5 and isolate x.

EXAMPLE 5.4.2

Solve $\frac{x}{3} = 15$.

Solution

$$3 \cdot \frac{x}{3} = 15 \cdot 3$$

$$x = 45$$

Comments

Undo division of x by 3 with multiplication of both sides by 3.

This isolates x and solves the equation.

EXAMPLE 5.4.3

Solve $2x - 3 = 9$.

Solution

$$\begin{aligned} 2x - 3 &= 9 \\ +3 &= +3 \\ \hline 2x &= 12 \end{aligned}$$

$$\frac{\not{2}x}{\not{2}} = \frac{12}{2}$$

$$x = 6$$

Comments

Add 3 to both sides to undo subtraction of 3.

Divide both sides of resulting equation by 2 to undo multiplication by 2.

This isolates x and solves the equation.

EXAMPLE 5.4.4

Solve $5x - 7 = 2x + 5$.

Solution

$$\begin{aligned} 5x - 7 &= 2x + 5 \\ -5x \quad &\quad -5x \\ \hline -7 &= -3x + 5 \end{aligned}$$

$$\begin{aligned} -7 &= -3x + 5 \\ -5 \quad &\quad -5 \\ \hline -12 &= -3x \end{aligned}$$

$$\frac{-12}{-3} = \frac{-\not{3}x}{-\not{3}}$$

$$4 = x$$

Comments

Subtract $5x$ from both sides in order to collect on the same side of the equals sign all the terms that contain x.

Subtract 5 from both sides to undo addition of 5 and separate, with the equals sign, the terms that contain the unknown from the terms that do not.

Divide both sides by -3 to undo multiplication by -3. This isolates x and solves the equation.

We can check our solution in the previous example by substituting $x = 4$ into the equation $5x - 7 = 2x + 5$:

$$5(4) - 7 = 2(4) + 5$$
$$20 - 7 = 8 + 5$$
$$13 = 13$$

EXAMPLE 5.4.5

Solve $3(y - 2) = 12$.

Solution	Comments
$3(y - 2) = 12$ $3y - 6 = 12$	Use the distributive rule to remove parentheses.
$3y - 6 = 12$ $+ 6 = + 6$ $3y = 18$	Add 6 to both sides to undo subtraction of 6.
$\frac{\not{3}y}{\not{3}} = \frac{18}{3}$	Divide both sides by 3 to undo multiplication by 3.
$y = 6$	This isolates y and solves the equation.

EXAMPLE 5.4.6

Solve $4(z - 5) + 3 = 2z - 7$.

Solution	Comments
$4(z - 5) + 3 = 2z - 7$ $4z - 20 + 3 = 2z - 7$	Use distributive rule to remove the parentheses.
$4z - 17 = 2z - 7$	Simplify the left side by combining -20 and 3.
$4z - 17 = 2z - 7$ $+ 17 \quad + 17$ $4z = 2z + 10$ $- 2z = - 2z$ $2z = 10$	By adding and subtracting the same terms to both sides, the terms containing z are separated from those that do not.
$\frac{\not{2}z}{\not{2}} = \frac{10}{2}$	Divide both sides by 2 to undo multiplication by 2.
$z = 5$	This isolates z and solves the equation.

EXAMPLE 5.4.7

Solve $3q - (q - 2) = 3(2q + 5) + 10$.

Solution	Comments
$3q - (q - 2) = 3(2q + 5) + 10$ $3q - q + 2 = 6q + 15 + 10$	Use the distributive rule to remove the parentheses on each side. Note that a minus sign in front of a parenthesis indicates that each term inside is to be multiplied by -1.
$2q + 2 = 6q + 25$	Combine the like terms to simplify both sides of the equation.
$2q + 2 = 6q + 25$ $- 2q \quad - 2q$ $2 = 4q + 25$ $- 25 = - 25$ $- 23 = 4q$	Subtract the same terms from each side of the equation to separate the terms that contain q from those that do not.
$\frac{-23}{4} = \frac{\not{4}q}{\not{4}}$	Divide both sides of the equation by 4 to undo multiplication by 4.
$\frac{-23}{4} = q$	This isolates q and solves the equation.

PROBLEM SET 2

Solve each of the following equations for the variable indicated.

1. $x - 3 = -4$
2. $-5 + x = 14$
3. $9 - x = 17$
4. $\frac{x}{6} = 9$
5. $7x = 2149$
6. $2x + 3 = 11$
7. $8 - 3x = 2$
8. $19 = 25 - 2x$
9. $-x = 121$
10. $3 - x = 8$
11. $5y - 4 = 7y + 10$
12. $9q - 7 = 3 - 2q$
13. $10 - 3r = 6r$
14. $15 + 3z = 16 - z$
15. $5u - 6 = 12u + 7$
16. $3.2p - 5.4 = 6.1p + 1$

(*Hint*: Multiply each term of the equation by 10 to remove decimal numbers.)

17. $5(k - 3) = 15$
18. $7t = 3t - 5(t + 6)$
19. $6v + 3(v - 1) = 5(v - 5) + 13$
20. $12 - (w - 2) = 7 + 5w$
21. $4 - (r + 5) = 5(r - 2) + 10$
22. $5(x - 3) + 9 = x + 3$
23. $6(x - 2) - (x - 4) = 8x + 2$
24. $10(y + 5) - (y + 3) = 3(y - 2) - 1$
25. $-3(h - 4) - (5 - h) = 4(h - 3) - 2(h + 6)$
26. $7(x - 1) + 8x = -(x + 3) + 10$
27. $12(x - 2) = -x + 8$
28. $29 - 3x = x + (10 - 3x)$
29. $(100 - x) - 7 = 10(x - 3)$
30. $x - (4 + 3x) - 12 = x + (7 - 2x)$

Answers to odd-numbered problems appear on page 232.

5.5 EQUATIONS WITH FRACTIONS

Fractions appear in equations in two ways. Sometimes they appear as constants or as coefficients of the variable. Examples of this are:

$$x + \frac{1}{3} = 5$$

$$\frac{1}{2}x = 28$$

$$\frac{1}{3}x - \frac{1}{4} = \frac{1}{2} + 2$$

$$\frac{2}{3}(x - 3) = 30$$

Fractions in an equation may also contain the variable in the denominator. Example of this are:

$$\frac{2}{x} = 45$$

$$\frac{1}{2x} + \frac{1}{x} = \frac{1}{2} - 4$$

$$\frac{3}{x-1} + \left(-\frac{2}{x}\right) = \frac{4}{x}$$

Regardless of how the fractions appear in an equation, the *first step* in the solution is usually to multiply each term by the **lowest common denominator** of all fractions in the equation.

We have already considered finding the lowest common denominator for arithmetic fractions such as $\frac{2}{3}$, $\frac{3}{10}$, and $\frac{7}{9}$.

For the sake of review, the lowest common denominator (lcd) of these fractions will be found.

Step 1. Express each of the denominators in terms of its prime factors, using exponents if possible.

$$3 = 3'$$
$$10 = 5 \cdot 2$$
$$9 = 3^2$$

Step 2. Form the product of all the different prime factors.

$$2 \cdot 3 \cdot 5$$

Step 3. On each of these factors place the largest exponent found on it in step 1 and multiply.

$$2 \cdot 3^2 \cdot 5 = 90$$

90 is the lcd of $\frac{2}{3}$, $\frac{3}{10}$, and $\frac{7}{9}$.

Remember that a number with no exponent indicated is understood to be the first power. For example, $2 = 2^1$.

We now consider a technique that will yield a lowest common denominator for fractions containing a variable.

Consider the fractions

$$\frac{2x}{x-1}, \frac{4}{3(x+3)}, \text{ and } \frac{5}{6x}.$$

Step 1. It is important that the student identify the different factors here. They are

$$6, 3, x, (x - 1), \text{ and } (x + 3).$$

Step 2. Find the lcd of the constant factors if there are any. In this example they are 6 and 3, which have 6 as the lcd.

Step 3. Form the product of the lcd found in step 2 and the variable factors from step 1. This product will be the lcd for all the fractions. In this case it is

$$6x(x - 1)(x + 3).$$

In some cases step 2 is unnecessary. Consider the fractions

$$\frac{1}{R_1}, \frac{2}{(R-2)}, \text{ and } \frac{8}{V}.$$

The different factors are R_1, $(R - 2)$, and V. There are no constant factors, so the lcd is simply the product of these factors, which is

$$R_1V(R - 2).$$

For convenience, we write R_1 and V first. This is possible because of the commutative rule.

The student will also notice that throughout this discussion we have treated sums and differences involving variables as single factors. For example, the product $x(x - 1)(x + 2)$ consists of three factors: x, $(x - 1)$, and $(x + 2)$.

When an equation contains fractions with a variable in the denominator, the student should substitute the possible solution in each denominator to make sure that zero does not result. If it does, then the value found is not a solution of the equation. Such a value found from solving the equation is called an **extraneous** root.

The following examples will help you to solve fractional equations.

EXAMPLE 5.5.1

Solve $x - \frac{3}{4} = \frac{7}{3}$.

Solution

$$x - \frac{3}{4} = \frac{7}{3}$$

$$12x - (\cancel{12})^{3} \cdot \frac{3}{\cancel{4}} = (\cancel{12})^{4} \cdot \frac{7}{\cancel{3}}$$

Comments

The first step is to multiply both sides of the equation by the lowest common denominator of $-\frac{3}{4}$ and $\frac{7}{3}$, which is 12.

$$12x - 9 = 28.$$

$$\begin{array}{rcr} 12x - 9 & = & 28 \\ +9 & = & +\ \ 9 \\ \hline 12x \quad\ & = & 37 \end{array}$$

Add 9 to both sides to undo the subtraction of 9.

$$\frac{\cancel{12}}{\cancel{12}}x = \frac{37}{12}$$

Divide both sides by 12 to undo multiplication by 12.

$$x = \frac{37}{12}$$

This isolates x and solves the equation.

EXAMPLE 5.5.2

Solve $\frac{1x}{2} + \frac{2}{3} = \frac{1x}{4} - 2$.

Solution

$$\frac{1x}{2} + \frac{2}{3} = \frac{1x}{3} - 2$$

$$(\cancel{6})^{3} \cdot \frac{1x}{\cancel{2}} + (\cancel{6})^{2}\,\frac{2}{\cancel{3}}$$

$$= (\cancel{6})^{2} \cdot \frac{1x}{\cancel{3}} - (6)2$$

Comments

The first step is to multiply both sides of the equation by the lowest common denominator of $\frac{1}{2}$, $\frac{2}{3}$, and $\frac{1}{3}$, which is 6.

$$3x + 4 = 2x - 12$$

$$\begin{array}{rcr} 3x + 4 & = & 2x - 12 \\ -\ 2x \qquad & = & -\ 2x \qquad \\ \hline x + \cancel{4} & = & -\ 12 \\ -\ \cancel{4} & = & -\ \ 4 \\ \hline x \qquad & = & -\ 16 \end{array}$$

By subtracting the same terms from both sides of the equation, the terms which contain x are separated from those which do not. This isolates x and solves the equation.

EXAMPLE 5.5.3

Solve $10 = \frac{5}{9}(F - 32)$.

Solution

$$10 = \frac{5}{9}(F - 32)$$

$$(9)10 = (9)\frac{5}{9}(F - 32)$$

$$90 = 5(F - 32)$$
$$90 = 5F - 160$$

$$\begin{array}{rcl} 90 &=& 5F - 160 \\ +160 && +160 \\ \hline 250 &=& 5F \end{array}$$

$$\frac{250}{5} = \frac{5F}{5}$$

$$50 = F$$

Comments

The first step is to multiply each term on both sides of the equation by the lowest common denominator of $\frac{5}{9}$, $(F - 32)$, and 10, which is 9.

Use the distributive rule to remove the parenthesis.

Add 160 to both sides to undo subtraction of 160.

Divide both sides by 5 to undo multiplication by 5.

This isolates F and solves the equation.

EXAMPLE 5.5.4

Solve $\frac{3}{x} - 7 = \frac{1}{2}$.

Solution

$$\frac{3}{x} - 7 = \frac{1}{2}$$

$$2x\frac{3}{x} - (2x)7 = (2x)\frac{1}{2}$$

$$6 - 14x = x$$

$$\begin{array}{rcl} 6 - 14x &=& x \\ +14x && +14x \\ \hline 6 &=& 15x \end{array}$$

$$\frac{6}{15} = \frac{15x}{15}$$

$$\frac{6}{15} = \frac{2}{5} = x$$

Comments

The first step is to multiply both sides of the equation by the lowest common denominator of $\frac{3}{x}$, $\frac{1}{2}$, and 7, which is $2x$.

Add $14x$ to both sides in order to separate the terms that contain x from those that do not.

Divide both sides by 15 in order to undo multiplication by 15.

This isolates x and, after $\frac{6}{15}$ is reduced to lowest terms, solves the equation.

Notice that if $x = \frac{2}{5}$ the term $\frac{3}{x}$ will not have a zero in its denominator.

EXAMPLE 5.5.5

Solve $\frac{2}{x+1} - \frac{1}{x} = \frac{2}{x}$.

Solution

$$\frac{2}{x+1} - \frac{1}{x} = \frac{2}{x}$$

$$x(x+1)\frac{2}{x+1} - x(x+1)\frac{1}{x}$$
$$= x(x+1)\frac{2}{x}$$

$$2x - (x + 1) = 2(x + 1)$$
$$2x - x - 1 = 2x + 2$$

Comments

The first step is to multiply both sides of the equation by the lowest common denominator of $\frac{2}{x+1}$, $\frac{1}{x}$, and $\frac{2}{x}$, which is $x(x + 1)$.

Use the distributive rule to remove parentheses on each side.

$x - 1 = 2x + 2$

Simplify the left side by combining like terms.

$$\begin{array}{rcl} x - 1 & = & 2x + 2 \\ -x & & -x \\ \hline -1 & = & x + 2 \\ -2 & & -2 \\ \hline -3 & = & x \end{array}$$

Subtract the same terms from each side in order to separate the terms that contain x from terms that do not. This isolates x and solves the equation.

Notice that if $x = -3$ none of the denominators of the original equation will be equal to zero.

EXAMPLE 5.5.6

Solve $\frac{2}{x} + \frac{5}{2x} = \frac{1}{x+2} - \frac{1}{x}$.

Solution

$\frac{2}{x} + \frac{5}{2x} = \frac{1}{x+2} - \frac{1}{x}$

Comments

The first step is to multiply both sides of the equation by the lowest common denominator of $2/x$, $5/2x$, $1/x + 2$, and $1/x$, which is $2x(x + 2)$.

$$2\cancel{x}(x + 2) \cdot \frac{2}{\cancel{x}} + \cancel{2x}(x + 2) \cdot \frac{5}{\cancel{2x}}$$

$$= 2x\cancel{(x + 2)} \cdot \frac{1}{\cancel{x + 2}} - 2\cancel{x}(x + 2) \cdot \frac{1}{\cancel{x}}$$

$4(x + 2) + 5(x + 2) = 2x - 2(x + 2)$

Use the distributive rule to remove the parentheses on each side.

$4x + 8 + 5x + 10$
$= 2x - 2x - 4$
$9x + 18 = -4$

Simplify each side by combining like terms.

$$\begin{array}{rcl} 9x + 18 & = & -4 \\ -18 & & -18 \\ \hline 9x & = & -22 \end{array}$$

Subtract 18 from each side in order to separate terms that contain x from terms that do not.

$\frac{\cancel{9}x}{\cancel{9}} = -\frac{22}{9}$

Divide both sides by 9 in order to undo multiplication by 9.

$x = -\frac{22}{9}$

This isolates x and solves the equation.

Notice that if $x = \frac{-22}{9}$ none of the denominators in the original equation will be equal to zero.

Summary of Procedures Necessary to Solve Equations

1. Remove fractions by multiplying each term by the lcd of all fractions in the equation.
2. Remove parentheses by applying the distributive rule.
3. Combine all like terms on the same side of the equals sign.
4. Separate the terms that contain the unknown (i.e., the variable to be isolated) from the terms that do not. This can be accomplished by adding (or subtracting) appropriate terms to both sides of the equation.
5. Divide each term in the equation by the coefficient of the unknown. This should leave the unknown isolated with a coefficient of positive one (+1), thus solving the equation.
6. Check for extraneous roots in cases where a variable appeared in one or more of the denominators of a fractional equation.

PROBLEM SET 3

Solve each of the following equations for the variable indicated.

1. $\frac{x}{2} = 34$
2. $\frac{5}{2}x = 15$
3. $2x - \frac{2}{3} = 4$
4. $\frac{x}{2} = \frac{8}{3}$
5. $\frac{1x}{3} + \frac{1}{2} = \frac{3}{4}$
6. $\frac{7a}{3} + \frac{3a}{4} = \frac{38}{6}$
7. $12x - \frac{3}{4} = \frac{2}{3}x + 2$
8. $\frac{3}{4}(x - 20) = 4x + 20$
9. $\frac{1}{10} - \frac{x-4}{x} = \frac{1}{x} + \frac{3}{20}$
10. $\frac{5b}{4} + \frac{b-1}{6} = -\frac{7}{12}$
11. $\frac{1}{2x} - \frac{3}{4x} = 12$
12. $1 - \frac{2}{x} = 10 - \frac{2}{3x}$
13. $\frac{2}{f} + \frac{4}{3} = \frac{6}{f}$
14. $\frac{1}{2}(x - 8) + 7x = 8$
15. $\frac{5}{y} = \frac{11}{72} - \frac{2}{y}$
16. $\frac{1}{a} + \frac{2}{3a} = 1$
17. $\frac{3}{x} + \frac{5}{x} = \frac{2}{x+1}$
18. $\frac{3}{x+1} + \frac{3}{x} = \frac{3}{4x}$
19. $\frac{9}{z-1} + \frac{8}{3z} = \frac{5}{6z} - \frac{1}{z}$

Answers to odd-numbered problems appear on page 232.

5.6 FORMULAS

A formula is an equation relating several variables. For example, consider the formula $D = RT$, where D is distance, R is average rate, and T is time. The distance you can go depends not only on how fast you go but also on how long you travel. The formula as given will tell you how far you have traveled given an average speed R and a time T. Suppose you are given a time and a distance and are asked to find the average speed R. This can be done if we take the formula $D = RT$, treat D and T as constants, and solve for R:

$$D = RT$$

$$\frac{D}{T} = \frac{R\not{T}}{\not{T}}$$ divide both sides by T to isolate R.

$$\frac{D}{T} = R$$ Now the equation is solved for R.

In a similar manner we can treat D and R as constants and solve for T:

$$D = RT$$

$$\frac{D}{R} = \frac{\not{R}T}{\not{R}}$$ Divide both sides by R to isolate T.

$$\frac{D}{R} = T$$ Now the equation is solved for T.

A formula can be solved for any of its component parts or variables by treating all the other parts of the formula as constants and following the rules already established for solving an equation.

We will now look at some examples. When solving a formula, sometimes called a **literal equation**, the part for which you are solving must be indicated.

EXAMPLE 5.6.1

Solve $\frac{R}{S} = V$ for R.

Solution

$\frac{\cancel{S}R}{\cancel{S}} = V \cdot S$

Multiply both sides of the equation by S to undo division by S.

$R = VS$

This isolates R and solves the equation for R.

EXAMPLE 5.6.2

Solve $\frac{R}{S} = V$ for S.

Solution

$\cancel{S} \cdot \frac{R}{\cancel{S}} = V \cdot S$

$R = VS$

As in any equation containing fractions, the first step is to remove them, with multiplication of both sides by the lowest common denominator, in this case S.

$\frac{R}{V} = \frac{\cancel{V}S}{\cancel{V}}$

Divide both sides by V in order to undo multiplication by V.

$\frac{R}{V} = S$

This isolates S and solves the equation for S.

EXAMPLE 5.6.3

Solve $a(q + r) = P$ for a.

Solution

$\frac{a\cancel{(q + r)}}{\cancel{(q + r)}} = \frac{P}{q + r}$

Divide both sides by $(q + r)$ to undo multiplication by $(q + r)$. [Note that the sum $(q + r)$ is treated as a *single variable*.]

$a = \frac{P}{q + r}$

This isolates a and solves the equation for a.

Notice that in this example the parentheses was not removed because it did *not* contain the variable for which we were solving.

EXAMPLE 5.6.4

Solve $a(q + r) = P$ for r.

Solution

$a(q + r) = P$

$aq + ar = P$

Use the distributive rule to remove the parentheses since it contains the variable for which we are solving.

$$\begin{array}{rcl} \cancel{aq} + ar &=& P \\ -\cancel{aq} & & -\ aq \\ \hline ar &=& P - aq \end{array}$$

By subtracting aq from both sides, we separate the terms that contain r from those that do not.

$\frac{\cancel{a}r}{\cancel{a}} = \frac{P - aq}{a}$

Divide both sides by a to undo multiplication by a.

$r = \dfrac{P - aq}{a}$ — This isolates r and solves the equation for r.

Observe the final answer in the previous example,

$$\frac{P - aq}{a}.$$

You will notice that the a's are *not* divided out; that is, we do *not* say

$$\frac{P - \not{a}q}{\not{a}} = P - q$$

Dividing into only part of a sum or difference is never correct *under any circumstances.* Look at this arithmetic example to see why this is true:

$\dfrac{18 + 12 - 8}{2}$ — This expression means that the entire combination of $18 + 12 - 8$ is divided by 2, *not* a part of it.

$= \dfrac{18}{2} + \dfrac{12}{2} - \dfrac{8}{2}$ — We must divide *each* and *every* part of this numerator by 2 to get the correct answer.

$= 9 + 6 - 4 = 11$

$\dfrac{18 + 12 - 8}{2} = \dfrac{22}{2} = 11$ — Of course since we know all of the values, we can simply combine the numerator and divide by 2.

$\dfrac{18 + 12 - \overset{4}{\not{8}}}{2} = 30 - 4 = 26$ — Notice, however, if we divide only one part of the numerator by 2, we get an incorrect result.

$26 \neq 11$

On the other hand, we may, in example 5.6.4, divide both parts of the numerator $P - aq$ by a, but not just the term aq:

Incorrect

$$\frac{P - aq}{a} = \frac{P - \not{a}q}{\not{a}} \neq P - q$$

Correct

$$\frac{P - aq}{a} = \frac{P}{a} - \frac{\not{a}q}{\not{a}} = \frac{P}{a} - 1$$

Please remember this as we continue with more examples.

EXAMPLE 5.6.5

Solve $\dfrac{1}{2}ax - \dfrac{b}{3} = 5$ for x.

Solution / **Comments**

$\overset{3}{\not{6}} \cdot \dfrac{1}{\not{2}}ax - \overset{2}{\not{6}} \cdot \dfrac{b}{\not{3}} = 5 \cdot 6$ — The first step is to remove fractions by multiplying both sides by the lowest common denominator, 6.

$3ax - 2b = 30.$

$$\begin{array}{rcl} 3ax - \not{2b} & = & 30 \\ + \not{2b} & & + 2b \\ \hline 3ax & = & 30 + 2b \end{array}$$

Add $2b$ to both sides to separate the terms that contain x from those that do not.

$\dfrac{\not{3}\not{a}x}{\not{3}\not{a}} = \dfrac{30 + 2b}{3a}$ — Divide both sides by $3a$ to undo multiplication by $3a$.

$x = \dfrac{30 + 2b}{3a}$ — This isolates x and solves the equation for x.

EXAMPLE 5.6.6

Solve $\frac{1}{V_1} = \frac{1}{V_2} - \frac{1}{V_3}$ for V_2.

Solution

$$\frac{1}{V_1} = \frac{1}{V_2} - \frac{1}{V_3}$$

Comments

Remove fractions with multiplication of both sides by the lowest common denominator of $1/V_1$, $1/V_2$, and $1/V_3$, which is $(V_1 V_2 V_3)$.

$$(\cancel{V_1} V_2 V_3)\frac{1}{\cancel{V_1}}$$

$$= (V_1 \cancel{V_2} V_3)\frac{1}{\cancel{V_2}} - (V_1 V_2 \cancel{V_3})\frac{1}{\cancel{V_3}}$$

$$V_2 V_3 = V_1 V_3 - V_1 V_2$$

$$\begin{array}{r} V_2 V_3 = V_1 V_3 - V_1 V_2 \\ + V_1 V_2 \qquad\qquad + V_1 V_2 \\ \hline V_1 V_2 + V_2 V_3 = V_1 V_3 \end{array}$$

Add $V_1 V_2$ to both sides in order to separate the terms that contain V_2 from those that do not.

$$V_2(V_1 + V_3) = V_1 V_3$$

Use the distributive rule in reverse to write the left side as a product of V_2 and $(V_1 + V_3)$. We do this to separate V_2 from the other variables.

$$\frac{V_2(\cancel{V_1 + V_3})}{(\cancel{V_1 + V_3})} = \frac{V_1 V_3}{V_1 + V_3}$$

Divide both sides by $(V_1 + V_3)$ in order to isolate V_2. This solves the equation for V_2.

$$V_2 = \frac{V_1 V_3}{V_1 + V_3}; (V_1 + V_3 \neq 0)$$

EXAMPLE 5.6.7

Solve $\frac{5}{3}(x - 8) = d$ for x.

Solution

$$\frac{5}{3}(x - 8) = d$$

Comments

Remove fractions with multiplication of both sides by the lowest common denominator of $\frac{5}{3}$, which is 3.

$$\cancel{3} \cdot \frac{5}{\cancel{3}}(x - 8) = 3 \cdot d$$

$$5(x - 8) = 3d$$
$$5x - 40 = 3d$$

Use distributive rule to remove the parentheses.

$$\begin{array}{r} 5x - 40 = 3d \\ + 40 \qquad + 40 \\ \hline 5x \qquad = 3d + 40 \end{array}$$

Add 40 to both sides in order to separate the terms that contain x from those that do not.

$$\frac{\cancel{5}x}{\cancel{5}} = \frac{3d + 40}{5}$$

Divide both sides by 5 in order to isolate x. This solves the equation for x.

$$x = \frac{3d + 40}{5}$$

or

$$x = \frac{3d}{5} + 8$$

EXAMPLE 5.6.8

Solve $\frac{3}{t - r} - 1 = \frac{4}{t - r}$ for t.

Solution

$(\cancel{t-r}) \cdot \frac{3}{\cancel{t-r}} - (t-r)\,1 = (\cancel{t-r}) \cdot \frac{4}{\cancel{t-r}}$

Comments
Remove fractions with multiplication of both sides by the lowest common denominator of $3/t - r$ and $4/t - r'$ which is $t - r$.

$3 - (t - r) = 4$
$3 - t + r = 4$

Use the distributive rule to remove the parentheses.

$$\begin{array}{rrcl} 3 & -\cancel{t} + r & = & 4 \\ & +\cancel{t} & & + t \\ \hline 3 & + r & = & \cancel{4} + t \\ -4 & & & -\cancel{4} \\ \hline -1 & + r & = & t \end{array}$$

Add t to both sides and subtract 4 from both sides in order to separate the terms that contain t from those that do not.

$r - 1 = t$

This isolates t and solves the equation for t. $(-1 + r = r - 1$ because of the Commutative Rule of Addition.)

EXAMPLE 5.6.9

Solve $\frac{1}{h} + \frac{q}{r-q} = \frac{2}{s}$ for q.

Solution

$\cancel{h}s(r-q)\frac{1}{\cancel{h}} + hs(\cancel{r-q})\frac{q}{\cancel{r-q}} = h\cancel{s}(r-q)\frac{2}{\cancel{s}}$

Comments
Remove the fraction with multiplication of both sides by the lcd of $\frac{1}{h}$, $\frac{q}{r-q}$, and $\frac{2}{s}$, which is $hs(r - q)$.

$s(r - q) + hsq = 2h(r - q)$
$sr - sq + hsq = 2hr - 2hq$
$2hq - sq + hsq = 2hr - sr$

Remove the parentheses using the distributive property.

$$\begin{array}{lcl} \cancel{sr} - sq + hsq & = & 2hr - \cancel{2hq} \\ +2hq - \cancel{sr} & & +\cancel{2hq} - sr \\ \hline q(2h - s + hs) & = & 2hr - sr \end{array}$$

Add $2hq$ to both sides and subtract sr from both sides to separate the terms that contain q from those that do not.

Using the distributive rule, write the left side as a product of q and $(2hs - s + hs)$.

$\frac{q(\cancel{2h - s + hs})}{(\cancel{2h - s + hs})} = \frac{2hr - sr}{(2h - s + hs)}$

Divide both sides of the equation by $(2h - s + hs)$ to solve for q.

$q = \frac{2hr - sr}{(2h - s + hs)}$

$(2h - s + hs) \neq 0.$

PROBLEM SET 4

Solve each of the following formulas for the variable indicated.

1. $P_1 = P_2P_3$, for P_3
2. $\frac{Q}{S} = L$, for S
3. $T = \frac{kq}{R}$, for q
4. $T = \frac{Kq}{R}$, for R
5. $C = 2\pi r$, for r
6. $A = \frac{1}{2}bh$, for h

7. $E = mc^2$, for m

8. $PV = nRT$, for T

9. $E = \frac{1}{2}mv^2$, for m

10. $\frac{P_1V_1}{T_1} = \frac{P_2V_2}{T_2}$, for V_2

11. $P = P_1 + P_2 + P_3$, for P_3

12. $F = \frac{GM_1M_2}{d^2}$, for M_2

13. $5(x + 3b) = 7 - b$, for x

14. $5(x + 3b) = 7 - b$, for b

15. $\frac{3}{4}(P - 2) = R$, for P

16. $C = \frac{5}{9}(F - 32)$, for F

17. $F = \frac{9}{5}C + 32$, for C

18. $D_1 = \frac{AD_2}{A + 12}$, for D_2

19. $M = \frac{28}{t + 2}$, for t

20. $M = \frac{2Q}{2 - q}$, for q

(*Note*: Q an q are two different variables.)

21. $\frac{1}{f} = \frac{1}{u} + \frac{1}{v}$, for u

22. $Y = \frac{vy}{v - s} - \frac{z}{v - s}$, for v

23. $\frac{1}{x} = \frac{2}{x - 2} + \frac{3}{wx}$, for w

Answers to odd-numbered problems appear on page 232.

5.7 RATIO AND PROPORTION

A **ratio** is simply a fraction. Examples of ratios are

$$\frac{3}{2}, \frac{6 \text{ pounds}}{10 \text{ pounds}}, \frac{5.2 \text{ miles}}{1 \text{ inch}}, \text{ 60 miles is to 3 hours, } \frac{500 \text{ mL}}{25 \text{ g}}$$

The word "ratio" in Latin means a "comparison." A fraction compares the size of one quantity to that of another. A **proportion** is the statement that two ratios are equal. For example,

$$\frac{3}{4} = \frac{6}{8}$$

is a proportion. Another way to state a proportion is to say, for example, "7 is to 5 as 35 is to what?" This can be written as $\frac{7}{5} = \frac{35}{x}$, where x is the unknown number. In this section we will deal with proportions that have unknown parts. We will find those missing parts, using the following rule:

RULE 10

$\frac{A}{B} = \frac{C}{D}$ if and only if $AD = BC$.

Rule 10 states that two ratios are equal only if the product of the first numerator and the second denominator is equal to the product of the second numerator and the first denominator. These products are called **cross products.** For example, if we look again at the proportion above we see that

$$\text{if } \frac{3}{4} = \frac{6}{8}$$

$$\text{then } 3 \cdot 8 = 4 \cdot 6$$

$$\text{or } 24 = 24$$

We use this rule and the rules for solving equations to find the missing parts of proportions. Some examples follow.

EXAMPLE 5.7.1

If $\frac{x}{5} = \frac{20}{50}$, find x.

Solution

If $\frac{x}{5} = \frac{20}{50}$

then $x \cdot 50 = 5 \cdot 20$
or $50x = 100$

$\frac{\cancel{50}x}{\cancel{50}} = \frac{100}{50}$

$x = 2$

Comments

Find the cross products and a simple equation results.

Solve by dividing both sides by 50.

We see that 2 is the same part of 5 that 20 is of 50.

EXAMPLE 5.7.2

If $\frac{25}{x} = \frac{15}{4}$, solve for x.

Solution

If $\frac{25}{x} = \frac{15}{4}$

then $25 \cdot 4 = 15 \cdot x$
or $100 = 15x$

$\frac{100}{15} = \frac{\cancel{15}x}{\cancel{15}}$

$\frac{20}{3} = x$

or $6\frac{2}{3} = x$

Comments

This example is solved exactly like example 5.7.1.

Find the cross products and a simple equation results.

Divide both sides by 15.

The answer is not always an integer. Sometimes it too will be a fraction.

EXAMPLE 5.7.3

Solve $\frac{40}{25} = \frac{10}{2x}$ for x.

Solution

If $\frac{40}{25} = \frac{10}{2x}$,

then $(40)(2x) = (25)(10)$
or $80x = 250$.

$\frac{\cancel{80}x}{\cancel{80}} = \frac{25\cancel{0}}{8\cancel{0}} = \frac{25}{8}$

$x = \frac{25}{8}$ or $3\frac{1}{8}$

Comments

Find the cross products.

A simple equation results, which is solved by division of *both sides* by 80.

Again, a fraction results.

EXAMPLE 5.7.4

If 12 is to 7 as x is to 21, find x.

Solution

$\frac{12}{7} = \frac{x}{21}$

Comments

"Is to" represents the fraction bar, and "as" represents an equal sign

$(12)(21) = 7(x)$
$252 = 7x$

$$\frac{252}{7} = \frac{\not{7}x}{\not{7}}$$

$36 = x$

The problem is solved as in the preceding examples.

Many word problems can be solved using ratio and proportion. Uses are found in making conversions, solution problems, radiology, and in working with the gas laws. Some examples follow.

EXAMPLE 5.7.5

If an architect's scale drawing of a new laboratory is such that $\frac{1}{2}$ inch = 6 feet, what is the length of the floor that measures $1\frac{3}{4}$ inches on the drawing?

Solution

$$\frac{\frac{1}{2}\text{ inch}}{6\text{ ft}} = \frac{1\frac{3}{4}\text{ inches}}{x\text{ ft}}$$

Comments

The ratios here compare inches to feet. If we compare inches to feet on one side, we must compare inches to feet on the other.

$$\left(\frac{1}{2}\right)(x) = (6)\left(1\frac{3}{4}\right).$$

Change mixed number to an improper fraction.

$$\frac{1}{2}x = 6 \cdot \frac{7}{4}$$

$$\frac{1}{2}x = \frac{42}{4}$$

$$\not{4}^{2} \cdot \frac{1}{2}x = \frac{42}{\not{4}} \cdot \not{4}$$

Multiply both sides by the lcd; then proceed as in the previous examples.

$2x = 42$

$x = 21$ ft

Be sure your answer carries the proper unit. The floor represented in the drawing is 21 ft in length.

EXAMPLE 5.7.6

If a laboratory assistant can order twenty Erlenmeyer flasks from Company A for \$30.00, or order the same kind of flasks from Company B at the rate of twelve for \$16.00, which is the best buy?

Hint: The best buy is found by determining the unit price, or the price of one flask. The company charging the lowest price per unit will provide the best buy.

Solution

Company A:

$$\frac{20\text{ flasks}}{\$30.00} = \frac{1\text{ flask}}{x}$$

Comments

x represents the price of one flask for each company.

$20x = \$30.00$

$$\frac{20}{20}x = \frac{\$30.00}{20}$$

$x = \$1.50$

Company A price: \$1.50 per flask.

Company B:

$$\frac{12 \text{ flasks}}{\$16.00} = \frac{1 \text{ flask}}{x}$$

$$\frac{12}{12}x = \frac{\$16.00}{12}$$

$x = \$1.33$

Company B price: \$1.33 per flask

Therefore Company B is providing the best buy.

5.8 PERCENTS

The word **percent** literally means "per 100." Percents are used in almost every field: business, mathematics, chemistry, physics, sports, and medicine. To change a percent to a fraction or decimal, say "per hundred" instead of percent.

$$25\% = 25 \text{ per hundred} = \frac{25}{100} = 0.25$$

$$1.2\% = 1.2 \text{ per hundred} = \frac{1.2}{100} = 0.012$$

$$0.020\% = 0.020 \text{ per hundred} = \frac{0.020}{100} = 0.00020$$

Notice that a ratio results when you divide by 100. Therefore, a basketball player that has a 84% free throw percentage makes

$$\frac{84}{100}, \text{ or 84 goals out of 100 shots}$$

If 4.2% of the patients who take an experimental drug develop a reaction to it, then 4.2 per hundred, or $\frac{4.2}{100}$, or 4.2 persons out of every 100 who take the drug develop a reaction.

EXAMPLE 5.8.1

If 4.2% of the patients who take an experimental drug develop a reaction to it, how many patients could be expected to develop a reaction if 3500 patients were treated with the drug?

We may solve this problem, or any percent problem, by deriving a general formula. A ratio is found consisting of the **part** (usually the smaller quantity) divided by the **whole** (the total amount, usually the larger quantity). It is written as

$$\frac{\text{Part}}{\text{Whole}}$$

We set this ratio equal to another ratio containing the percent (or per 100). It is then written as

$$\frac{\text{Part}}{\text{Whole}} = \frac{\%}{100}$$

The number represented by the percent symbol (%) will be your percent. This one proportion may be solved for the unknown part. The solution to example 5.8.1 follows.

Solution	**Comments**
$\frac{\%}{100} = \frac{\text{Part}}{\text{Whole}}$	Write down the basic percent formula.
$\frac{4.2}{100} = \frac{x}{3500}$	The part is the number of patients that develop a reaction. The whole is the total number of patients who took the drug.

$(3500)(4.2) = 100x$

$14{,}700 = 100x$

$\frac{14{,}700}{100} = \frac{\cancel{100}x}{\cancel{100}}$

4.2 is the percent.

$147 = x$

147 persons out of 3500 will probably develop a reaction. This is 4.2% of the sample.

EXAMPLE 5.8.2

The sales tax in a certain city is 7%. If a person buys merchandise worth \$82.50, how much sales tax must be paid?

Solution

$\frac{\$0.07}{\$1} = \frac{x}{\$82.50}$

$\$5.78 = 1x$

Comments

7% means 7 cents per 100 cents or 7 cents per 1 dollar. Seven cents can be written as \$0.07. The "part" here is the sales tax, which is unknown. The "whole" is \$82.50. The sales tax is \$5.78.

EXAMPLE 5.8.3

A patient is placed on a strict diet and is told to lose 35 lb. The patient loses 28 lb over a period of 3 months. What percent of the weight loss goal has the patient met?

Solution

$\frac{\text{Part}}{\text{Whole}} = \frac{\%}{100}$

Write down the formula.

$\frac{28}{35} = \frac{\%}{100}$

Substitute: % = ?; part = 28; whole = 35.

$(28)(100) = (\%)(35)$

Solve for %.

$\frac{2800}{35} = \%$

$80 = \%$

The patient has lost 80% of the weight goal.

EXAMPLE 5.8.4

The patient in example 5.8.3 originally weighed 225 lb. Find the percent decrease in weight.

Solution

$\frac{\text{Part}}{\text{Whole}} = \frac{\%}{100}$

$\frac{\text{Amount of decrease}}{\text{Whole}} = \frac{\%}{100}$

Comments

To find the percent decrease, we must first find the amount of decrease, which is given in example 5.31 as 28 lb. This is the part. The whole is the total weight (225 lb).

$\frac{28}{225} = \frac{\%}{100}$

$(28)(100) = (225)(\%)$

$\frac{2800}{225} = \%$

$12.4 = \%$

$12 \approx \%$

The patient lost 12% of the total body weight.

PROBLEM SET 5

Solve each of the following proportions.

1. $\frac{3}{5} = \frac{21}{x}$
2. $\frac{x}{17} = \frac{8}{34}$
3. $\frac{6}{13} = \frac{x}{72}$
4. $\frac{4}{x} = \frac{1}{8}$
5. $\frac{3x}{30} = \frac{10}{50}$
6. $\frac{40{,}000}{12} = \frac{70{,}000}{x}$
7. $\frac{\frac{1}{2}}{5} = \frac{x}{40}$
8. $\frac{\frac{1}{3}}{6} = \frac{x}{8}$
9. $\frac{27}{30} = \frac{5}{4x}$
10. $\frac{30}{9} = \frac{175}{5x}$
11. If, on a map, $\frac{1}{4}$ inch = 2 miles, how many inches would represent 10 miles?
12. A patient breathes a gas with a total pressure of 1280 mm Hg. Nitrous oxide, an anesthetic, accounts for 900 mm Hg of the total pressure. What percent of the total pressure is due to nitrous oxide?
13. A contest sponsored by a fast food franchise has rules that state that there is only 1 chance in 250,000 to win the first prize. What is the percent chance of winning the first prize?
14. If 50 gallons of paint can cover 25,000 square feet of surface, how much paint is needed to cover 6,000 square feet?
15. A drug used to treat patients with diarrhea, doxycycline, was found to help 34 out of 36 patients treated. What percent of patients were helped?
16. A laboratory assistant can order 22 kg of aluminum chloride from Company A for $202.00 and can order the same grade of substance from Company B at a price of $29.00 for 3 kg. Which is the best buy?
17. The atmosphere is composed of approximately 0.031% carbon dioxide (CO_2). How many grams of CO_2 would be contained in a 12,500-g sample of air?
18. An automobile lists for $9,200, but the dealer is offering a 5.5% discount for 1 week only. How much is the discount? What is the selling price of the automobile?
19. A drug is found to have serious side effects for 0.70% of all patients that took the drug. If 2000 patients took the drug, how many patients experienced serious side effects?
20. If a car is rated to get 35 miles per 1 gallon of gasoline, how many miles can it run on its 12-gallon tank?
21. A sample of polluted air contains 300 molecules of NO_2 (nitrogen dioxide) for every billion molecules of air sampled. What percent of the air is NO_2?
22. A rookie baseball player made 12 hits in his first 42 times at bat. What is his hitting percent?
23. A chemist can get 8 oz of potassium hydroxide pellets for $4.60 from Caustic Chemical Company. The chemist can order 15 lb of the same substance from Acrid Chemical Company for $162.00. Which company is offering the best buy?

    (*Hint*: 16 oz = 1 lb.)

Answers to odd-numbered problems appear on page 232.

5.9 VARIATION

An equation or formula relates one quantity to another, such as the formula for the area of a circle:

$$A = \pi r^2$$

As the value of r changes, so does the value of A. How variables change with respect to each other is called **variation.**

There are three types of variation. The first is called **direct variation.** We say that one quantity, call it A, "varies directly" or "varies as" or is "proportional to" a second quantity, B, if, as B increases, so does A. We can mathematically write

$$A = kB$$

where k is called the **proportionality constant.** This constant tells us specifically how A is changing with respect to B. For example, if A represents a weekly wage, and B represents the hours worked, then A varies directly as B. If the proportionality constant here was \$4.00 per hour, we would write the equation as follows:

$$A = \$4.00(B)$$

For every 1 hour worked, your wages, A, will increase by \$4.00.

The second type of variation is **inverse variation.** We say that A "varies inversely" as B, if, as B increases, A decreases. We write this mathematically as

$$A = k \cdot \frac{1}{B}$$

or

$$A = \frac{k}{B}$$

Note that B is the denominator of a fraction where the numerator is constant. If B gets bigger, the fraction, equal to A, gets smaller. As an example, consider a gas trapped in a cylinder with a movable piston. As pressure (P) is applied to the piston, it moves downward, forcing the gas into a smaller volume (V). As shown in the figure below, with a decrease in the pressure the volume increases:

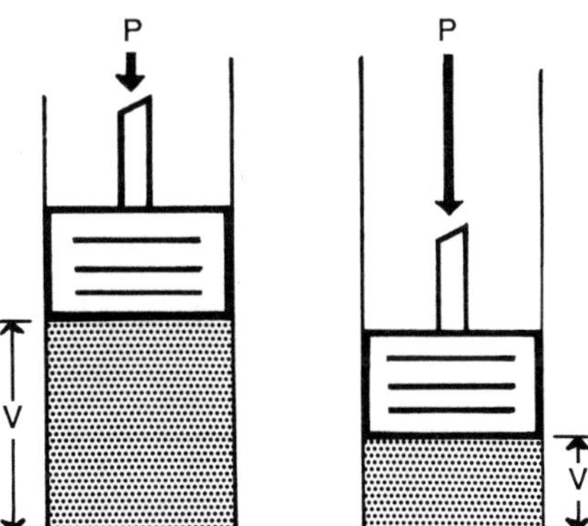

We say that the volume of the gas is inversely proportional to the pressure of the gas:

$$V = k\frac{1}{P}$$

$$V = \frac{k}{P}.$$

The third type of variation is called **joint variation.** Joint variation occurs when one quantity varies directly as *two* or *more* quantities. This is written mathematically as

$$C = k \cdot A \cdot B$$

If, as B and A increase, so does C, then C "varies jointly" as B and A. An example is seen in the formula for simple interest:

$$I = PRT$$

where I is interest, P is principal, or the amount of the loan, R is the annual rate of interest (%), and T is the term of the loan. The interest due on a loan varies jointly as the principal, the rate, and the term of the loan. Example 5.9.1 illustrates the three types of variation.

EXAMPLE 5.9.1

Translate the following statements into algebraic equations.

Statement	Equations
P varies directly as U.	$P = kU$
C varies inversely as t.	$C = k \cdot \frac{1}{t} = \frac{k}{t}$
G varies jointly as r and q.	$G = krq$
M varies directly as 1 and inversely as $3v$.	$M = k \cdot \frac{1}{3v} = \frac{k}{3v}$
N varies directly as the square of x.	$N = kx^2$
T varies directly as the square of y and the fourth power of b.	$T = ky^2b^4$
H varies jointly as a and the square root of d and inversely as the third power of L.	$H = \frac{ka\sqrt{d}}{L^3}$
E varies jointly as M and the square of V.	$E_k = kMV^2$

EXAMPLE 5.9.2

If P varies directly as R, and $P = 20$ when $R = 5$, what is the value of the proportionality constant k?

Solution	Comments
$P = kR$	Write the equation.
$\frac{P}{R} = k$	Solve the equation for k.
$\frac{20}{5} = k$	Substitute the given values for P and R, and solve for k. You then find the value for k.
$4 = k$	
$P = 4R$	Now you can rewrite the equation with the specific value of the constant. This equation can now be used to find any value of P given R.

EXAMPLE 5.9.3

If Z varies directly as U and inversely as the third power of t, find the proportionality constant k if $Z = 4$ when $U = 2$ and $t = 3$.

Solution	Comments
$Z = \frac{kU}{t^3}$	Write the equation. Note that the equation involves both direct and inverse variation.

$4 = \frac{k(2)}{3^3}$	Substitute values for Z, U, and t.
$\frac{(4)(27)}{2} = k$	Solve for k.
$54 = k$	
$Z = \frac{54U}{t^3}$	Rewrite the formula with 54 substituted for k.

EXAMPLE 5.9.4

The volume of a cylinder varies jointly as the square of the radius of its circular top and its height. A certain cylinder has a radius of 2 and a height of 10. What would happen to the volume of the cylinder if its radius were doubled and its height were increased to 5 times its original height?

Note: Since this problem does not specifically ask for the new volume, we can concern ourselves with only how much the volume changes. This means we do not have to know the value of the constant k.

Solution	**Comments**
$V = kr^2h$	Write the formula (r = radius, h = height).
$V = k(2)^2(10)$	Find the volume when $r = 2$ and $h = 10$.
$V = 40k$	The volume is 40 times the constant.
old radius = 2; old height = 10 new radius = 4; new height = 50	Now, find the volume when the radius and height are changed.
$V = k(4)^2(50)$ $V = k(16)(50)$	Substitute into the equation: $r = 4$, $h = 50$.
$V = 800k$	The new volume is 800 times the constant.
$\frac{800\not{k}}{40\not{k}} = 20$	To find how much the volume changes, divide the new volume by the old.
	The new volume is 20 times greater than the old volume.

As you can see, we can predict what will happen to one variable if others are changed. In the foregoing example, we did not even need to know the value of the constant to make the comparison. The next example further illustrates this method of making predictions from equations.

EXAMPLE 5.9.5

The area enclosed by a triangle varies jointly as the length of its base and height. If $k = \frac{1}{2}$, what happens to the area when the length of the base is tripled and the length of the height is doubled?

Solution	**Comments**
$A = \frac{1}{2}bh$	Write the formula for the area of the triangle. Let b = original base and h = original height.
$A = \frac{1}{2}(3b)(2h)$	Now, rewrite the formula, letting $3b$ = base after it is tripled and $2h$ = height after it is doubled.
$A = (3)(2)\left(\frac{1}{2}bh\right)$	Using the commutative and associative properties, move the expression $(\frac{1}{2}bh)$ to the end.

$$A = 6\left(\frac{1}{2}bh\right)$$

The area before was $\frac{1}{2}bh$, but now it has become 6 times $\frac{1}{2}bh$. The area of the triangle has increased to 6 times its original area.

Our next example is an application from the gas laws. Again, we will make use of simple algebraic substitution to make our predictions.

EXAMPLE 5.9.6

The pressure of a gas trapped inside a steel cylinder is 10 atmospheres (atm). If the cylinder is damaged in a fire by being crushed, thus having its volume lowered by half, and is heated, increasing its temperature by 500 times, what will happen to the pressure of the gas trapped inside the cylinder?

Given:

$$\frac{P_1V_1}{T_1} = \frac{P_2V_2}{T_2}$$

where P, V, and T represent pressure, volume, and temperature. The subscript "1" represents the original conditions and the subscript "2" represents the final conditions.

Solution	**Comments**
$P_2 = ?$ $V_2 = \frac{1}{2}V_1$	Represent the final conditions in terms of the original conditions. P_2 is what you are trying to find.
$T_2 = 500T_1$ V_1 T_1 $P_1 = 10$ atm	V_2 is one half of the original volume, and the final temperature, T_2, is 500 times the original temperature, T_1. The original pressure (P_1) is 10 atm. Let V_1 and T_1 represent themselves.
$\frac{P_1V_1}{T_1} = \frac{P_2V_2}{T_2}$	Write down the given formula.
$\frac{P_1V_1}{T_1} = \frac{P_2(V_1/2)}{500T_1}$	Substitute $\frac{1}{2}V_1$ for V_2 and 500 T_1 for T_2. Solve for P_2.
$500T_1(P_1)(V_1) = P_2(V_1/2)T_1$	Find cross products.
$\frac{(500T_1)(P_1)(V_1)}{(V_1/2)T_1} = P_2$	Divide both sides by $(V_1/2)T_1$.
$\frac{(500\not{T}_1)(P_1)(\not{V}_1)}{(\not{V}_1/2)(\not{T}_1)} = P_2$	The "V_1s" and "T_1s" cancel out.
$\frac{500\ P_1}{\frac{1}{2}} = P_2$	Simplify completely.
$2 \cdot 500P_1 = P_2$ $1000\ P_1 = P_2$ $1000 \cdot 10 \text{ atm} = P_2$	The final pressure (P_2) will be 1000 times the original pressure.
$10{,}000 \text{ atm} = P_2$	The final pressure is actually 10,000 atm.

PROBLEM SET 6

Translate the following statements into algebraic equations.

1. V varies directly as R.
2. v varies directly as R.
3. W varies inversely as L.
4. J varies jointly as L, M, and Z.
5. X varies directly as N and inversely as L.
6. Y varies directly as the square of b and inversely as the fourth power of A.
7. D varies jointly as r and the square root of t and inversely as $4e$.

Find the proportionality constant and the specific formula for the following conditions.

8. Problem 1 with $R = 4$ and $v = 28$.
9. Problem 3 with $L = 0.2$ and $W = 10$.
10. Problem 5 with $N = 12$, $L = 0.2$, and $X = 5$.
11. Problem 7 with $r = 5$, $t = 25$, $e = 0.5$, and $D = 100$.
12. The volume of a gas varies directly with its absolute temperature and inversely with its pressure. If a gas in an elastic container occupies a volume of 20 L when the temperature is 200°K and the pressure is 50 atm, find the volume when the temperature is 300K and the pressure is lowered to 10 atms.
    (*Hint:* Use the gas law from example 5.9.6.)
13. A dosage of a particular medicine varies directly with the patient's weight. Suppose that 10 cc of medicine is given to a 200-lb patient. What dosage should be given to an 180-lb patient?
14. Z varies jointly as q and the third power of t, and inversely as the square of y. If $Z = 25$ when $q = 4$, $t = 2$, and $y = 2$, find Z when $q = 2$, $t = 4$, and $y = 4$.
15. The area of a triangle is given by the formula $A = \frac{1}{2}bh$. If the base of a triangle is cut by half, and the height is increased to 4 times its original height, what happens to the area of the triangle?
16. The radius of a lithium atom is three times larger than the radius of a fluorine atom. If an atom is considered to be a sphere, how much greater is the volume of a lithium atom than a fluorine atom? (Volume of a sphere $= \frac{4}{3}\pi r^3$.)
17. The rate of diffusion of a gas is inversely proportional to the square root of its molecular weight:

$$R = \frac{k}{\sqrt{\text{mol wt}}}$$

    If oxygen gas is 16 times heavier than hydrogen gas, which gas will diffuse faster, and by how much?
18. A quantity of oxygen exerts a pressure of 3 atm. What is the pressure if the same amount of oxygen occupies twice the volume at one half the original temperature?
19. The strength of the gravitational force between two heavenly bodies is given by the formula

$$F = \frac{GM_1M_2}{d^2}$$

where d is the distance between the two bodies. If the distance between the earth and the moon were 4 times greater than at present, what would happen to the force of gravity between them?

Answers to odd-numbered problems appear on page 233.

CHAPTER REVIEW

(5.3)

Indicate which rules of algebra justify each of the following statements. More than one rule may apply to the same statement.

1. $7x \cdot \frac{1}{7x} = 1$
2. $3(x - y + r) = 3x - 3y + 3r$
3. $q(2p)(3x) = (6x)(pq)$

(5.4–5.5)

Solve each of the following equations for the variable indicated.

4. $3r - 5 = 46$
5. $9(y + 3) = 2(y - 4)$
6. $\frac{1}{3}(x - 3) = 7 - 2x$
7. $\frac{1x}{2} + \frac{2}{3} = \frac{3x}{4} - 1$
8. $\frac{5}{y} - \frac{2}{y} = -1$
9. $\frac{2}{x + 2} - \frac{3}{2x} = \frac{1}{5x}$

(5.6)

Solve each of the following formulas for the variable indicated.

10. $A = \frac{1}{2}bh$, for b
11. $PV = nRT$, for R
12. $\frac{P_1V_1}{T_1} = \frac{P_2V_2}{T_2}$, for T_2
13. $\frac{1}{t} = \frac{2}{q} - \frac{3}{R}$, for R
14. $\frac{1}{t} = \frac{2}{q} - \frac{3}{R}$, for q
15. $\frac{x}{24} = \frac{10}{80}$
16. $\frac{15}{2x} = \frac{3}{2}$
17. $\frac{50{,}000}{15} = \frac{10x}{3}$
18. $\frac{\frac{1}{3}}{7} = \frac{x}{9}$

19. A map scale reads 2 inches = 1.5 miles. How many miles does 3.5 inches on the map represent?
20. A chemist can get 12 oz of sodium phosphate from Company A for \$5.50. He can order 10 lb of the same substance from Company B for \$175.00. Which company is offering the best buy?
21. If a car's mileage is rated at 32 miles per 1 gal of gasoline, how many miles can it run with a 16-gal tank?
22. A drug has been determined to have serious side effects for 0.15% of all patients who take it. If 6000 patients take the drug, how many can expect to experience serious side effects?

(5.8)

Translate the following statements into algebraic equations.

23. W varies directly as x.

24. Z varies inversely as Y.

25. Q varies jointly as P, R, and S, and inversely as T.

Find the proportionality constant and the specific formula for the following conditions.

26. Problem 23 with $W = 12$ and $x = 4$.

27. Problem 24 with $Z = 4$ and $Y = 0.5$.

28. Problem 25 with $P = 2$, $R = 8$, $S = 1$, $T = \frac{1}{4}$, and $Q = 32$.

29. If G varies jointly as h and the square of t, and inversely as q, find a specific formula for G if $G = 100$ when $h = 4$, $t = 2$, and $q = 16$.

30. Using problem 29, find G when $h = 10$, $t = 8$, and $q = 64$.

Answers to all problems appear on page 233.

chapter 6

Solution Mathematics

OBJECTIVES

After studying this chapter, the student should be able to:

1. Perform calculations involving all percent concentration forms, including milligram percent.
2. Relate the concept of parts per million and parts per billion to other concentration units.
3. Convert from ratio strength to percent strength.
4. Identify the solute and solvent components of a solution.
5. Interchange gram mass to molar mass, and vice versa.
6. Perform calculations involving molarity and normality.
7. Interchange from gram mass to equivalent mass, and vice versa.
8. Perform the mathematics of dilutions.

6.1 INTRODUCTION

Blood plasma is a solution; so is the air we breathe and many of the liquid beverages we drink. Most of the fluids and medicines used in the health field are solutions. The strength of these solutions must be measured in some way to enable us to predict their properties, both physical and chemical. In this chapter, we concentrate upon the mathematics of solution strengths, and upon some of the chemistry involved.

6.2 DEFINITIONS

A solution is a uniform mixture of two or more substances.. It may be thought of as having two components: a **solute**—the substance that is dissolved, or the substance present in the smaller quantity; and a **solvent**—the substance that does the dissolving, or that is present in the larger quantity. The strength of a solution is referred to as its **concentration.**

Some simple solutions are presented in example 6.2.1.

EXAMPLE 6.2.1

Table sugar and water	Solute—table sugar Solvent—water
Salt and water (saline solution)	Solute—salt Solvent—water

Alcohol and water	Solute—alcohol Solvent—water (if there is more water in the solution than alcohol)
Aqueous KCl	Solute—KCl (potassium chloride) Solvent—water ("aqua" means water)

In this chapter, we examine several concentration measuring formulas. All of these formulas will have the same general form:

$$\text{Concentration} = \frac{\text{Amount of solute (mass or volume)}}{\text{Total amount of solution (mass or volume)}}$$

In other words, all of the concentration formulas will be ratios of amount of solute to amount of solution. In the case of "percents," this ratio will be multiplied by 100.

A solution with a high ratio of solute to solvent will have a high concentration level and is said to be **concentrated.** A solution with a low ratio of solute to solvent will have a low concentration level and is said to be **dilute.** In example 6.2.2, the volume of the solution is held constant and the level of solute varied in order to show the distinction between a concentrated and a dilute solution.

EXAMPLE 6.2.2

$$\frac{5.0 \text{ g salt}}{100 \text{ mL solution}} = \text{a dilute solution}$$

$$\frac{35.0 \text{ g salt}}{100 \text{ mL solution}} = \text{a concentrated solution}$$

If a certain amount of solvent holds all of the solute that it can possibly hold at a certain temperature (say, laboratory temperature), then the solution is said to be **saturated.** If the solvent can hold more solute, then the solution is said to be **unsaturated.** Obviously, the amount of solute a solvent can hold depends upon certain chemical properties of both the solute and solvent as well as the temperature of each.

6.3 PERCENT CONCENTRATIONS

Percent Weight for Weight (% w/w)

In certain concentrated solutions, percent weight for weight (% w/w) is used to express the concentration of the solution. Recall from Chapter 5 that percent may be defined as

$$\% = \frac{\text{Part}}{\text{Whole}} \cdot 100$$

Adapting this formula to percent weight for weight, we may write

$$\%\ \text{w/w} = \frac{\text{Weight of solute}}{\text{Weight of solution}} \cdot 100$$

The weight may be in any weight unit, but in laboratory work, the gram unit is most often used.

EXAMPLE 6.3.1

What is the percent weight for weight concentration of a solution containing 25.0 g of glucose in 250.0 g of solution? How much solvent (water) is in the solution?

Solution	**Comments**
$\%\ \text{w/w} = \frac{25.0 \text{ g}}{250.0 \text{ g}} \cdot 100$	Substitute weight of solute into the numerator and weight of solution into denominator.

$\%\ w/w = 0.100 \cdot 100$	Divide numerator by denominator; multiply by 100. Note that units divide out.
$\%\ w/w = 10.0$	The solution is 10% w/w.
Amount of solvent = amount of solution − amount of solute = 250.0 g − 25.0 g = 225.0 g	To find the weight of the solvent, subtract the weight of the solute from the total weight of the solution.

Note that the formula

$$\% = \frac{\text{Part}}{\text{Whole}} \cdot 100$$

may be rearranged to obtain the following:

$\frac{1}{100} \cdot \% = \frac{\text{Part}}{\text{Whole}} \cdot \cancel{100} \cdot \frac{1}{\cancel{100}}$	Multiply both sides by the inverse of 100.
$\frac{\%}{100} = \frac{\text{Part}}{\text{Whole}}$	This is the same formula we used in Chapter 5.

You may use cross multiplication to solve any part of this formula, as in 6.3.2.

EXAMPLE 6.3.2

A sample of a 5% w/w dextrose (glucose) and water solution has a mass of 152.4 g. How much dextrose (solute) is present, and how much solvent (water) is present?

Solution	**Comments**
$\frac{5}{100} = \frac{x}{152.4\ \text{g}}$	Substitute into formula: % w/w = 5; part = x; and whole = 152.4 g.
$(5)(152.4\ \text{g}) = 100x$ $\frac{(5)(152.4\ \text{g})}{100} = \frac{100x}{100}$	Cross multiply and then divide both sides by 100 to solve for x.
$7.62\ \text{g} = x$	There are 7.62 g of dextrose present.
Amount solvent = 152.4 g − 7.62 g = 144.8 g	There are 144.8 g of solvent present.

Percent weight for weight is not often used in calculating solution concentrations, but it is the most accurate means of measuring concentration, since weight (or mass) is not dependent upon temperature, whereas volume measurement (discussed below) is dependent upon temperature.

Percent Weight for Volume (% w/v)

The most common method of expressing percent concentrations is using the weight of a solute per volume of solution. We saw in Chapter 4 that 1 mL of water has a mass approximately equal to 1 g. For dilute water solutions, we may assume that 1 mL of the solution has a mass very close to 1 g. Drug solutions and other dilute solutions with a concentration of 10% or less are usually written in percent weight for volume (% w/v). We may use a variation of the weight for weight formula we used in the last section for these kinds of solution problems.

$$\%\ w/v = \frac{\text{Weight of solute (usually grams)}}{\text{Volume of solution (usually milliliters)}} \cdot 100$$

EXAMPLE 6.3.3

What is the percent weight for volume concentration of a solution made by dissolving 16.2 g of potassium chloride (KCl) in 842 mL of solution?

Solution	Comments
$\% \text{ w/v} = \frac{16.2 \text{ g}}{842 \text{ mL}} \cdot 100$	Substitute into formula: weight of solute = 16.2 g; and volume of solution = 842 mL.
$\% \text{ w/v} = 1.92\%$	Note that the units here do not actually divide out. But since the density of most dilute water solutions is about 1 g = 1 mL, we may consider the units as dividing out.

The percent w/v formula may be rearranged by multiplying both sides by $\frac{1}{100}$ to obtain

$$\frac{\% \text{ w/v}}{100} = \frac{\text{Weight of solute}}{\text{Volume of solution}}$$

Use this formula to solve for values other than percent.

EXAMPLE 6.3.4

How much solute do you need to make $25\bar{0}$ mL of a 1.75% w/v aqueous solution of potassium permanganate ($KMnO_4$)?

Solution	Comments
$\frac{1.75}{100} = \frac{x}{25\bar{0}}$	Substitute into formula: % w/v = 1.75; weight of solute = x; and volume of solution = $25\bar{0}$ mL.
$100x = (1.75)(25\bar{0})$	Cross multiply.
$\frac{100x}{100} = \frac{(1.75)(25\bar{0})}{100}$	Divide both sides by 100.
$x = 4.38$ g	The weight of the solute is 4.38 g. The weight of the solute is always in grams if the volume of the solution is expressed in milliliters. Recall: For water solutions, 1 g ≈ 1 mL.

To prepare the solution in example 6.3.4, you would measure out 4.38 g of the solute, place it in a volumetric flask, and add enough water to bring the entire volume up to $25\bar{0}$ mL. Do not add $25\bar{0}$ mL of water, as this would make more than 250 mL of solution.

EXAMPLE 6.3.5

How much 3.0% w/v solution can be made from 38.6 g of NaOH (sodium hydroxide)?

Solution	Comments
$\frac{3.0}{100} = \frac{38.6 \text{ g}}{x \text{ mL}}$	Substitute into the formula: % w/v = 3.0; weight of solute = 38.6 g; and volume of solution = x mL.
$3.0x = (38.6)(100)$	Solve for x by cross multiplying.
$\frac{3.0x}{3.0} = \frac{(38.6)(100)}{3.0}$	Divide both sides by 3.0.
$x = 1287$ ml $x = 1300$ mL	Round off your answer to two significant digits.

To prepare this solution, follow these steps.

1. Measure out 38.6 g of NaOH.
2. Add to a beaker or similar container.
3. Add enough water to make the entire volume of the solution up to 1300 mL.
4. The resulting solution has a concentration of 3.0% w/v. Be sure to label it as such.

Milligram Percent (mg %)

Milligram percent (mg %) is a variation of the percent weight for volume solution concentration method:

$$\begin{aligned} \text{mg \%} &= \text{milligrams per hundred} \\ &= \text{milligrams per hundred milliliters} \end{aligned}$$

But since 100 mL = 1 dL,

$$\text{mg \%} = \frac{\text{Milligrams of solute}}{\text{Deciliters of solution}}$$

Many clinical laboratory test results are reported with these units. Listed below are typical blood components and their normal concentrations:

Component	Normal Blood Level
Cholesterol	150–300 mg/dL
Triglycerides	10–195 mg/dL
Creatinine	0.5–1.5 mg/dL
Calcium	8.6–10.7 mg/dL
Bilirubin	0.2–1 mg/dL

It may be necessary to convert from a percent weight for volume concentration measurement to milligram percent, or vice versa. A review of dimensional analysis may be helpful for these types of problems.

EXAMPLE 6.3.6

A patient has a blood cholesterol level of 225 mg/dL. Refigure this as percent weight for volume.

Solution	**Comments**
$\frac{225\text{ mg}}{1\text{ dL}} \cdot \frac{1\text{ dL}}{100\text{ mL}} = \frac{225\text{ mg}}{100\text{ mL}} = \frac{2.25\text{ mg}}{\text{mL}}$	Use dimensional analysis to change milligrams per deciliter to milligrams per milliliter.
$\frac{2.25\text{ mg}}{\text{mL}} \cdot \frac{1\text{ g}}{1000\text{ mg}} = \frac{2.25\text{ g}}{1000\text{ mL}} = \frac{0.00225\text{ g}}{\text{mL}}$	Now, use dimensional analysis to convert from milligrams per milliliter to grams per milliliter.
$\frac{\text{\% w/v}}{100} = \frac{\text{Weight of solute}}{\text{Volume of solution}}$; $\frac{\text{\% w/v}}{100} = \frac{0.00225}{1\text{ mL}}$; % w/v = (0.00225)(100); % w/v = 0.225%	Change to percent weight for volume using the percent formula. Weight of solute = 0.00225 g; volume of solution = 1 mL.

Percent Volume for Volume (% v/v)

This method of expressing solution concentrations is usually reserved for liquid–liquid solutions, or gas–gas solutions. We may use still another variation of the percent formula for these type concentrations. Any volume units may be used in this formula as long as the solute and solution units are the same:

$$\% \text{ v/v} = \frac{\text{Volume of solute}}{\text{Volume of solution}} \cdot 100$$

EXAMPLE 6.3.7

What is the percent volume for volume strength of a solution made by dissolving 25.0 mL of alcohol in enough water to make 400.0 mL of solution?

Solution	Comments
$\% \text{ v/v} = \frac{25.0 \text{ mL}}{400.0 \text{ mL}} \cdot 100$	Substitute into the formula: % v/v = x; volume of solute = 25.0 mL; and volume of solution = 400.0 mL.
$x = \frac{(25.0)(100)}{400.0}$	Solve for percent volume for volume. Units divide out.
$x = 6.25\% \text{ v/v}$	
Proof = 6.25 · 2 = 12.5	Alcohol solutions may have their concentrations expressed as "proof." Proof = % v/v · 2.

PROBLEM SET 1

1. Calculate the percent weight for weight of a solution made by dissolving 5.0 g of NaCl in 500.0 g of solution.
2. Calculate the percent weight for weight of a solution made by dissolving 12.2 g of magnesium sulfate in 250 g of solution.
3. A solution made by dissolving 26.4 g of Glauber's salt in 168.0 g of water has what percent weight for weight?
4. Find the percent weight for weight of a solution made by dissolving 50.00 g of glucose in 5000.0 g of water.
5. Calculate the percent weight for volume of a solution made by dissolving 15.0 g of dextrose in 300.0 mL of solution.
6. Calculate the percent weight for volume of a solution made by dissolving 5.4 g of NaCl in 600.0 mL of solution.
7. How would you prepare 500.0 mL of a 12% w/v solution of benzalkonium chloride?
8. How would you prepare 1.2 L of a 2.0% w/v solution of $KMnO_4$?
9. If you were asked to make as much sodium bicarbonate solution at 3.0% w/v strength from 32.0 g of sodium bicarbonate, how much could you make?
10. A label on a drug bottle states that there is 0.25 mg of drug per 2.0 mL of solution. What is the percent weight for volume?
11. If 12.5 g of isopropyl alcohol are dissolved in $5.00 \cdot 10^2$ mL of water solution, what is the percent weight for volume of alcohol?
12. A popular bourbon is 86 proof. The bottle holds 1.00 L of the alcohol–water solution. Roughly, how many milliliters of alcohol are in the bottle?
13. A tipsy bar patron consumes 4 glasses of 80-proof whiskey in 1 hour. If each glass contains 50.0 mL of the straight whiskey, how much alcohol did the bar patron consume?
14. What volume of 0.5% w/v boric acid solution can be made from 98.2 g of boric acid?

15. How would you prepare $85\bar{0}$ g of 4.00% w/w solution of $FeSO_4$? How much water would you add?
16. An injectable solution of digoxin is labeled 0.025% w/v. How much should be injected to administer a dose of 0.020 mg?
17. A patient is found to have a creatinine level of 12.0 mg/L. What is the creatinine level in milligram percent?
18. A patient has a blood albumin concentration of 0.47 g/L. Normal albumin levels range from 35 to 50 mg %. Does the patient have a normal albumin level?
19. Normal blood levels of iron range from 50 to 180 μg/dL. Recalculate these levels in milligram percent.

Answers to odd-numbered problems appear on page 233.

6.4 CONCENTRATION BY PARTS

The simplest method of measuring solution concentrations, especially when measuring concentrations of toxic chemicals or chemicals present in very small quantities, is that of parts per million (ppm) and parts per billion (ppb).

Parts per million is defined as

$$\text{ppm} = \frac{\text{Parts of solute}}{10^6 \text{ Parts of solution}}$$

Parts per billion is defined

$$\text{ppb} = \frac{\text{Parts of solute}}{10^9 \text{ Parts of solution}}$$

The "parts" referred to here may be any unit we wish in the weight for weight and volume for volume modes, as long as the unit in the numerator matches the unit in the denominator. Study these examples:

$$5 \text{ ppm w/w} = \frac{5 \text{ g of solute}}{1{,}000{,}000 \text{ g of solution}}$$

$$5 \text{ ppm v/v} = \frac{5 \text{ L of solute}}{1{,}000{,}000 \text{ L of solution}}$$

In the weight for volume mode, we use the same units we used in the percent problems:

$$5 \text{ ppm w/v} = \frac{5 \text{ g of solute}}{1{,}000{,}000 \text{ mL of solution}}$$

EXAMPLE 6.4.1

The concentration of gaseous nitrogen in the air is 780,000 ppm v/v. What is the percent volume for volume N_2 in the air?

Solution	**Comments**
$\frac{780{,}000 \text{ parts } N_2}{10^6 \text{ parts air}} = \frac{x \text{ parts } N_2}{10^2 \text{ parts air}}$	Note that percent volume for volume is really parts per hundred. Set up a proportion. Let x = parts N_2 in one hundred parts air.
$\frac{(780{,}000 \text{ parts } N_2)(10^2 \text{ parts air})}{(10^6 \text{ parts air})} = x$	Cross multiply and solve for x.
$(780{,}000 \text{ parts } N_2)(10^{2-6}) = x$ $780{,}000 \cdot 10^{-4} \text{ parts } N_2 = x$	Subtract exponents.
$78 \text{ parts } N_2 = x$	Rewrite as a decimal number.
78 parts N_2 per 10^2 parts air	The level of N_2 in the air is 78% v/v.

EXAMPLE 6.4.2

Carbon monoxide (CO) may cause death when the level reaches 750 ppm v/v in the air. A garage has a CO level of $6.54 \cdot 10^4$ ppb v/v. Is the concentration of CO within the lethal range?

Solution	Comments
$\frac{6.54 \cdot 10^4 \text{ parts CO}}{10^9 \text{ parts air}} = \frac{x}{10^6 \text{ parts air}}$	Set up a ratio and proportion to convert the current concentrations of CO to parts per million, which is the units in which the lethal level (750 ppm v/v) is expressed. Let x = parts CO in 10^6 parts of air.
$\frac{(6.54 \cdot 10^4)(10^6)}{10^9} = x$	Solve for x.
$\frac{6.54 \cdot 10^{10}}{10^9} = x$	Add exponents in the numerator.
$6.54 \cdot 10^1 = x$	Subtract exponents.
65.4 parts CO per 10^6 parts air.	Rewrite as a decimal number. The measured level is 65.4 ppm.
65.4 ppm $<$ 750 ppm	The measured concentration in the garage is less than the lethal level.

To help us realize how small the units ppm and ppb really are, imagine 1 Dodger fan sitting among a total of 70,000 fans at a World Series game in Yankee Stadium. The concentration of Dodger fans expressed in parts per million is

$$\frac{1 \text{ Dodger fan}}{7 \cdot 10^4 \text{ fans}} = \frac{x \text{ Dodger fans}}{10^6 \text{ fans}}$$

$$\frac{1 \cdot 10^6}{7 \cdot 10^4} = x$$

$$0.14 \cdot 10^{6-4} = x$$

$$0.14 \cdot 10^2 = x$$

$$14 = x.$$

The concentration of Dodger fans would be approximately 14 ppm.

6.5 RATIO STRENGTH

Occasionally, a solution will have its concentration written as a ratio instead of a percent. For example, a 1:300 w/v Lysol solution (read "one to three hundred weight per volume") is made up of 1 part (gram) Lysol in 300 parts (milliliters) of solution. Ratio strength may also be expressed as weight for weight and volume for volume. The units allowed for parts solute and parts solution are the same here as for percent strength.

For the purposes of our study, it is best to change from a ratio strength to the decimal (or percent) form when using the concentration in a calculation. The 1:300 w/v solution may be changed to a percent concentration in this manner:

$$\text{If } 1:300 = \frac{1 \text{ g}}{300 \text{ mL}}$$

$$\text{then } \frac{1 \text{ g}}{300 \text{ mL}} = \frac{x}{100 \text{ mL}} \text{ (the percent formula)}$$

$$\text{Solving for } x\text{: } \frac{1 \cdot 100}{300} = x$$

$$0.33 = x$$

The 1:300 solution has a percent weight for volume concentration of 0.33%.

EXAMPLE 6.5.1

A 2:250 w/v saline solution is used as a gargle for a sore throat. Is this solution equivalent to a physiological saline solution?

Solution	Comments
$\frac{\text{Part}}{\text{Whole}} = \frac{\%}{100}$	Write down the percent formula.
$\frac{2\text{ g}}{250\text{ mL}} = \frac{x}{100}$	Substitute part = 2 g and whole = 250 mL into the formula, and solve for x.
$0.008 \cdot 100 = x$	
$0.8 = x$	The gargle has a percent weight for volume concentration of 0.8%. Physiological saline has a concentration of 0.9%.

PROBLEM SET 2

1. The concentration of neon in the air is approximately 18 ppm v/v. What is the percent volume for volume concentration of neon in the air?
2. The concentration of carbon dioxide in the air is approximately 0.314 ppb. Recalculate this as parts per million.
3. Sulfur dioxide (SO_3) is a noxious air pollutant. Lung irritation may be caused when the concentration is as low as 20 ppm. What is this concentration in percent volume for volume?
4. Which is more concentrated: An 0.10% v/v alcohol solution or one with a concentration of 750 ppm v/v?
5. Which is larger: a concentration of 820 ppb or 1.2 ppm?
6. Most states rule that a person is legally intoxicated if the blood alcohol level is at least 0.10 percent weight for volume. What is this concentration in parts per million?
7. Tetraethyl lead is added to gasoline to make it burn more efficiently. If 3.0 mL of this substance is added per gallon of gasoline, this would increase the octane rating significantly. What is the percent volume for volume concentration of tetraethyl lead in this solution? (*Hint:* Be sure not to use mixed units.)
8. Can you show that 1 mg of solute in 1 L of solution is the same as 1 g of solute in $1 \cdot 10^6$ mL of solution?
9. During surgery, patients often receive a mixture of gases consisting of $7.4 \cdot 10^5$ ppm nitrous oxide (N_2O), $2.5 \cdot 10^5$ ppm oxygen, and $1 \cdot 10^4$ ppm halothane. Recalculate those concentrations as percent volume for volume.
10. In the entire state of Tennessee, there are 128 people with the last name "Highers." If the state of Tennessee has a population of approximately $4.2 \cdot 10^6$ people, what is the concentration of "Highers'" in parts per million?
11. We have already seen that parts per million weight for volume can have the units "grams per milliliter." Can parts per million weight for volume also have the units "kilograms per liter"? Prove your answer. (*Hint:* 1 g water solution ≈ 1 mL.)
12. A solution of dilute NaOH is labeled 1:20 w/v. What is the concentration in percent weight for volume?
13. A laboratory has 750 mL of a 1:5000 w/v potassium permanganate solution. What is the percent weight for volume of this solution?
14. An alcohol solution is labeled 3:50 v/v. How many milliliters of alcohol are in 1 L of this solution?

15. How much 1:1000 weight for volume epinephrine solution can be made from 750 mg of epinephrine?

16. How much solid boric acid is needed to make 2000 mL of 1:50 w/v boric acid solution?

Answers to odd-numbered problems appear on page 233.

6.6 MOLARITY

In laboratory work, we often encounter solution concentrations measured in a unit called **molarity**. Molarity is defined as follows:

$$\text{Molarity} = \frac{\text{Moles of solute}}{\text{Liters of solution}}$$

You may notice that this formula is just another variation of the basic ratio:

$$\text{Concentration} = \frac{\text{Amount of solute}}{\text{Amount of solution}}$$

The "amount of solute" in this case is "moles of solute." Mole is abbreviated "mol."

The Mole

Chemists often measure the amount of a substance in terms of the **mole**. For our purposes, the mole may be defined in these two ways:

A mole of an element is that amount of substance equal to the atomic weight expressed in grams. This amount is also known as the **gram atomic weight.**

1 mole of a compound is that amount of the substance equal to the formula weight of the substance expressed in grams. This is also known as the **gram formula weight**.

The **formula weight** of a compound is the sum of all the weights of the atoms indicated in the formula of the compound. Formula weights, as atomic weights, are expressed in atomic mass units (a.m.u.).

Before we can begin making calculations with the mole, we need to examine the method for finding atomic weight and formula weight. There is a periodic table for your use in Appendix E.

EXAMPLE 6.6.1

Find the atomic or formula weights of these substances:
a. Cu (copper) **b.** H_2O (water) **c.** $MgSO_4$ (magnesium sulfate)
d. $C_6H_{12}O_6$ (glucose)

Solution	Comments
a. Cu = 63.5 a.m.u.	**a.** Consulting the periodic table, the atomic weight of copper is 63.54 atomic mass units (a.m.u.). Round off all atomic weights to the nearest tenth.
b. H_2O: H = 2 · 1.0 = 2.0 a.m.u. O = 1 · 16.0 = 16.0 a.m.u. F.W. = 18.0 a.m.u.	**b.** Make a table for the elements in the formula. Multiply the atomic weight of each element by the number of atoms of that element, then find the total.
c. $MgSO_4$: Mg = 1 · 24.3 = 24.3 a.m.u. S = 1 · 32.1 = 32.1 a.m.u. O = 4 · 16.0 = 64.0 a.m.u. F.W. = 120.4 a.m.u.	**c.** Repeat the preceding process for each element in the compound.

d. $C_6H_{12}O_6$:

$$\begin{aligned} C &= 6 \cdot 12.0 = 72.0 \text{ a.m.u.} \\ H &= 12 \cdot 1.0 = 12.0 \text{ a.m.u.} \\ O &= 6 \cdot 16.0 = \underline{96.0} \text{ a.m.u.} \\ \text{F.W.} &= 180.0 \text{ a.m.u.} \end{aligned}$$

d. The formula weights for H_2O and $C_6H_{12}O_6$ may also be called molecular weights. Consult a chemistry text for the difference between the two terms. For our explanation, we will stick with formula weight.

We can easily change from atomic and formula weights to molar quantities by using our definition of the mole. For example,

1 atom of Cu = 63.5 a.m.u.; then 1 mol Cu = 63.5 g

1 molecule of H_2O = 18.0 a.m.u.; then 1 mol H_2O = 18.0 g

1 particle of $MgSO_4$ = 120.4 a.m.u.; then 1 mol $MgSO_4$ = 120.4 g

1 particle $C_6H_{12}O_6$ = 180.0 a.m.u.; then 1 mol $C_6H_{12}O_6$ = 180.0 g

You may be wondering why we need a concept such as the mole. Imagine this situation: One molecule of water has a weight of 18.0 a.m.u. This is *very* small. We cannot see, feel, or taste this quantity of water, let alone work with it in the laboratory. However, if we have 18.0 g of water, enough for a couple of small swallows, we can see it, feel it, weigh it, or measure its volume. Remember, 18.0 g of water would be about 18.0 mL of water.

The mole is also a quantity similar to the familiar "dozen," which is always "12" of anything. By definition, 1 mol of a substance is equal to $6.022 \cdot 10^{23}$ particles of the substance in question, regardless of its atomic or formula weight. In our discussion of the mole, we will not be using this part of the definition, although it is often used in chemistry.

The examples that follow will illustrate other calculations involving the mole.

EXAMPLE 6.6.2

A beaker of water contains 36.0 g of water. How many moles of water are present?

Solution	**Comments**
$H = 2 \cdot 1.0 = 2.0$ a.m.u. $O = 1 \cdot 16.0 = \underline{16.0}$ a.m.u. F.W. = 18.0 a.m.u.	Find the weight of 1 mol of H_2O.
1 mol = 18.0 g	We will use this as our conversion factor.
$36.0 \cancel{\text{g H}_2\text{O}} \cdot \dfrac{1 \text{ mol}}{18.0 \cancel{\text{g H}_2\text{O}}}$	Use dimensional analysis to convert from grams to moles.
= 2.00 mol	The beaker contains 2.00 mol of water.

EXAMPLE 6.6.3

Find the weight of 2.50 mol of KNO_3 (potassium nitrate).

Solution	**Comments**
$K = 1 \cdot 39.1 = 39.1$ a.m.u. $N = 1 \cdot 14.0 = 14.0$ a.m.u. $O = 3 \cdot 16.0 = \underline{48.0}$ a.m.u. F.W. = 101.1 a.m.u.	Find the weight of 1 mol of KNO_3.
1 mol = 101.1 g	Use this as your conversion factor.
$2.50 \cancel{\text{mol}} \cdot \dfrac{101.1 \text{ g}}{1 \cancel{\text{mol}}}$	Use dimensional analysis to convert from moles to grams.
= 252.75 g	
≈ 253 g	2.50 mol of KNO_3 weighs 253 g.

From examples 6.6.2 and 6.6.3, we can see that given moles, we can find the gram quantity, and given grams, we can find the quantity of moles. Now, let us consider a few problems where molarity can be calculated. Recall the earlier definition:

$$\text{Molarity } (M) = \frac{\text{Moles of solute}}{\text{Liters of solution}}$$

If we make a solution where the amount of solute is known (in grams), and the amount of solution (usually in milliliters or liters) is known, we can then determine the molarity of the solution. Consider the following examples.

EXAMPLE 6.6.4

A chemist prepares a solution by dissolving 42.0 g of KCl in 150.0 mL of solution. What is the molarity of the solution?

Solution	**Comments**
$M = \frac{\text{Moles of solute}}{\text{Liters of solution}}$	Write down the molarity formula.
$M = \frac{\text{Moles of solute}}{0.1500 \text{ L}}$	We have 150.0 mL of solution, which is 0.1500 L. Substitute into the formula.
$K = 1 \cdot 39.1 = 39.1$ a.m.u. $Cl = 1 \cdot 35.5 = \underline{35.5}$ a.m.u. F.W. = 74.6 a.m.u.	To find moles of solute, we must first find the formula weight of KCl.
1 mol KCl = 74.6 g	
$42.0 \text{ g} \cdot \frac{1 \text{ mol}}{74.6 \text{ g}} = 0.563 \text{ mol}$	Change 42.0 g to moles using dimensional analysis.
$M = \frac{0.563 \text{ mol}}{0.1500 \text{ L}}$	Complete substitution into formula.
$M = 3.75$ mol/L	The molarity is 3.75 M.

EXAMPLE 6.6.5

A solution is made by dissolving 8.55 g of Fe_2SO_4 in enough water to make 375 mL of solution. What is the resulting molarity of the solution?

Solution	**Comments**
$M = \frac{\text{Moles of solute}}{0.375 \text{ L}}$	Write down the basic formula, substitute in 0.375 L for the volume of the solution.
$Fe = 1 \cdot 55.8 = 55.8$ a.m.u. $S = 1 \cdot 32.1 = 32.1$ a.m.u. $O = 4 \cdot 16.0 = \underline{64.0}$ a.m.u. F.W. = 151.9 a.m.u.	Find the formula weight of $FeSO_4$.
1 mol $FeSO_4$ = 151.9 g	
$8.55 \text{ g} \cdot \frac{1 \text{ mol}}{151.9 \text{ g}} = 0.0563 \text{ mol}$	Change grams of $FeSO_4$ to moles using dimensional analysis.
$M = \frac{0.0563 \text{ mol}}{0.375 \text{ L}}$	Substitute molar amount into the basic formula. Solve for M.
$M = 0.150$ mol/L	The molarity of the solution is 0.150 M.

In certain situations we may know the molarity of the solution we want to make, and how much solution we want to make. We will need to solve the basic molarity formula for the moles of solute needed, which can be converted into grams of solute.

EXAMPLE 6.6.6

A lab technician needs $15\bar{0}0$ of a 6.0-*M* solution of NaOH (sodium hydroxide). How much NaOH is needed to make the solution?

Solution	Comments
$6.0\ M = \dfrac{x}{0.150\ \text{L}}$	Write down the basic formula. Substitute in the molarity (6.0 *M*) and the volume (0.150 L). Let x equal the moles of solute.
$6.0\ \dfrac{\text{mol}}{\text{L}} = \dfrac{x}{0.150\ \text{L}}$	To make the units cancel out properly, express molarity (*M*) in moles per liter.
$(0.150\ \cancel{\text{L}})\ \dfrac{6.0\ \text{mol}}{\cancel{\text{L}}} = \dfrac{(x)}{0.150\ \cancel{\text{L}}}\ (0.150\ \cancel{\text{L}})$	Solve for x. Multiply both sides of the equation by 0.150 L. Notice that "liters" cancels out on both sides.
$0.90\ \text{mol} = x$	There are 0.90 mol of NaOH needed.
$\text{Na} = 1 \cdot 23.0 = 23.0$ a.m.u. $\text{O} = 1 \cdot 16.0 = 16.0$ a.m.u. $\text{H} = 1 \cdot 1.0 = \underline{1.0}$ a.m.u. F.W. $= 40.0$ a.m.u.	Find the formula weight of NaOH, and determine the weight of 1 mol.
1 mol NaOH $= 40.0$ g	
$0.90\ \cancel{\text{mole}} \cdot \dfrac{40.0\ \text{g}}{1\ \cancel{\text{mole}}} = 36\ \text{g}$	Use dimensional analysis to change from moles to grams.
	We need to dissolve 36 g of NaOH in enough water to make 1500 mL of solution. The resulting solution will be 6.0 *M*.

Another variation of the molarity concept occurs when both the molarity of the solution and the amount of solute we have available are known, and we need to determine how much solution we will have. Example 6.6.7 illustrates this type of problem.

EXAMPLE 6.6.7

How much of a 0.40-*M* solution of Na_2SO_4 can be made from 55.0 g of Na_2SO_4?

Solution	Comments
$0.40\ \dfrac{\text{mol}}{\text{L}} = \dfrac{\text{Moles of solute}}{\text{Liters of solution}}$	Write down the formula. Substitute in 0.40 mol/L and let x represent liters of solution.
$\text{Na} = 2 \cdot 23.0 = 46.0$ a.m.u. $\text{S} = 1 \cdot 32.1 = 32.1$ a.m.u. $\text{O} = 4 \cdot 16.0 = \underline{64.0}$ a.m.u. F.W. $= 142.1$ a.m.u.	We must convert 55.0 g of Na_2SO_4 to moles of Na_2SO_4 before substituting into the formula.
1 mol $Na_2SO_4 = 142.1$ g	
$55.0\ \cancel{\text{g}} \cdot \dfrac{1\ \text{mol}}{142.1\ \cancel{\text{g}}} = 0.387\ \text{mol}$	
$0.40\ \dfrac{\text{mol}}{\text{L}} = \dfrac{0.387\ \text{mol}}{x}$	Substitute moles Na_2SO_4 into the formula. Solve for x.
$(x)\ 0.40\ \dfrac{\text{mol}}{\text{L}} = \dfrac{0.387\ \text{moles}}{\cancel{x}}\ (\cancel{x})$	Multiply both sides by x.
$\dfrac{(x)\ \cancel{0.40\ \text{mol/L}}}{\cancel{0.40\ \text{mol/L}}} = \dfrac{0.387\ \text{mol}}{0.40\ \text{mol/L}}$	Divide both sides by 0.40 mol/L.

$$x = \frac{0.387 \text{ mol}}{0.40 \text{ mol/L}}$$

$x = 0.97$ L

We can make 0.97 L, or 970 mL, of the 0.40-M solution.

EXAMPLE 6.6.8

A student has a jug of sulfuric acid (H_2SO_4) labeled "20% w/w," and determines by experiment that the density of the solution is 1.20 g/mL.
a. What is the weight of H_2SO_4 in 1.00 L of this solution?
b. What is the molarity of the solution?

Solution

a. $1000 \cancel{\text{mL}} \cdot \frac{1.20 \text{ g}}{\cancel{\text{mL}}} = 1200 \text{ g}$

$$\frac{20.0 \text{ g}}{100 \text{ g}} = \frac{x}{1200 \text{ g}}$$

$100\,x = 24{,}000$
$x = 240$ g

b. H = 2 · 1.0 = 2.0 a.m.u.
S = 1 · 32.1 = 32.1 a.m.u.
O = 4 · 16.0 = 64.0 a.m.u.
F.W. = 98.1 a.m.u.

1 mol = 98.1 g

$$240 \cancel{\text{g}} \cdot \frac{1 \text{ mol}}{98.1 \cancel{\text{g}}} = 2.45 \text{ mol}$$

$$M = \frac{2.45 \text{ mol}}{1.00 \text{ L}}$$

$= 2.45\ M$

Comments

a. First, find the weight of 1 L of the H_2SO_4 solution. The density may be used as a conversion factor.

Find the actual weight of H_2SO_4 in 1200 g of the solution: 20% = 20 g/100 g. Solve for x.

There are 240 g of H_2SO_4 in 1000 mL of the solution. To use the molarity formula, change grams of H_2SO_4 to moles, which we do in **b**.

b. Find the weight of 1 mol of H_2SO_4.

Use dimensional analysis to change from grams to moles.

There are 2.45 mol of H_2SO_4 in 1.00 L of the solution. Substitute this into the molarity equation.

PROBLEM SET 3

1. Find the weight of 1 mol of each of the following substances.
   a. Hg (mercury)
   b. CO_2 (carbon dioxide)
   c. $Fe(OH)_3$ (ferric hydroxide)
   d. $Mg(OH)_2$ (magnesium hydroxide, or Milk of Magnesia)
   e. Br_2 (bromine gas)
   f. KNO_3 (potassium nitrate)
   g. NH_4NO_3 (ammonium nitrate)
   h. H_2CO_3 (carbonic acid)
   i. $NaHCO_3$ (sodium bicarbonate)
   j. $CaCO_3$ (calcium carbonate)

k. C_2H_6O (ethyl alcohol)
l. H_3PO_4 (phosphoric acid)

2. Determine the number of moles of each of the following substances.
   a. 16.2 g of HCl
   b. 0.253 g of KCl
   c. 81.02 g of $NaNO_3$
   d. 55.5 g of H_2O
   e. 0.0022 g of Cu
   f. $5.0 \cdot 10^4$ g of CaO
   g. 9.06 g of H_2
   h. 76.7 mg of SO_3
   i. 3.0 kg of $C_6H_{12}O_6$
   j. 100.0 g of $C_{12}H_{22}O_{11}$
   k. 88.00 g of $(NH_4)_3PO_4$
   l. $4.02 \cdot 10^{-10}$ kg of NaOH
3. Find the molarity of a solution made by dissolving 4.9 mol of KCl in 1 L of solution.
4. Find the molarity of a solution made by dissolving 2.72 mol of H_2SO_4 in 1000 mL of solution.
5. Exactly 500 mL of solution contains 2.0 mol of $Mg(OH)_2$. What is the molarity of this solution?
6. If 24.8 g of NaOH is placed in a beaker and enough water is added to bring the total volume up to 840 mL, what is the resulting molarity of the solution?
7. A laboratory technician places 37.20 g of potassium permanganate ($KMnO_4$) into a 100.0-mL volumetric flask and adds distilled water up to the mark. What is the molarity of the solution?
8. A 500-mL graduated cylinder is exactly half full of a $MgSO_4$ solution. If 8.75 g of $MgSO_4$ is in the solution, what is the molarity?
9. A service station attendant places 158.0 g of ethylene glycol ($C_2H_6O_2$) in the radiator of a car so that the total volume of the solution in the radiator after water is added is 7.54 L. What is the molarity of this solution?
10. How would you prepare 755 mL of a 2.00-*M* solution of $AgNO_3$ (silver nitrate)?
11. How would you prepare 250 mL of a 6.0-*M* solution of NaOH (sodium hydroxide)?
12. An ethyl alcohol–water solution has a concentration of 8.02 mol/L. If there are 337 mL of the solution, how many grams of ethyl alcohol (C_2H_6O) are in the solution?
13. The concentration of salt (NaCl) in body fluids is about 0.154 *M*. How much salt is present in 2.50 L of body fluid?
14. How much 1.00 M KCl solution can be made from 25.0 g of KCl?
15. Dr. Florence Flask needs a 2.00-*M* solution of $SnCl_2$ for a laboratory she is conducting. Each student needs at least 25.0 mL of the solution, and the laboratory has 16 students. To her dismay, she finds only 130.0 g of $SnCl_2$ on her shelf. Will she be able to make enough 2.00-*M* $SnCl_2$ for all of her students?
16. Which is stronger—a 20.0% w/v solution of NaOH or a 2.00-*M* solution?
17. A 6.00% w/w solution of H_2SO_4 has a density of about 1.04 g/mL. Find the molarity of this solution.

18. A solution made by dissolving 11.2 g of an alkaline substance in 820 mL of solution has a molarity of 0.224 *M*. Find the formula weight of the substance. $\left(\textit{Hint: } \text{moles of solute} = \dfrac{\text{grams of solute}}{\text{molar weight}}\right)$

Answers to odd-numbered problems appear on page 234.

6.7 CONCENTRATION OF IONIC SUBSTANCES

The concept of molarity becomes inadequate when we begin working with acids and bases. In this section we study another concentration unit used for these kinds of solutions. First, however, we look at the classical definition of the terms "acid" and "base":

1. An **acid** is a chemical substance that breaks apart in a water solution to yield hydrogen ions (H^+).
2. A **base** is a chemical substance that breaks apart in a water solution to yield hydroxide ions (OH^-).

It will be helpful in understanding why molarity is inadequate to measure concentrations of acids and bases to consider the following illustrations:

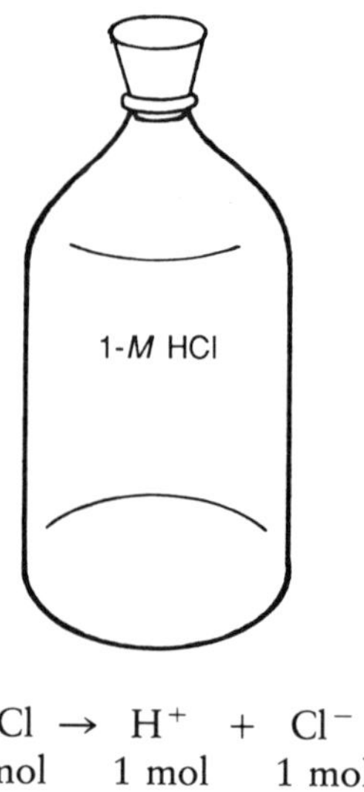

$$\underset{1\text{ mol}}{HCl} \rightarrow \underset{1\text{ mol}}{H^+} + \underset{1\text{ mol}}{Cl^-}$$

In the 1-L bottle of 1-*M* HCl shown above, there is 1 mol of HCl molecules breaking apart (dissociating) to yield 1 mol of hydrogen ions and 1 mol of chloride ions.

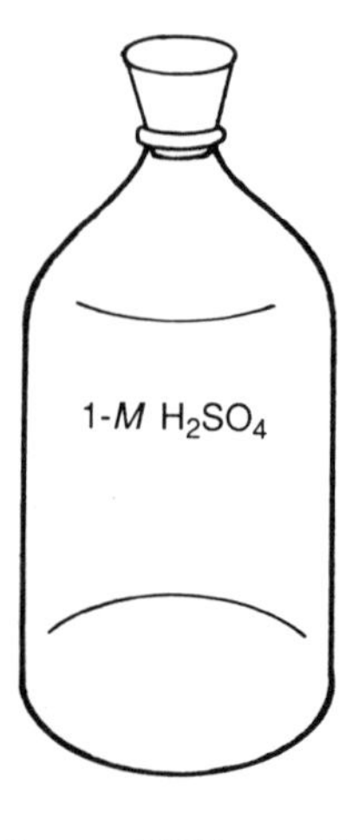

$$\underset{1\text{ mol}}{H_2SO_4} \rightarrow \underset{2\text{ mol}}{2H^+} + \underset{1\text{ mol}}{SO_4^{2-}}$$

In the 1-L bottle of 1-M H_2SO_4 shown above, there is 1 mol of H_2SO_4 dissociating to yield 2 mol of hydrogen ions and 1 mol of sulfate ions.

These illustrations show that two acids with the same molarity can yield hydrogen ions with two different molarities. What we need is a concentration unit that will assure that equal quantities of these ions are present when the concentration units are the same.

Before we define that unit, let us first examine the concept of equivalence. An **equivalent** of an acid or base will yield 1 mol of hydrogen ions or hydroxide ions in a water solution. The weight in grams of an equivalent (the **equivalent weight**) can be determined by the following equations:

For an acid:

$$\text{Equivalent weight} = \frac{\text{Gram formula weight (molar weight)}}{\text{Number of hydrogen ions in formula}}$$

For a base:

$$\text{Equivalent weight} = \frac{\text{Gram formula weight (molar weight)}}{\text{Number of hydroxide ions in formula}}$$

Some common acids and bases are shown in the table below:

Acid		Base	
HCl	Hydrochloric acid	NaOH	Sodium hydroxide
H_2SO_4	Sulfuric acid	KOH	Potassium hydroxide
HNO_3	Nitric acid	$Ca(OH)_2$	Calcium hydroxide
$HC_2H_3O_2$	Acetic acid	$Mg(OH)_2$	Magnesium hydroxide

Acidic and basic reactions are important in chemistry and in biomedical reactions. The hydrogen ions (H^+) and the hydroxide ions (OH^-) are the ions that interact during the process of neutralization, such as when an antacid (usually a weak base) neutralizes excess stomach acid (HCl) to form a salt and water. This process is illustrated by the following simplified reaction:

$$H^+ + OH^- \rightarrow H_2O$$

We will study in greater detail the phenomena of ionization of water in Chapter 7.

EXAMPLE 6.7.1

Find the equivalent weights of the following acids and bases:
a. HNO_3 **b.** $Mg(OH)_2$ **c.** H_3PO_4

Solution

a.
$$\begin{aligned} H &= 1.0 \text{ a.m.u.} \\ N &= 14.0 \text{ a.m.u.} \\ O_3 &= \underline{48.0} \text{ a.m.u.} \\ \text{F.W.} &= 63.0 \text{ a.m.u.} \end{aligned}$$

$$1 \text{ mol} = 63.0 \text{ g}$$

$$\text{Eq wt} = \frac{63.0 \text{ g}}{1}$$

$$\text{Eq wt} = 63.0 \text{ g}$$

b.
$$\begin{aligned} Mg &= 24.3 \text{ a.m.u.} \\ O_2 &= 32.0 \text{ a.m.u.} \\ H_2 &= \underline{2.0} \text{ a.m.u.} \\ \text{F.W.} &= 58.3 \text{ a.m.u.} \end{aligned}$$

$$1 \text{ mole} = 58.3 \text{ g}$$

Comments

a. Find the formula weight of HNO_3.

To find the equivalent weight, divide the molar weight by the number of hydrogens in the formula, which is 1.

In this case, the equivalent weight is the same as the molar weight, 63.0 g.

b. Find the formula weight of the compound.

$$\text{Eq wt} = \frac{58.3 \text{ g}}{2}$$

Divide the molar weight of the compound by the number of hydroxide ions in the formula.

$$\text{Eq wt} = 29.2 \text{ g}$$

The equivalent weight is 29.2 g of magnesium hydroxide, and this amount will yield 1 mol of hydroxide ions in solution.

c. H_3 = 3.0 a.m.u.
P = 31.0 a.m.u.
O_4 = 64.0 a.m.u.
F.W. = 98.0 a.m.u.

c. Find the formula weight.

1 mol = 98.0 g

$$\text{Eq wt} = \frac{98.0 \text{ g}}{3}$$

Divide the molar weight by the number of hydrogens in the formula.

$$\text{Eq wt} = 32.7 \text{ g}$$

One mole of hydrogen ions is produced by 32.7 g of H_3PO_4 (phosphoric acid) when dissolved in water.

In the case of H_3PO_4, $\frac{1}{3}$ mol of the acid will yield 1 mol of hydrogen ions in solution.

$$\begin{aligned} H_3PO_4 &\rightarrow 3\ H^+ + PO_4^{3-} \\ \text{If } 1 \text{ mol} &\rightarrow 3 \text{ mol} + 1 \text{ mol} \\ \text{then } \tfrac{1}{3} \text{ mol} &\rightarrow 1 \text{ mol} + \tfrac{1}{3} \text{ mol} \end{aligned}$$

Equivalents of Electrolytes

The definition of the equivalent we have just studied may be extended to ions other than H^+ and OH^- ions. Keeping in mind that 1 Eq of an acid or a base will yield 1 mol of these ions in solution, we can now say that 1 Eq of an ion will yield 1 mol of unit charge of that ion. To arrive at the weight of an equivalent for any ionic substance, we can use the following formula:

$$1 \text{ Eq} = \frac{\text{Molar weight of the ion}}{\text{Numerical charge of the ion}}$$

Ions in a water solution will carry an electric current; hence they are called **electrolytes.** Many electrolytes of the kind shown below are also found in the blood and are significant in maintaining good health:

$1 \text{ mol } Na^+ = 23.0 \text{ g}$ $\qquad 1 \text{ Eq } Na^+ = \frac{23.0 \text{ g}}{1} = 23.0 \text{ g}$

$1 \text{ mol } Cl^- = 35.5 \text{ g}$ $\qquad 1 \text{ Eq } Cl^- = \frac{35.5 \text{ g}}{1} = 35.5 \text{ g}$

$1 \text{ mol } Ca^{+2} = 40.1 \text{ g}$ $\qquad 1 \text{ Eq } Ca^{+2} = \frac{40.1 \text{ g}}{2} = 20.05 \text{ g}$

$1 \text{ mol } (SO_4^{-2}) = 96.1 \text{ g}$ $\qquad 1 \text{ Eq } (SO_4^{-2}) = \frac{96.1 \text{ g}}{2} = 48.05 \text{ g}$

The guiding principle here is that 1 Eq of any positive ion or 1 Eq of negative ion will yield 1 mol of charge. By 1 mol of charge we mean the same amount of charge as 1 mol of H^+ ions.

The ions found in body fluids are usually reported in laboratory tests in milliequivalents per liter (mEq/L). Since the prefix "milli" means 1/1000, then

$$1000 \text{ mEq} = 1 \text{ Eq}$$

EXAMPLE 6.7.2

Find the number of milliequivalents of each of the following ions:
a. 14.2 mg Cl^- ions **b.** 8.34 mg HCO_3^- (bicarbonate ion) **c.** 23.19 mg Fe^{2+}

Solution	Comments
a. $1 \text{ Eq } Cl^- = \frac{35.5 \text{ g}}{1} = 35.5 \text{ g}$	**a.** Find the weight of 1 Eq of Cl^-.
$35.5 \text{ g} = 35{,}500 \text{ mg}$	Change from grams to milligrams.
$\frac{1 \text{ Eq}}{1000} = \frac{35{,}500 \text{ mg}}{1000}$	Change from equivalents to milliequivalents by dividing both sides of this equation by 1000.
$1 \text{ mEq} = 35.5 \text{ mg}$	
$14.2 \cancel{\text{mg}} \cdot \frac{1 \text{ mEq}}{35.5 \cancel{\text{mg}}} = 0.400 \text{ mEq}$	Use dimensional analysis to find the number of milliequivalents.
b. $H = 1.0$ a.m.u. $C = 12.0$ a.m.u. $O_3 = \underline{48.0}$ a.m.u. F.W. $= 61.0$ a.m.u.	**b.** Find the weight of 1 Eq of (HCO_3^-).
$1 \text{ mol} = 61.0 \text{ g}$	
$1 \text{ Eq} = \frac{61.0 \text{ g}}{1} = 61.0 \text{ g}$	Change from grams to milligrams.
$= 61{,}000 \text{ mg}$ $1 \text{ mEq} = 61.0 \text{ mg}$	Change from equivalents to milliequivalents (divide by 1000).
$8.34 \cancel{\text{mg}} \cdot \frac{1 \text{ mEq}}{61.0 \cancel{\text{mg}}} = 0.137 \text{ mEq.}$	Use dimensional analysis to find the number of milliequivalents.
c. $Fe^{2+} = \frac{55.8 \text{ g}}{2} = 27.9 \text{ g}$	**c.** Find the weight of 1 Eq of Fe^{-2}.
$1 \text{ Eq} = 27.9 \text{ g} = 27{,}900 \text{ mg}$	Change from grams to milligrams.
$1 \text{ mEq} = 27.9 \text{ mg}$	Change from equivalents to milliequivalents.
$23.19 \cancel{\text{mg}} \cdot \frac{1 \text{ mEq}}{27.9 \cancel{\text{mg}}} = 0.831 \text{ mEq.}$	Use of dimensional analysis to find the number of milliequivalents.

Normality

Now that we have defined the equivalent, the concept of **normality** may be defined as follows:

$$\text{Normality} = \frac{\text{Equivalents of solute}}{\text{Liters of solution}}$$

A 1-*N* solution of NaOH will contain 1 Eq of NaOH for every 1 L of solution. A 2-*N* solution of H_2SO_4 will contain 2 Eq of H_2SO_4 for every 1 L of solution.

It can be stated, then, that equal volumes of acids and bases with the same normalities will neutralize each other, since they produce equal molar quantities of H^+ and OH^- ions.

EXAMPLE 6.7.3

Find the normality of each of the following solutions:
a. 38.2 g of NaOH in 2.00 L of solution **b.** 16.94 g of H_2SO_4 in 450 mL of solution.

Solution	Comments
a. Na = 23.0 a.m.u. O = 16.0 a.m.u. H = 1.0 a.m.u. F.W. = 40.0 a.m.u.	**a.** Find the equivalent weight of NaOH.
1 mol = 40.0 g	
$1\ \text{Eq} = \frac{40.0\ \text{g}}{1} = 40.0\ \text{g}$	Recall that 1 Eq of a base is the molar weight divided by the number of hydroxide ions in the formula.
$38.2\ \text{g NaOH} \cdot \frac{1\ \text{Eq}}{40.0\ \text{g}}$ $= 0.955\ \text{Eq}$	Use dimensional analysis to change from grams to equivalents.
$N = \frac{\text{Eq}}{\text{L}}$	Substitute appropriate values into the normality formula.
$N = \frac{0.955\ \text{Eq}}{2.00\ \text{L}} = 0.478\ \text{Eq/L}$ or 0.478 *N*	
b. H_2 = 2.0 a.m.u. S = 32.1 a.m.u. O_4 = 64.0 a.m.u. F.W. = 98.1 a.m.u.	**b.** Find the equivalent weight of H_2SO_4.
1 mol = 98.1 g	
$1\ \text{Eq} = \frac{98.1\ \text{g}}{2} = 49.0\ \text{g}$	Recall that 1 Eq of an acid is the molar weight divided by the number of hydrogens in the formula.
$16.94\ \text{g} \cdot \frac{1\ \text{Eq.}}{49.0\ \text{g}} = 0.346\ \text{Eq}$	Use dimensional analysis to change from grams to equivalents.
$N = \frac{0.346\ \text{Eq}}{0.450\ \text{L}} = 0.768\ \text{Eq/L}$ or 0.768 *N*	Substitute appropriate values into the normality formula.

Since the normality definition, as in molarity, contains three variables, we can solve for any of the three. If we are given the normality of a solution and the volume of the solution, we can then solve for equivalents of solute (and also the gram quantity of the solute).

EXAMPLE 6.7.4

A technician uses 38.2 mL of a 2.00-*N* HCl solution in making a test. How many equivalents of HCl did the technician use? How many grams?

Solution	Comments
$N = \frac{\text{Eq}}{\text{L}}$	First determine the number of equivalents of HCl. Substitute known quantities into the normality formula (changing milliliters to liters).

$$2.00\ \frac{\text{Eq}}{\text{L}} = \frac{x}{0.0382\ \text{L}}$$

Solve for x.

$$2.00\ \frac{\text{Eq}}{\cancel{\text{L}}}(0.0382\ \cancel{\text{L}}) = x$$

Note that "liters" cancels out.

$$0.0764\ \text{Eq} = x$$

$$1\ \text{Eq HCl} = \frac{36.5\ \text{g}}{1} = 36.5\ \text{g}$$

$$0.0764\ \cancel{\text{Eq}} \cdot \frac{36.5\ \text{g}}{1\ \cancel{\text{Eq}}} = 2.79\ \text{g}$$

Use dimensional analysis to convert from equivalents to grams. The technician used 0.0764 Eq of HCl or 2.79 g.

Another type of problem arises when both the normality of the solution and the equivalents (or grams) of the acid or base are known and we wish to find the volume of the solution.

EXAMPLE 6.7.5

An experiment requires 2.033 g of HNO_3 dissolved in a 6.00-N HNO_3 solution to neutralize a certain base. How many milliliters of HNO_3 solution is required?

Solution

H = 1.0 a.m.u.
N = 14.0 a.m.u.
O_3 = <u>48.0</u> a.m.u.
F.W. = 63.0 a.m.u.

Comments

First, change grams of HNO_3 to equivalents. Find the equivalent weight of HNO_3.

$$1\ \text{mol} = 63.0\ \text{g}$$

$$1\ \text{Eq} = \frac{63.0\ \text{g}}{1} = 63.0\ \text{g}$$

$$2.033\ \cancel{\text{g}} \cdot \frac{1\ \text{Eq}}{63.0\ \cancel{\text{g}}} = 0.0323\ \text{Eq}$$

Use dimensional analysis to change from grams to equivalents.

$$6.00\ \frac{\text{Eq}}{\text{L}} = \frac{0.0323\ \text{Eq}}{x}$$

Substitute 0.0323 Eq and 6.00 Eq/L into the normality formula. Let "x" be equal to the volume.

$$x = \frac{0.0323\ \cancel{\text{Eq}}}{6.00\ \cancel{\text{Eq}}/\text{L}}$$

Solve for x.

$$x = 0.00538\ \text{L} = 5.38\ \text{mL}$$

Changing from Molarity to Normality

There is a convenient method for changing from molarity to normality that will save time, and involves a simple formula.

$$\text{Normality} = \text{Molarity} \cdot \begin{cases} \text{number of hydrogens in formula (acid)} \\ \text{or} \\ \text{Number of hydroxides in formula (base)} \end{cases}$$

For example:

$$1\ M\ \text{HCl} \cdot 1 = 1\ N\ \text{HCl}$$
$$16\ M\ H_2SO_4 \cdot 2 = 32\ N\ H_2SO_4$$
$$0.1\ M\ HNO_3 \cdot 1 = 0.1\ N\ HNO_3$$
$$1.5\ M\ Mg(OH_2) \cdot 2 = 3.0\ N\ Mg(OH_2)$$

Always remember: normality is always a whole number multiple of molarity.

PROBLEM SET 4

1. Find the equivalent weights of the following acids and bases:
   a. H_3PO_4
   b. $H(C_2H_3O_2)$
   c. $Ca(OH)_2$
   d. $Al(OH)_3$
   e. HF
   f. $Mg(OH)_2$
   g. $H_2(SO_3)$
2. Find the number of milliequivalents of each of the ionic substances below:
   a. 2300 mg Na^+
   b. 9.00 g of $(CO_3)^-$
   c. 16.0 g of $(PO_4)^{3-}$
   d. 170 mg of Fe^{2+}
   e. 0.150 mol of Cl^-
   f. 0.300 mol of K^+
   g. 0.350 mol of $(HCO_3)^-$
3. Find the number of equivalents in each of the following acids and bases:
   a. 350.0 g of HCl
   b. 2.79 g of H_3PO_4
   c. 12.82 g of H_2SO_4
   d. 3.33 g of $Al(OH)_3$
   e. 8972 mg of $Mg(OH)_2$
   f. 40.0 g of H_2CO_3
   g. $2.7 \cdot 10^{-2}$ kg of $HC_2H_3O_2$
4. Determine the normality of each of the following solutions:
   a. 85.0 g of $Mg(OH)_2$ in 2.00 L of solution
   b. 67.4 g of HCl in 2.50 L of solution
   c. 197.2 g of H_2SO_4 in 4500 mL of solution
   d. $4.76 \cdot 10^4$ mg of HNO_3 in 2500 mL of solution
   e. 98.7 g H_3BO_3 in 458 mL of solution
5. A 6.0 *N* solution of NaOH contains 445.2 mEq of NaOH. What is the volume of the solution?
6. A 12.0 *N* solution of HCl contains 12.2 g of HCl. What is the volume of the solution?
7. A chemist has 2.5 L of a 16.0 *N* H_2SO_4 solution. How many equivalents of H_2SO_4 are present?
8. A laboratory has two bottles of 18.0-*M* $HC_2H_3O_2$. Each bottle contains 4.2 L of solution. How many grams of $HC_2H_3O_2$ are in the bottles?
9. Dr. Millie Graham has 1.80 L of 96.2% w/w H_2SO_4 on hand. The density of the acid is 1.84 g/mL. Find the normality of the acid.
10. Dr. Bea Kerr needs some 20.0% w/v NaOH for an experiment. She wants to calculate the normality of the NaOH solution, so she turns to you, the lab assistant. Can you do it for her?

Answers to odd-numbered problems appear on page 234.

6.8 DILUTIONS

One of the most common tasks performed in the laboratory is that of preparation of solutions from pre-existing solutions, that is, diluting a preexisting solution using water. It need not be a complicated job, however. There are a couple of points to keep in mind when making dilutions.

1. The molar quantity of a substance in the solution is not changed when making a dilution; only the volume of the solution, and therefore, the concentration, of the solution, is changed.
2. A solution cannot be made stronger (more concentrated) by diluting it.

Let us examine the first statement. What happens when 100 mL of 12-*M* HCl is diluted to 1000 mL? Using dimensional analysis, we can calculate the number of moles of HCl present in the original solution:

$$(0.100 \text{ L}) \frac{12 \text{ mol HCl}}{1 \text{ L}} = 1.2 \text{ mol HCl present}$$

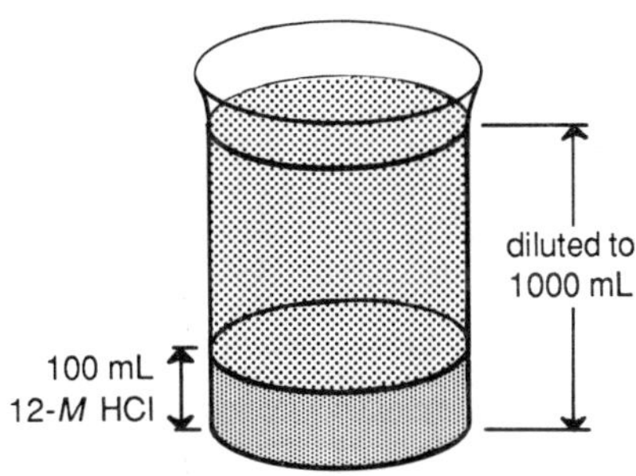

Water is added to the existing HCl. No more HCl is added, there are still 1.2 mol of HCl in the beaker. Therefore,

$$\text{Number of moles before dilution} = \text{number of moles after dilution}$$

Substituting,

$$(\text{Volume before}) \cdot (\text{molarity before}) = (\text{volume after}) \cdot (\text{molarity after})$$

Letting the subscript 1 = before, and the subscript 2 = after, and letting V = volume, and M = molarity, the equation becomes

$$V_1 \cdot M_1 = V_2 \cdot M_2$$

This is called the "dilution formula." Actually, the concentration of the solution may be any concentration unit, such as percent, molarity, or normality. The formula may be rewritten to let C stand for the concentration unit:

$$V_1 \cdot C_1 = V_2 \cdot C_2.$$

EXAMPLE 6.8.1

What is the final concentration of a solution made by dissolving 50.0 mL of 6.0-*M* H_2SO_4 in enough water to make 1000.00 mL of solution?

Solution	**Comments**
$V_1C_1 = V_2C_2$	Write the basic formula. Note that two volumes are given, which is an indication to use the dilution formula. In other dilution problems, two concentration units may be given.
$V_1 = 50.0$ mL; $C_1 = 6.0\ M$ $V_2 = 1000.0$ mL; $C_2 = ?$	Make a table from the information given.
$(50.0 \text{ mL})(6.0\ M) = (1000.0 \text{ mL})(C_2)$	Substitute into the formula. Solve for C_2.
$\frac{(50.0 \cancel{\text{mL}})(6.0\ M)}{1000.0 \cancel{\text{mL}}} = C_2$	
$0.30\ M = C_2$	The final concentration is 0.30 *M*.

Keep in mind the following pointers concerning dilutions:

1. The original concentration of a solution is always greater than the final concentration.
2. The original volume of the solution is always smaller than the final volume.

Example 6.8.2 illustrates how the formula may be used with percent concentrations.

EXAMPLE 6.8.2

How would you prepare 520 mL of a 5.0% w/v solution of NaOH from a 20.0% w/v solution?

Solution	**Comments**
$V_1C_1 = V_2C_2$	Write down the formula. Note that two concentrations are given.
$V_1 = ?;\ C_1 = 20.0\%\ \text{w/v}$ $V_2 = 520\ \text{mL};\ C_2 = 5.0\%\ \text{w/v}$	Make a table of values.
$(V_1)(20.0\%) = (520\ \text{mL})(5.0\%)$	Substitute into the formula.
$V_1 = \dfrac{(520\ \text{mL})(5.0\cancel{\%})}{20.0\cancel{\%}}$	Solve for V_1. The "percents" cancel.
$V_1 = 130\ \text{mL}$	To prepare 520 mL of a 5.0% w/v NaOH solution, measure out 130 mL of the 20.0% NaOH solution, and then add enough distilled water to make 520 mL of the solution.

Any concentration unit and any volume unit may be used in the formula, provided the same units are used on *both* sides of the formula. *Never mix units.*

EXAMPLE 6.8.3

A teacher has 16 students in a chemistry laboratory. Each student needs 75.0 mL of a 0.100-*N* NaOH solution. The teacher has only 6.00-*N* NaOH solution in stock. How should the teacher go about making the solution for the students?

Solution	**Comments**
$16\ \cancel{\text{students}} \cdot \dfrac{75.0\ \text{mL}}{1\ \cancel{\text{student}}} = 1200\ \text{mL}$	First, calculate the amount of solution the teacher needs for all of the students.
$V_1V_2 = V_2C_2$	Write down the dilution formula.
$V_1 = ?;\ C_1 = 6.00\ N$ $V_2 = 1200\ \text{mL};\ C_2 = 0.100\ N$	Make a table of values.
$(V_1)(6.00\ N) = (1200\ \text{mL})(0.100\ N)$	Substitute values into the formula. Solve for V_1.
$V_1 = \dfrac{(1200\ \text{mL})(0.100\ N)}{(6.00\ N)}$	
$V_1 = 20.0\ \text{mL}$	The teacher should measure out 20.0 mL of the 6.0-*N* solution, and dilute it to 1200 mL. This amount would be enough for exactly 16 students. There is none to waste, however, and it might be smart to make more than 1200 mL to begin with.

Serial Dilutions

There are occasions when a series of dilutions must be made. The dilution formula may be used to calculate the resulting concentrations of these dilutions. The following example illustrates the process of serial dilutions.

EXAMPLE 6.8.4

A laboratory instructor wishes to illustrate how the pH of an acid varies with the concentration of the acid. The teacher measures out 100.0 mL of a 0.100-*M* HCl solution. This is placed in a beaker marked number 1. The teacher then takes 10.0 mL of this solution and dissolves it in enough distilled water to make 100.0 mL of solution. This is placed in beaker number 2. The teacher measures out 10.0 mL of the solution in beaker number 2, and places it in beaker number 3, and adds enough distilled water to make 100.0 mL of solution. Calculate the concentrations of beaker numbers 2 and 3.

Below is an illustration of the problem:

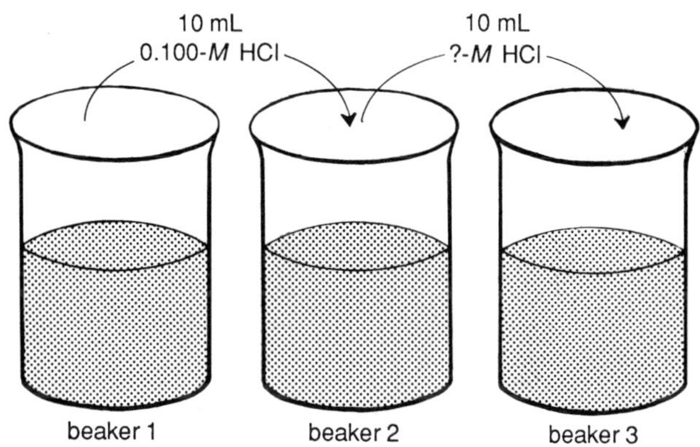

Solution	**Comments**
$V_1C_1 = V_2C_2$	Start with the dilution formula. We know the concentration of beaker number 1. It is 0.100 *M*. Calculate the concentration of beaker number 2.
$V_1 = 10.0\text{ mL};\ C_1 = 0.100\ M$ $V_2 = 100.0\text{ mL};\ C_2 = ?$	Make a table of values.
$(10.0\text{ mL})(0.100\ M) = (100.0\text{ mL})(C_2)$	Substitute values into the formula.
$\dfrac{(10.0\ \cancel{\text{mL}})(.100\ M)}{100.0\ \cancel{\text{mL}}} = C_2$	Solve for C_2.
$0.0100\ M = C_2$	The final concentration of solution number 2 is 0.0100 *M*. This becomes the initial concentration of solution number 3, since we took 10.0 mL of it to make the third solution.
$V_1 = 10.0\text{ mL};\ C_1 = 0.0100\ M$ $V_2 = 100.0\text{ mL};\ C_2 = ?$	Make another table of values.
$(10.0\text{ mL})(0.0100\ M) = (100.0\text{ mL})(C_2)$	Substitute into the formula.
$\dfrac{(10.0\ \cancel{\text{mL}})(.0100\ M)}{100.0\ \cancel{\text{mL}}} = C_2$	Solve for C_2.
$0.00100\ M = C_2$	The final concentration of solution number 3 is 0.00100 *M*.

Solution number 1 = 0.100 *M* (original)
Solution number 2 = 0.0100 *M*
Solution number 3 = 0.00100 *M*

There is a shortcut of working the preceding problem. Since 10 mL of the original solution was dissolved in 100 mL of solution the ratio of solute to solution is

$$\frac{10\ \cancel{\text{mL}}}{100\ \cancel{\text{mL}}} = \frac{1}{10}$$

The concentration of the solution in beaker number 2 is $\frac{1}{10}$ that of beaker number 1. Also, 10 mL of the solution in beaker number 2 was dissolved in enough water to make 100 mL of solution and placed into beaker number 3. The ratio of solute to solution here is

$$\frac{10\ \cancel{\text{mL}}}{100\ \cancel{\text{mL}}} = \frac{1}{10}$$

The concentration of the solution in beaker number 3 is

$$\frac{1}{10} \cdot \frac{1}{10} = \frac{1}{100}$$

of the concentration of beaker number 1:

$$\frac{1}{100} \cdot 0.100\ M = 0.00100\ M \text{ (the concentration of beaker number 3)}$$

PROBLEM SET 5

1. How would you make 250.0 mL of a 2.0-M HCl solution from a 12-M solution?
2. How would you make 75.0 mL of a 25% isopropyl alcohol solution from a 95% solution of isopropyl alcohol?
3. Ten milliliters of a 75% ethyl alcohol solution diluted to 25 mL has what strength?
4. One liter of 86-proof whiskey diluted to 1.5 L has what strength?
5. How much water is needed to prepare a 40.0% w/v solution from 400 mL of 100% w/v ethyl alcohol (absolute alcohol)?
6. How much water is needed to add to 5.00 mL of a 14.0% w/v benzalkonium chloride solution to make a 0.040% w/v solution?
7. How would you make $4.2 \cdot 10^2$ mL of a 3.00-M H_2SO_4 solution from a 9.00-N H_2SO_4 solution?
8. Forty-eight milliliters of a hydrochloric acid (HCl) solution were diluted to make 0.5 L of a hydrochloric acid solution that was tested by titration to have a concentration of 0.100 M. What was the strength of the initial hydrochloric acid solution?
9. A laboratory instructor has 18 students in a class. Each student is to do a procedure twice that requires 25.0 mL of 0.200-M HCl each time the procedure is performed. The instructor has only concentrated (12-M) HCl in stock. How should the instructor prepare the hydrochloric acid solution for the students?
10. A student delivers 2.0 mL of 0.200-M NaOH into a volumetric flask, and adds water to the 100.0-mL mark; then 5.0 mL of this solution is pipetted into a beaker and water up to 100.0 mL of solution is added. This beaker number is 1. Then 5.0 mL of this solution is transfered to another beaker, and water up to 100.0-mL mark is added. This beaker is labeled number 2. Find the concentrations of the sodium hydroxide in beakers 1 and 2.
11. A laboratory technician sets up four test tubes, each containing 9.9 mL of distilled water; 0.10 mL of 20.0% NaOH is pipetted into test tube 1, and mixed. Then 0.10 mL of the solution in test tube 1 is transfered to test tube 2, and mixed. This process is repeated with test tubes 3 and 4. Find the concentrations (in percent) of NaOH in all four test tubes. (*Hint:* Find the total volume of solution in each test tube.)

Answers to odd-numbered problems appear on page 234.

CHAPTER REVIEW

(6.3)

1. Find the percent weight for weight of a solution made by dissolving 18.2 g of Glauber's salt in 250.0 g of water.
2. A label states that there is 0.45 mg of drug per 4.0 mL of solution. What is the percent weight for volume?
3. How much ethyl alcohol is contained in 500.0 mL of a 43.0% v/v solution of ethyl alcohol?
4. How would you prepare 2.6 L of a 2.5% w/v solution of $KMnO_4$?
5. If a patient has a blood cholesterol level of 199 mg %, how much cholesterol would be contained a 1-pt sample of the patient's blood?
6. If the concentration of DDT in lake trout in Lake Michigan averages 6.96 ppm w/w, how many grams of DDT would be found in a lake trout weighing 4.2 lb?
7. A solution of Lysol has a concentration of 5:250 v/v. What is the concentration in parts per million?

(6.4)

8. Fifteen hundred milliliters of a 6.00-*M* solution of NaOH contains how many grams of NaOH?
9. What is the molarity of a D_5W (5% dextrose and water) solution? Dextrose is $C_6H_{12}O_6$.

(6.5)

10. A solution of HCl is made by dissolving 28.6 g of HCl in enough water to make 2077 mL of solution. What is the normality of the solution?
11. Find the number of milliequivalents of each of these ions:
    a. 3.75 g of (HCO_3^-)
    b. 4.52 g of Na^+

(6.6)

12. How would you prepare 320.0 mL of a 70.0% v/v ethyl alcohol solution from 95.0% v/v stock solution?
13. How much 1:5000 v/v solution can be made from 250 mL of a 1:250 stock solution?
14. A technician obtains 2.50 mL of 6.00 *M* HCl, dilutes it to 50.0 mL, and labels this solution as solution number 1. The technician then takes 2.50 mL of this solution and dilutes it to 50.0 mL, and labels it as solution number 2; then 5.0 mL of solution number 2 are diluted to 100.0 mL, and labels it as solution number 3. Find the concentrations of the three solutions.

Answers to all problems appear on page 234.

chapter 7

Logarithms and Their Applications

OBJECTIVES

After studying this chapter, the student should be able to:

1. Define logarithm.
2. Take the logarithm of a number using either a log table or calculator, as directed by the instructor.
3. Compute the inverse logarithm using either a log table or calculator, as directed by the instructor.
4. Perform simple calculations using logarithms.
5. Use logarithms in solving certain formulas containing them.

7.1 INTRODUCTION

Certain formulas, such as the pH formula, the Henderson–Hasselbach equation, and calculations involving absorbance and transmittance of light, make use of a concept called the logarithm. In this chapter, we define the logarithm, learn to find the logarithm of a number, and perform calculations with logarithms.

7.2 THE LOGARITHM AND POWERS OF TEN

If $10^3 = 1000$, we say that the logarithm of 1000 in base 10 is 3. A **logarithm** is an exponent placed on a base (most commonly 10) in order to obtain a given number. When 10 is the base, this exponent is called a **common logarithm**. Common logarithms are indicated by the symbol "log." We define a common logarithm as follows:

$$\log A = E \quad \text{if and only if} \quad 10^E = A$$

To define a logarithm in general we say

$$\log_b A = E \quad \text{if and only if} \quad b^E = A.$$

However, we will confine our study of logarithms to base 10. The following examples will clarify the definitions.

EXAMPLE 7.2.1

Find the logarithms of the following numbers: **a.** 0.001 **b.** 0.01 **c.** 0.1 **e.** 10 **f.** 100 **g.** 1000

Solution	Comments
a. $0.001 = 10^{-3}$ $\log 0.001 = -3$	**a.** Write 0.001 as a power of 10. The "exponent" of base 10 is -3.

b. $0.01 = 10^{-2}$
$\log 0.01 = -2$

b. Write 0.01 as a power of 10. The "exponent" of base 10 is -2.

c. $0.1 = 10^{-1}$
$\log 0.1 = -1$

c. Write as a power of 10. The "exponent" of base 10 is -1.

d. $1 = 10^0$
$\log 1 = 0$

d. Write 1 as a power of 10. The "exponent" of base 10 is 0.

e. $10 = 10^1$
$\log 10 = 1$

e. Write 10 as a power of 10. The "exponent" of base 10 is 1.

f. $100 = 10^2$
$\log 100 = 2$

f. Write 100 as a power of 10. The "exponent" of base 10 is 2.

g. $1000 = 10^3$
$\log 1000 = 3$

g. Write 1000 as a power of 10. The "exponent" of base 10 is 3.

Remember that the common logarithm is the exponent placed on 10 to obtain the given number.

7.3 PROPERTIES OF THE LOGARITHM

The algebraic properties that apply to exponents apply to logarithms. These properties are outlined here.

Property	**Explanation**
1. $\log(AB) = \log A + \log B$	The logarithm of a product is the sum of the logarithms of each factor. Recall: When bases are multiplied, their "exponents" are added.
2. $\log \frac{A}{B} = \log A - \log B$	The logarithm of a quotient is the difference of the logarithms of the numerator and the denominator. Recall: When bases are divided, their "exponents" are subtracted.
3. $\log A^p = p \log A$	The logarithm of an exponential quantity (a base raised to a power) is equal to the product of the exponent or power and the logarithm of the base.

EXAMPLE 7.3.1

Rewrite the following logarithms using the properties of logarithms: a. $\log \frac{15}{6}$ b. $\log (1.24)(4.8)$ c. $\log \frac{(5.2)(6.8)}{(2.7)}$ d. $\log [(1.2)(4.8)]^2$ e. $\log \frac{1.2}{(4.8)^2}$

Solution

Comments

a. $\log \frac{15}{6} = \log 15 - \log 6$

a. The log of a quotient is equal to the difference of the logarithms of the numerator and denominator (property 2).

b. $\log (1.24)(4.8)$
$= \log 1.24 + \log 4.8$

b. The log of a product is equal to the sum of the logarithms of the factors (property 1).

c. $\log \frac{(5.2)(6.8)}{(2.7)}$
$= \log 5.2 + \log 6.8 - \log 2.7$

c. Combine properties 1 and 2.

d. $\log [(1.2)(4.8)]^2$ $= 2 \log (1.2)(4.8)$ $= 2 (\log 1.2 + \log 4.8)$	**d.** Move exponent (property 3). Write log of product as sum of logs (property 1).
e. $\log \left(\frac{1.2}{4.8}\right)^2$	**e.** Use property 3 to move exponent.
$= 2 \log \frac{1.2}{4.8}$ $= 2(\log 1.2 - \log 4.8)$	Use property 2 to write the log of a quotient as a difference of the logs of the numerator and denominator.

It will simplify your work with logarithms to remember the following equations:

$$\log 10 = 1 \quad (\text{since } 10^1 = 10)$$
$$\log 1 = 0 \quad (\text{since } 10^0 = 1)$$

7.4 FINDING LOGARITHMS

Most numbers are not integral powers of 10. The question arises of how to write a number such as 286 as a power of 10? Let us examine following method.

EXAMPLE 7.4.1

Find the logarithm of 286 (i.e., $10^? = 286$).
(*Note:* A logarithm is composed of a whole number called the **characteristic** and a decimal part called the **mantissa.** If the number is the result of a measurement, the *mantissa* portion of the logarithm should contain the same number of significant digits as the measurement.)

Step 1. Write in scientific notation. $2.86 \cdot 10^2$

Step 2. Find the log of the product using the properties of the logarithm. $\log (2.86 \cdot 10^2) = \log 2.86 + \log 10^2$

Step 3. Take the log of 10^2. $= (\log 2.86) + 2$

$(\log 10^2 = 2)$

Step 4. In order to find the logarithm of number between 1 and 10, we must consult a logarithm table. There is one provided in Appendix C. We find the first two digits of the number in the left-hand column, and the third digit across the top row. The figure at the right illustrates that the logarithm is located where these two columns intersect.

	4	5	6	7	8	9
2.3	.3692	.3711	.3729	.3747	.3766	.3784
2.4	.3874	.3892	.3909	.3927	.3945	.3962
2.5	.4048	.4065	.4082	.4099	.4116	.4133
2.6	.4216	.4232	.4249	.4265	.4281	.4298
2.7	.4378	.4393	.4409	.4425	.4440	.4456
2.8	.4533	.4548	.4564	.4579	.4594	.4609
2.9	.4683	.4698	.4713	.4728	.4742	.4757
3.0	.4829	.4843	.4857	.4871	.4886	.4900

$\log 2.86 = 0.456$

Step 5. Add the logarithms together. $(\log 2.86) + 2 = 0.456 + 2 = 2.456$

Therefore, $\log 286 = 2.456$. This is the same as saying "the exponent of base 10 to obtain 286 must be 2.456," or $10^{2.456} = 286$.

EXAMPLE 7.4.2

Find the logarithm of 1590.

Solution	**Comments**
$1.59 \cdot 10^3$	Write number in scientific notation.

$\log (1.59 \cdot 10^3)$ $= \log 1.59 + \log 10^3$	Take the logarithm of this product, and rewrite it using property 1.
$= (\log 1.59) + 3$	Take the log of 10^3.
$= 0.201 + 3$	Using the log table, find 1.5 under the *N* column, and the 9 across the top row. The row and column intersect at 0.2014. Round off to three significant digits.
$= 3.201$ $\log 1590 = 3.201$, or $10^{3.201} = 1590$	Add the logarithms together.

EXAMPLE 7.4.3

Find the logarithm of 0.0799.

Solution	**Comments**
$7.99 \cdot 10^{-2}$	Write in scientific notation.
$\log 7.99 + \log 10^{-2}$	Rewrite $\log (7.99 \cdot 10^{-2})$ using property 1.
$(\log 7.99) + (-2)$	Take the logarithm of 10^{-2}.
$0.902 + (-2)$	Using the log table, find the log 7.99.
-1.098 $\log 0.0799 = -1.098$ or $10^{-1.098} = 0.0799$	Add the logarithms together.

7.5 FINDING LOGARITHMS USING A CALCULATOR

A faster method to find the logarithm of a number is to use a hand held calculator. In laboratory work, or on homework, it is likely that a calculator will be available. It is still important, however, that you understand the concept of the logarithm, and understand all of its properties before relying on the calculator.

One of the advantages of using a calculator is that the logarithm of any number with up to eight significant digits may be easily computed. When using the tables, only the logarithms of numbers with three or fewer significant digits may be found easily.

EXAMPLE 7.5.1

Find the logarithm of 82.24 using a calculator.

Solution	**Comments**
Enter 82.24	We do not have to write the number in scientific notation to find its logarithm when using a calculator.
[LOG]	Press the LOG key. The logarithm should appear in the display.
Answer = 1.9151	
$\log 82.24 = 1.9151$	

EXAMPLE 7.5.2

Find the logarithm of 0.000201.

Solution	**Comments**
Enter 0.000201	Enter the number.
[LOG]	Press the LOG key.
Answer = -3.697	
$\log 0.000201 = -3.697$	

EXAMPLE 7.5.3

Find the logarithm of $4.79 \cdot 10^{-3}$.

Solution	**Comments**
Enter 4.79	To enter a number in exponential notation, enter the significant digit portion of the number first and then enter the exponent.
[EXP] or [EE]	Some calculators have an EXP key and some have an EE key.
Enter 3	
[+/−]	To make the 3 negative, you must press the +/− key.
[LOG]	Press the LOG key.

Answer = −2.320

$\log (4.79 \cdot 10^{-3}) = -2.320$

PROBLEM SET 1

Using either the log tables in Appendix C or a calculator (as directed by your instructor), find the logarithms of the following numbers. Assume numbers are the result of a measurement.

1. 4.56
2. 9.42
3. 0.0736
4. 31.7
5. 0.00394
6. 0.0000111
7. 8950
8. 101,000
9. 979,000
10. 1.01
11. 0.9015
12. 2.557
13. 38.91
14. 573.2
15. 6791
16. 3,427,000
17. $4.821 \cdot 10^{-3}$
18. $7.822 \cdot 10^{4}$
19. $1.044 \cdot 10^{0}$
20. $2.77 \cdot 10^{2}$

Rewrite, using the properties of logarithms, each of the following. Do not evaluate answers.

21. $\log (2.3)^4$
22. $\log (5.2)(7.1)$
23. $\log \dfrac{(2.3)(4.2)}{1.5}$
24. $\log \left(\dfrac{7.5}{2.3}\right)^4$

Answers to odd-numbered problems appear on page 235.

7.6 FINDING INVERSE LOGARITHMS

The process of taking logarithms can be reversed by finding the **inverse logarithm**, or, as it is sometimes called, the **antilogarithm**. We use the term "inverse logarithm" (abbreviated inv log) throughout the remainder of the chapter.

The process can be shown symbolically:

$$\text{If} \quad \log 10^N = N, \quad \text{then} \quad \text{inv log } N = 10^N$$
$$\text{If} \quad \log 10^4 = 4, \quad \text{then} \quad \text{inv log } 4 = 10^4 = 10{,}000.$$

N will always be a rational number.

EXAMPLE 7.6.1

Find the inverse logarithm of **a.** 3 **b.** 0 **c.** −4

Solution	**Comments**
a. If $\log 10^N = 3$ then $\text{inv log } 3 = 10^3 = 1000$	**a.** Remember: 3 is the exponent on the base 10.
b. If $\log 10^N = 0$ then $\text{inv log } 0 = 10^0 = 1$	**b.** Zero is the exponent on the base 10.
c. If $\log 10^N = -4$ then $\text{inv log } -4 = 10^{-4} = 0.0001$	**c.** Negative 4 is the exponent on the base 10.

EXAMPLE 7.6.2

Find the inverse logarithm of 2.4048.

Solution	**Comments**
$2.4048 = 2 + 0.4048$	Write 2.4048 as the sum of the characteristic and the mantissa.
$\text{inv log } 2 + \text{inv log } 0.4048$	Find the inverse logarithm of both the characteristic and the mantissa.
$10^2 \cdot \text{inv log } 0.4048$	If $\log (ab) = \log a + \log b$, then: $\text{inv log } a + \text{inv log } b = a \cdot b$. The inverse logarithm of 2 is 10^2.
$10^2 \cdot 2.54$	To find the inverse logarithm of 0.4048, find this value in the table of mantissas, and locate the corresponding value of N in the table at the left, and the third digit from the corresponding number along the top row.

	0	1	2	3	4
2.1	.3222	.3243	.3263	.3284	.3304
2.2	.3424	.3444	.3464	.3483	.3502
2.3	.3617	.3636	.3655	.3674	.3692
2.4	.3802	.3820	.3838	.3856	.3874
2.5	.3979	.3997	.4014	.4031	.4048

In this case $N = 2.54$. Therefore the inverse logarithm of 2.4048 is 2.54×10^2 or 254.

$\text{inv log } 2.4048 = 2.54 \cdot 10^2 = 254$

That is, $10^{2.4048} = 254$.

EXAMPLE 7.63

Find the inverse logarithm of −3.8861.

The entire logarithm in this problem is negative. Since all of the mantissas in the table are positive, we must make this logarithm positive. This is done by adding the next largest positive integer greater than the absolute value of the characteristic of the logarithm, and then subtracting this positive value from the entire logarithm:

$$|-3| = 3;\ \text{the next larger positive integer is } 4$$
$$4 + (-3.8861) - 4 = 0.1139 - 4$$

By adding and subtracting 4, we are able to make the mantissa positive without changing the value of the logarithm.

Solution	**Comments**
$-3.8861 = 0.1139 - 4$	Rewrite the logarithm so that the mantissa is positive as described previously
$\text{inv log } 0.1139 + \text{inv log } (-4)$ $= (\text{inv log } 0.1139) \cdot 10^{-4}$	Take the inverse logarithm of each part.

N	0	1	2	3	4
1.0	.0000	.0043	.0086	.0128	.0170
1.1	.0414	.0453	.0492	.0531	.0569
1.2	.0792	.0828	.0864	.0899	.0934
1.3	.1139	.1173	.1206	.1239	.1271
1.4	.1461	.1492	.1523	.1553	.1584
1.5	.1761	.1790	.1818	.1847	.1875

The inverse logarithm of 0.1139 is shown in the table on the left. The inverse logarithm of 0.1139 = 1.30.

$= 1.30 \cdot 10^{-4}$
$= 0.000130.$

That is, $10^{-3.8861} = 0.000130$.

EXAMPLE 7.6.4

Find the inverse logarithm of -1.0888.

Solution

$-1.0888 = 2 + (-1.0888) - 2$
$= 0.9112 - 2$

Comments

Write the logarithm as a positive logarithm. Since $|-1| = 1$, and the next larger positive integer is 2, add 2 and then subtract 2 from the logarithm.

inv log 0.9112 + inv log (-2)

Take the inverse logarithm of both the characteristic and mantissa.

$= \text{inv log } 0.9112 \cdot 10^{-2}$

The inverse logarithm of -2 is 10^{-2}.

$= 8.15 \cdot 10^{-2}$
inv log $(-1.0888) = 8.15 \cdot 10^{-2}$
$= 0.0815$

The inverse logarithm of 0.9112 is $8.15 \cdot 10^{-2}$.
That is, $10^{-1.0888} = 0.0815$.

7.7 FINDING INVERSE LOGARITHMS USING A CALCULATOR

The calculator may also be used to find inverse logarithms, and it has several advantages over the traditional log table:

1. The calculator is quicker.
2. The mantissa you need may lie somewhere between two adjacent mantissas. To find the inverse logs of these mantissas with the tables involves the use of interpolation, which we will not study because the calculator does this for us more quickly.

Most calculators have an inverse operation button marked INV. To find an inverse logarithm with this kind of calculator, press the inverse key and then the log key, as outlined below.

ENTER NUMBER → [INV] → [LOG] → ANSWER

Some calculators use a second function key, marked 2nd. This key forces the calculator to use certain keys in a mode that is usually marked in the same color as the 2nd key. To find the inverse logarithm with these calculators, do the following:

ENTER NUMBER → [2nd] → [10^x] → ANSWER

For the sake of simplicity, our examples will make use of the keystrokes used in the first type of calculator.

EXAMPLE 7.7.1

Find the inverse logarithm of 4.3711.

Solution

Enter 4.3711

[INV]

Comments

Enter the number.

Press the INV key.

LOG	Press the LOG key.
Answer = 23501.739 ≈ 23,500	Round off your answer.

EXAMPLE 7.7.2

Find the inverse logarithm of −3.2796.

Solution	**Comments**
Enter 3.2976	The calculator does not care whether the number is positive or negative. Enter as is.
+/−	Change the sign by pressing the +/− key.
INV	Press the INV key.
LOG	Press the LOG key.
Answer = 0.0005253 = $5.253 \cdot 10^{-4}$	

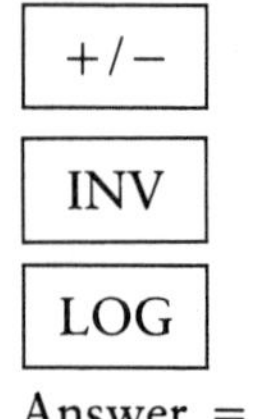

PROBLEM SET 2

Use the tables or a calculator to find the inverse logarithm of the following numbers. Assume that each number is a logarithm; each answer may have three digits if using a table.

1. 1.7059
2. 2.3345
3. 3.5105
4. 3.0000
5. −4.0000
6. 4.7980
7. −1.0278
8. −3.1397
9. −2.2700
10. −5.5591
11. 0.7397
12. −1.3505
13. 6.7777
14. −3.5366
15. 2.1987
16. −0.5505
17. 1.3284
18. 5.0021
19. −2.0048
20. −3.9739

Answers to odd-numbered problems appear on page 235.

7.8 CALCULATIONS WITH LOGARITHMS

Calculations may be carried out with logarithms; indeed, before the advent of the hand-held calculator, the use of logarithms often simplified many otherwise laborious computations. Now, however, the logarithm is used mainly in certain formulas, some of which we study in the following section. In this section we examine the techniques used to perform simple calculations involving multiplication and division.

Recall the three properties of logarithms studied previously:

1. $\log (AB) = \log A + \log B$
2. $\log \left(\frac{A}{B}\right) = \log A - \log B$
3. $\log A^p = p \log A$

We will use these three properties to perform our calculations.

EXAMPLE 7.8.1

Multiply (4.17)(2.08) using logarithms.

Solution	Comments
$\log[(4.17)(2.08)]$ $= \log(4.17) + \log(2.08)$	$\log(AB) = \log A + \log B$
$= 1.620 + 0.318$ $= 1.938$	Using a calculator, find the logarithm of each number: log 4.17 = 1.6201; and log 2.08 = 0.3181. Add the logarithms.
$\text{inv log } 1.9382 = 86.7$	To find the solution, take the inverse logarithm of 1.9382 to get 86.7, rounded to three significant digits.

EXAMPLE 7.8.2

Divide $\frac{0.4704}{10.77}$ using logarithms.

Solution	Comments
$\log \frac{0.4704}{10.77} = \log 0.4704 - \log 10.77$	$\log \frac{A}{B} = \log A - \log B$
$= -0.3275 - (1.0322)$	Find the logarithm of each number: log 0.4704 = −0.3275; and log 10.77 = 1.0322. Subtract the logarithms.
$= -1.3597$ $\text{inv log}(-1.3597) = 0.04386$	Find the inverse logarithm of −1.3597 to obtain the solution.

EXAMPLE 7.8.3

Simplify $\frac{(0.384)(6.72 \cdot 10^{-4})}{9.77}$ using logarithms.

Solution	Comments
$\log \frac{(0.384)(6.72 \cdot 10^{-4})}{9.77}$	$\log \frac{AB}{C} = (\log A + \log B) - \log C$
$= \log 0.384 + \log(6.72 \cdot 10^{-4}) - \log 9.77$	Find the logarithm of each number: log 0.384 = −0.416; log $(6.72 \cdot 10^{-4})$ = −3.173; and log 9.77 = 0.990.
$= -0.416 + (-3.173) - (0.990)$ $= -4.579$	Add the first two logs together, and then subtract the third.
$\text{inv log}(-4.579) = 0.0000264$	Find the inverse logarithm of −4.579.
$= 2.64 \cdot 10^{-5}$	Write the answer in scientific notation.

The next example shows how you can find the roots of any rational number using logarithms.

EXAMPLE 7.8.4

Find $\sqrt[3]{33.2}$ using logarithms.

Solution	Comments
Let $n = \sqrt[3]{33.2}$	
$n = (33.2)^{1/3}$	Property of rational exponents. (See Chap. 2.)

$$\log n = \log (33.2)^{1/3}$$
$$\log n = \frac{1}{3} (\log 33.2)$$

Take the logarithm of $(33.2)^{1/3}$ and apply property 3.

$$\log n = \frac{1}{3} (1.52)$$

$\log 33.2 = 1.52$

$$\log n = 0.507$$
$$n = 3.21$$

To find n, take the inverse logarithm of 0.507. This will equal $\sqrt[3]{33.2}$. Round off your answer to three significant digits.

PROBLEM SET 3

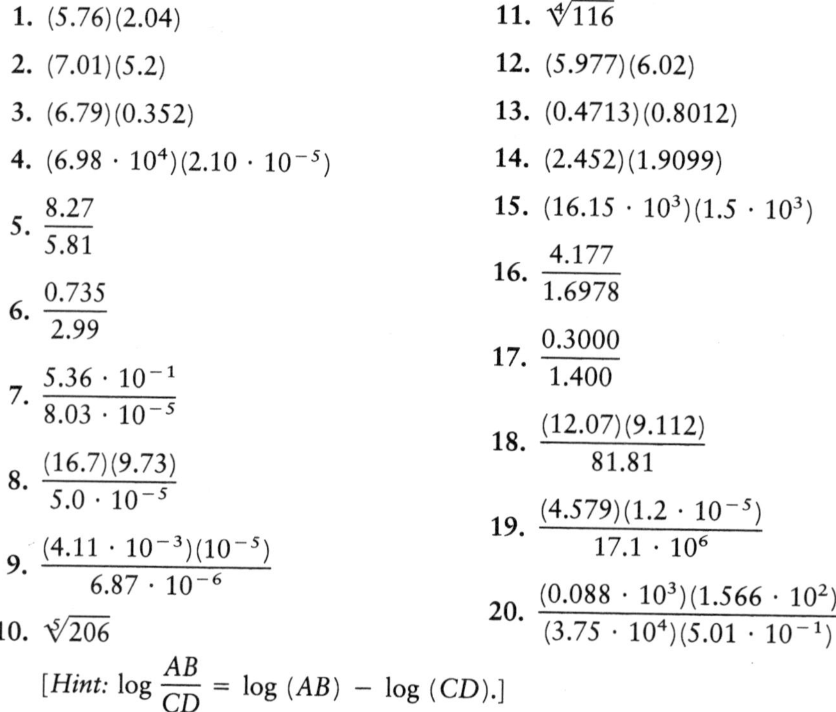

Compute the following using either a calculator or a table of logarithms. Assume that each number is the result of a measurement.

1. $(5.76)(2.04)$
2. $(7.01)(5.2)$
3. $(6.79)(0.352)$
4. $(6.98 \cdot 10^{4})(2.10 \cdot 10^{-5})$
5. $\dfrac{8.27}{5.81}$
6. $\dfrac{0.735}{2.99}$
7. $\dfrac{5.36 \cdot 10^{-1}}{8.03 \cdot 10^{-5}}$
8. $\dfrac{(16.7)(9.73)}{5.0 \cdot 10^{-5}}$
9. $\dfrac{(4.11 \cdot 10^{-3})(10^{-5})}{6.87 \cdot 10^{-6}}$
10. $\sqrt[5]{206}$
11. $\sqrt[4]{116}$
12. $(5.977)(6.02)$
13. $(0.4713)(0.8012)$
14. $(2.452)(1.9099)$
15. $(16.15 \cdot 10^{3})(1.5 \cdot 10^{3})$
16. $\dfrac{4.177}{1.6978}$
17. $\dfrac{0.3000}{1.400}$
18. $\dfrac{(12.07)(9.112)}{81.81}$
19. $\dfrac{(4.579)(1.2 \cdot 10^{-5})}{17.1 \cdot 10^{6}}$
20. $\dfrac{(0.088 \cdot 10^{3})(1.566 \cdot 10^{2})}{(3.75 \cdot 10^{4})(5.01 \cdot 10^{-1})}$

[*Hint:* $\log \dfrac{AB}{CD} = \log (AB) - \log (CD)$.]

Answers to odd-numbered problems appear on page 235.

7.9 APPLICATIONS OF LOGARITHMS

pH

Most of the solutions encountered in the laboratory are dissolved in water. The water molecules ionize (breaks apart) according to the following equation:

$$H_2O \rightarrow H^+ + OH^-$$

When pure water ionizes, it does so very weakly. Indeed, for every 1 mole of water (at 25°C) present in a sample, only $1 \cdot 10^{-7}$ mol of H^+ ions and OH^- ions are present. This is a very small quantity of these ions—one ten millionth of a mole each.

If we multiply the concentrations of these two ions together, we obtain a constant, called the **ion-product constant of water** (K_w).

$$K_w = [H^+][OH^-]$$
$$K_w = (1 \cdot 10^{-7})(1 \cdot 10^{-7})$$
$$K_w = 1 \cdot 10^{-14} \text{ mol}^2/\text{L}^2$$

An acid, by the classical definition, is any substance that releases hydrogen ions in solution, and a base is any substance that releases hydroxide ions in solution. If we know the concentration of one of these ions in a water solution, we can calculate the concentration of the other. Any change in the concentration of hydrogen ions in a water solution will cause a corresponding change in the concentration of hydroxide ions, since the product of the two must be equal to $1 \cdot 10^{-14}$.

EXAMPLE 7.9.1

If $[H^+] = 1 \cdot 10^{-3}$ mol/L, find $[OH^-]$.

Solution	**Comments**
$1 \cdot 10^{-14} = [H^+][OH^-]$	Write down the ion-product equation.
$= \dfrac{1 \cdot 10^{-14}}{[H^+]} = [OH^-]$	Solve for $[OH^-]$.
$= \dfrac{1 \cdot 10^{-14}}{1 \cdot 10^{-3}} = [OH^-]$	Substitute in value of $[H^+]$.
$= 1 \cdot 10^{-11}$	Divide.
$[OH^-] = 1 \cdot 10^{-11}$ mol/L	

To simplify matters, the hydrogen ion concentration of a water solution may be expressed as pH, which is defined as the negative of the logarithm of the hydrogen ion concentration in moles per liter.

$$pH = -\log[H^+]$$

If we know the H^+ concentration, we can find the pH of the solution. The pH scale ranges from 0 for very acid solutions, to 14 for very basic (or alkaline) solutions:

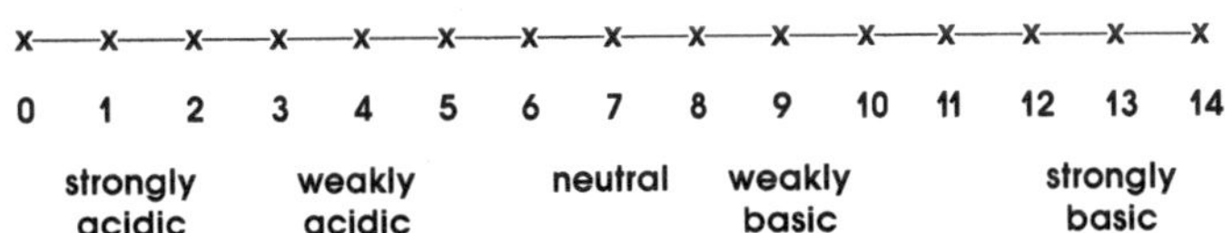

The pH values of some common solutions are given in the table below:

Substance	pH
1-*M* HCl	0
Gastric juice	1–3
Soft drinks	2.0–4.0
Lemons	2.2–2.4
Urine	4.5–8.0
Pure water	7
Saliva	6.5–7.5
Blood	7.35–7.45
Soap	8–10
Milk of Magnesia	9.9–10.1
1-*M* NaOH	14

EXAMPLE 7.9.2

Find the pH of a solution with a hydrogen concentration of $[H^+] = 2.30 \cdot 10^{-5}$.

Solution	**Comments**
$pH = -\log [H^+]$	Write down the pH formula.
$pH = -\log (2.30 \cdot 10^{-5})$	Substitute value for $[H^+]$.
$pH = -(\log 2.30 + \log 10^{-5})$	Leave the minus sign outside of the parenthesis for the time being.

$pH = -[0.362 + (-5)]$	Find the logarithm of each number: log 2.30 = 0.362; and log $10^{-5} = -5$.
$pH = -(-4.638)$	Add the logarithms together and simplify by multiplying this sum by -1.
$pH = 4.638$	

EXAMPLE 7.9.3

Find the pH of a solution with a hydroxide concentration of $[OH^-] = 7.83 \cdot 10^{-11}$.

Solution	**Comments**
$K_w = [H^+][OH^-]$ $1 \cdot 10^{-14} = [H^+](7.83 \cdot 10^{-11})$	Find $[H^+]$ by substituting the given value of $[OH^-]$ into the ion-product formula.
$\dfrac{1 \cdot 10^{-14}}{7.83 \cdot 10^{-11}} = [H^+]$	Solve for $[H^+]$.
$0.128 \cdot 10^{-14-(-11)} = [H^+]$ $0.128 \cdot 10^{-3} = [H^+]$ $1.28 \cdot 10^{-4} = [H^+]$	Write answer in scientific notation.
$pH = -\log(1.28 \cdot 10^{-4})$	Substitute the value for $[H^+]$ into the pH formula.
$pH = -(\log 1.28 + \log 10^{-4})$ $pH = -[0.107 + (-4)]$	Take the logarithm of each number: log 1.28 = 0.107; and log $10^{-4} = -4$.
$pH = -(-3.893)$	Add the logarithms together.
$pH = 3.893$	Simplify.

If $pH = -\log[H^+]$, then $pOH = -\log[OH^-]$. As we learned while studying the ion-product formula, the product of the concentration of hydrogen and hydroxide ions in water must be equal to $1 \cdot 10^{-14}$:

$$1 \cdot 10^{-14} = [H^+][OH^-]$$

Take the negative logarithm of both sides:

$$\begin{aligned} -\log(1 \cdot 10^{-14}) &= -\log([H^+][OH^-]) \\ -\log 1 + (-\log 10^{-14}) &= -\log[H^+] + (-\log[OH^-]) \\ 0 + 14 &= pH + pOH \\ 14 &= pH + pOH \end{aligned}$$

We can use this formula to determine the pH when the pOH is known, and vice versa.

EXAMPLE 7.9.4

The pOH of a solution of magnesium hydroxide was found to be 4.60. Find the pH of the solution.

Solution	**Comments**
$pH + pOH = 14$	Write down the formula relating pH to pOH.
$pH + 4.60 = 14$	Substitute in the value given.
$pH = 14 - 4.60$ $pH = 9.40$	Solve for pH.

Finding $[H^+]$ When Given pH

There will be circumstances when we know the pH of a solution and need to know the corresponding $[H^+]$. Inverse logarithms are used in these cases to find the concentration of hydrogen ions.

EXAMPLE 7.9.5

The pH of a blood sample was found to be 7.43. Find the corresponding $[H^+]$.

Solution	Comments
$pH = -\log [H^+]$	Write down the pH formula.
$7.43 = -\log [H^+]$	Substitute in the pH value.
$-1(7.43) = \log [H^+]$ $-7.43 = \log [H^+]$	Multiply both sides of the equation by -1.
$\text{inv log } (-7.43) = [H^+]$ $\text{inv log } [8 + (-7.43) - 8] = [H^+]$ $\text{inv log } (0.57 - 8) = [H^+]$ $\text{inv log } 0.57 \cdot \text{inv log } (-8) = [H^+]$ $3.7 \cdot 10^{-8} = [H^+]$	Take the inverse logarithm of the pH. You may either use a calculator or the log tables at this point.

EXAMPLE 7.9.6

The pOH of a soft drink was found to be 10.7. Find the $[H^+]$ of the solution.

Solution	Comments
$pH + pOH = 14$ $pH + 10.7 = 14$ $pH = 14 - 10.7$ $pH = 3.3$	Find the pH of the solution using the equation relating pH to pOH.
$pH = -\log [H^+]$ $-pH = \log [H^+]$	Using the pH formula, solve for $[H^+]$.
$-3.3 = \log [H^+]$	Substitute the value of the pH.
$[4 + (-3.3) - 4] = \log [H^+]$ $(0.7 - 4) = \log [H^+]$ $\text{inv log } (0.7 - 4) = [H^-]$	Make the pH positive if using the log tables. Otherwise, enter directly into a calculator.
$\text{inv log } 0.7 + \text{inv log } (-4) = [H^+]$ $5 \cdot 10^{-4} = [H^+]$	Take the inverse logarithm.

The Henderson–Hasselbach Equation

Solutions may be prepared so that they resist any change in pH when a small amount of acid or a base is added. These solutions are called **buffer** solutions. They are usually prepared by adding a weak acid to water along with a salt containing the **conjugate base** of the acid. A conjugate base is the negative portion of the acid molecule after the hydrogen ion dissociates.

H_2CO_3	$\rightarrow$	H^+	+	HCO_3^-
weak acid (carbonic acid)		hydrogen ion		conjugate base

The salt that would be added in the carbonic acid–bicarbonate ion buffer system would be sodium bicarbonate ($NaHCO_3$). This is the buffer system found in the blood to maintain a very narrow pH range.

An equation that deals with buffer calculations is called the **Henderson–Hasselbach equation.** This equation relates the relative concentrations of the weak acid and the conjugate base to the pH of the buffer solution needed. It is not our purpose here to go deeply into the chemistry of the equation, but to study the mathematics involved. Below is the mathematical statement of the equation:

$$pH = pK_a + \log \frac{[\text{conjugate base}]}{[\text{weak acid}]}$$

where $pK_a = -\log K_a$ and K_a is the ionization constant of the given acid.

EXAMPLE 7.9.7

What would be the pH of a buffer solution that, after mixing, has a sodium bicarbonate (the conjugate base) concentration of 0.10 M and a carbonic acid concentration of 0.14 M. Assume the K_a for carbonic acid to be $4.16 \cdot 10^{-7}$.

Solution	Comments
$K_a = 4.16 \cdot 10^{-7}$ $pK_a = -\log(4.16 \cdot 10^{-7})$ $pK_a = (-\log 4.16 + \log 10^{-7})$ $pK_a = -[0.619 + (-7)]$ $pK_a = -(-6.381)$ $pK_a = 6.381$	Before substituting into the equation, change K_a to pK_a. ($pK_a = -\log K_a$.)
$\text{pH} = 6.381 + \log \frac{0.10}{0.14}$	Substitute pK_a, [conjugate base], and [acid] into the Henderson–Hasselbach equation. Divide out the fraction.
$\text{pH} = 6.381 + \log 0.71$ $\text{pH} = 6.381 + (-0.15)$	Find the logarithm of 0.71.
$\text{pH} = 6.23$	The pH of the buffer solution would be 6.23, very close to the pK_a of the acid.

EXAMPLE 7.9.8

The pH of a buffer solution containing sodium formate (the conjugate base) and formic acid was found to be 4.22. If the concentration of the conjugate base is 0.300 mol/L, and if the K_a of formic acid is $1.8 \cdot 10^{-4}$, find the concentration in moles per liter of formic acid in the buffer.

Solution	Comments
$\text{pH} = pK_a + \log \frac{[\text{conjugate base}]}{[\text{acid}]}$	Write down the Henderson–Hasselbach equation.
$pK_a = -\log(1.8 \cdot 10^{-4})$ $pK_a = -(\log 1.8 + \log 10^{-4})$ $pK_a = -[0.26 + (-4)]$ $pK_a = -(-3.74)$ $pK_a = 3.74$	Find the pK_a of the acid.
$4.22 = 3.74 + \log \frac{(0.300)}{x}$	Substitute all given values into the equation. Let x = [acid].
$4.22 = 3.74 + (\log 0.300 - \log x)$ $4.22 = 3.74 + \log 0.300 - \log x$	Recall: $\log \frac{A}{B} = \log A - \log B$.
$4.22 - 3.74 - \log 0.300 = -\log x$	Solve for $\log x$.
$4.22 - 3.74 - (-0.523) = -\log x$	Take the logarithm of 0.300.
$1.00 = -\log x$	Multiply both sides by -1.
$-1.00 = \log x$ $\text{inv} \log(-1.00) = x$ $0.10 \text{ mol/L} = x = [\text{formic acid}]$	Take the inverse logarithm.

Absorbence Versus Transmittance of Light

An instrument very much in evidence in the medical laboratory is the **spectrophotometer**, often called the **colorimeter.** This instrument is designed to measure the amount of light that passes through a clear glass sample holder. The higher the concentration of a solution, the more light it will absorb. The light passing through the sample holder is detected by a photocell, which sends an electrical current to a meter. There are usually two scales on the meter—an **absorbance** scale, and a **transmittance** scale. Transmittance is defined as follows:

$$T = \frac{I_f}{I_0}$$

where I_f is equal to the intensity of the light leaving the sample holder, and I_0 is equal to the intensity of the light before entering the sample holder. Absorbence is inversely related to transmittance by the equation:

$$A = \log \frac{1}{T}.$$

If all of the light is absorbed, then the transmittance would be equal to zero, and if no light is absorbed, then the transmittance would be equal to one. Most instruments are calibrated in percent T rather than T. To obtain percent T, we would multiply the transmittance by 100.

The relationship between absorbance and transmittance is illustrated by the following examples.

EXAMPLE 7.9.9

If the transmittance of a sample of cholesterol solution is 0.321, find the corresponding absorbance of the sample.

Solution	Comments
$A = \log \frac{1}{T}$	Start with the basic equation.
$A = \log \frac{1}{(0.321)}$	Substitute into the equation $A = 0.321$. Divide out the fraction.
$A = \log 3.1$ $A = 0.49$	Take the logarithm of 3.1.

EXAMPLE 7.9.10

A spectrophotometer is used to find the absorbence of a bacterial growth in a test tube containing the bacteria in a broth medium. The absorbance of the broth was found to be 0.78. What is the corresponding percent T?

Solution	Comments
$A = \log \frac{1}{T}$	Start with the basic equation.
$A = \log 1 - \log T$	Solve for T. Use $\log \frac{A}{B} = \log A - \log B$.
$A = 0 - \log T$	Log $1 = 0$.
$A = -\log T$ $-A = \log T$	Multiply both sides by -1.
$-0.78 = \log T$	Substitute in the given value of A.
$\text{inv} \log (-0.78) = T$	Take the inverse logarithm.
$0.17 = T$ $17 = \%T$	Change to percent T by multiplying by 100.

PROBLEM SET 4

1. Find the pH of each solution indicated.
   a. Lime juice: $[H^+] = 1 \cdot 10^{-2}$ mol/L
   b. Beer: $[H^+] = 5.25 \cdot 10^{-5}$ mol/L
   c. Tomato juice: $[H^+] = 7.94 \cdot 10^{-5}$ mol/L
   d. Household ammonia: $[H^+] = 7.94 \cdot 10^{-13}$ mol/L
   e. Milk: $[H^+] = 2.60 \cdot 10^{-7}$ mol/L
2. Find the $[H^+]$ of each solution indicated.

a. Urine: pH = 6.77

b. Gastric acid: pH = 2.54

c. Wine: pH = 3.21

d. Blood: pH = 7.321

e. Lye: pH = 13.22

3. If the pH of black coffee is 4.99, what is the $[OH^-]$ in the coffee?
4. The pOH of a borax solution is 9.0. Find the pH of the solution, and the $[H^+]$.
5. The $[OH^-]$ of a soft drink is found to be $4.00 \cdot 10^{-12}$ mol/L. Find the pH of the soft drink.
6. Calculate the pH of a buffer solution made by dissolving 1.00 L of a 0.600-M sodium bicarbonate solution in 1.00 L of a 0.200-M solution of carbonic acid. K_a carbonic acid $= 4.30 \cdot 10^{-7}$.
7. What is the pH of a 0.667 M acetic acid solution that contains 0.133 mol of sodium acetate per liter? K_a acetic acid $= 1.75 \cdot 10^{-5}$.
8. The pH of a buffer solution made by dissolving 2.00 mol of sodium acetate in 1 L of carbonic acid was found to be 6.48. Find the concentration in moles per liter of the carbonic acid. (See Problem 6.)
9. A sample of $NiNO_3$ was placed in a spectrophotometer, and the percent T was found to be 38.2%. Find the corresponding absorbence of the solution.
10. A sample cell containing serum cholesterol mixed with the necessary reagents was placed in a spectrophotometer, and the resulting absorbence was found to be 0.472. What is the corresponding percent T of the sample?
11. The meters on most spectrophotometers has an absorbence scale that ranges from 0 to 4. Calculate the percent T that corresponds to these numbers.

Answers to odd-numbered problems appear on page 235.

CHAPTER REVIEW

(7.2, 7.4, 7.5)

1. Find the logarithms of the following numbers (assume they are the result of measurements):

   a. 28.2

   b. 142.7

   c. 0.00781

   d. 1,280

2. Find the inverse logarithm of the following numbers:

   a. 2.6972

   b. 3.4087

   c. −1.9614

   d. −3.8138

(7.8)

3. Compute the following using logarithms:

   a. (6.83)(1.97)

   b. $\dfrac{(15.4)}{(9.03)}$

   c. (1.593)(7.008)

   d. $\dfrac{(4.082)(1.97)}{(31.14)}$

(7.9)

4. Find the pH of the following:
   a. $[H^+] = 5.12 \cdot 10^{-6}$ mol/L
   b. $[OH^-] = 3.27 \cdot 10^{-12}$ mol/L
5. Find the $[H^+]$ of solutions that have:
   a. pH = 8.41
   b. pOH = 11.7
6. What is the pH of a 0.300 *M* formic acid (HCO_2H) solution that contains 0.24 mol of sodium formate ($NaCO_2H$) per liter? K_a formic acid = $1.78 \cdot 10^{-4}$.
7. A sample cell containing bacteria growing in a nutrient broth was placed in a spectrophotometer and found to have an absorbence of 1.8. What percent *T* corresponds to this absorbence?

Answers to odd-numbered problems appear on page 235.

chapter 8

Geometry

OBJECTIVES

After studying this chapter, the student should be able to:

1. Identify lines, line segments, rays, and angles.
2. Identify lines of intersection, parallel lines, parallel planes, and perpendicular lines.
3. Identify acute, obtuse, and right angles.
4. Use a protractor to draw and measure angles.
5. Identify complementary and supplementary angles.
6. Identify triangle types based upon side and angle measure.
7. Determine the unknown side of a right triangle given the other two sides.
8. Determine the perimeter and area of any triangle.
9. Determine the perimeter and area of any parallelogram.
10. Determine the circumference and area of a circle given its radius or diameter.
11. Determine the area of a figure made up of various plane figures given appropriate measurements.
12. Determine the surface area of cubes, prisms, spheres, and right circular cylinders given appropriate measurements.
13. Determine the volumes of prisms, pyramids, spheres, right circular cylinders, and right circular cones given the appropriate measurements.
14. Solve any area and volume formula for any unknown part given the other parts.
15. Solve problems that apply the concept of perimeter, area, and volume of those plane and solid figures discussed.

8.1 INTRODUCTION

A basic understanding of various geometric shapes is necessary in certain health fields. In this chapter we study some of the most common geometric figures and examine applications of their perimeters, areas, and volumes.

8.2 LINES AND ANGLES

The shortest distance between two points is along a line. It extends in both directions. A line is usually represented with arrows at both ends. The line displayed below is named line *AB* ($\overleftrightarrow{AB}$). Only two points are necessary to determine a unique line.

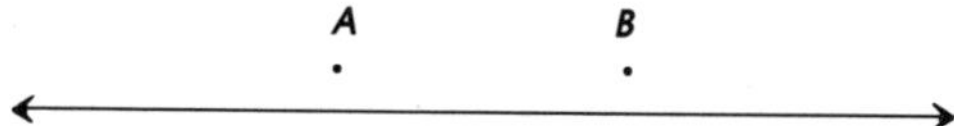

If the line does not have the arrows at either end, it is called a **line segment.** If the line segment connects two points that are identified by letters, then we name the line segment by using the two letters. For example, the line segment below

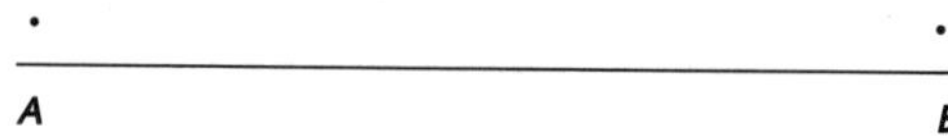

is labeled $\overline{AB}$ (line segment AB). A line segment is that portion of the line containing only its endpoints and all points in between.

In this example,

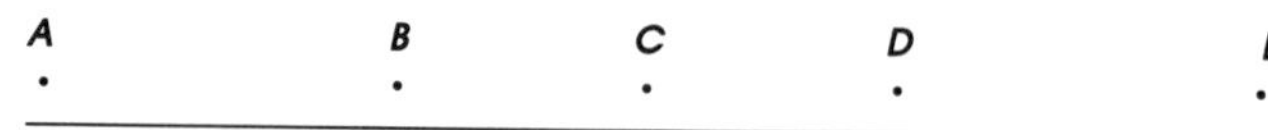

there are six line segments: $\overline{AB}$, $\overline{AC}$, $\overline{AD}$, $\overline{BC}$, $\overline{BD}$, $\overline{CD}$.

EXAMPLE 8.2.1

How many different line segments are there in the following figure?

A B C D E

Solution

There are ten different line segments:

$\overline{AB}$, $\overline{AC}$, $\overline{AD}$, $\overline{AE}$,
$\overline{BC}$, $\overline{BD}$, $\overline{BE}$,
$\overline{CD}$, $\overline{CE}$,
$\overline{DE}$,

Notice that line segment $\overline{ED}$ is the same segment as $\overline{DE}$, $\overline{EC}$ is the same as $\overline{CE}$, and so on.

If a line extends from a point (A) to infinity only in one direction, it is called a **ray**:

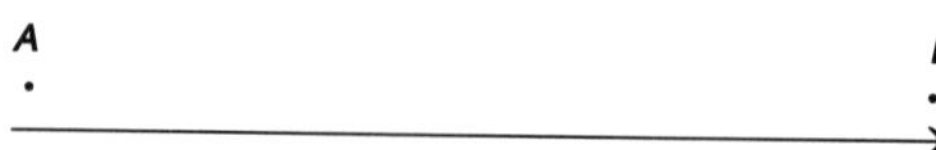

The ray shown above is named $\overrightarrow{AB}$. If we begin at point B and continue to the left through point A, we obtain the ray $\overrightarrow{BA}$:

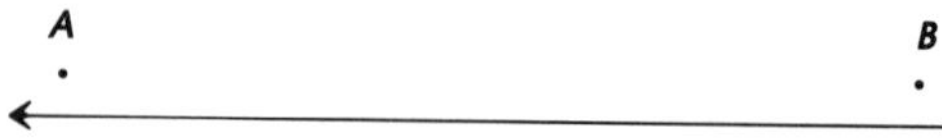

Notice that ray $\overrightarrow{BA}$ contains some but not all the same points that are contained in $\overrightarrow{AB}$. Notice too that the symbol for a ray is an arrow (→).

If two lines have one point in common, we say the lines **intersect.** Lines may intersect in varying ways, as we shall see later. Two lines that never intersect and lie in the same **plane** are called **parallel lines.** A **plane** can be thought of as a flat surface, such as a desk top or a blackboard surface, which has infinite length and width. While a line is determined by two distinct points, a plane is determined by three distinct points that are not all on the same line. Three such points determine a unique plane, just as two points determine a unique line. Two planes that never intersect are called **parallel planes.**

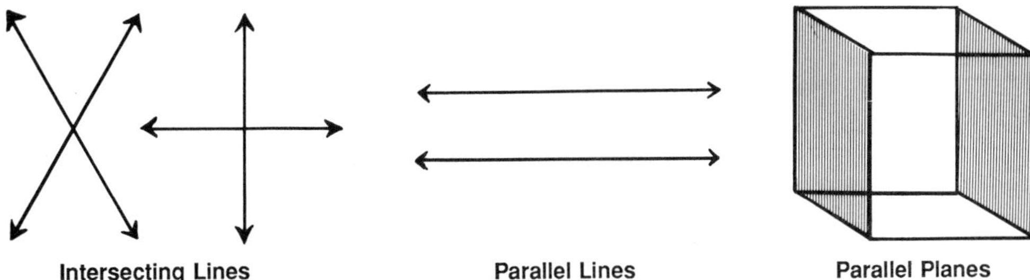

When two rays have a common end point, they form an **angle**. The rays that form the angle are called the **sides** of the angle. The point that the two rays have in common is called the **vertex**.

The angles are named by the points that form the two rays. For example, the angle in the figure below is named "angle CAB," which is written $\angle CAB$.

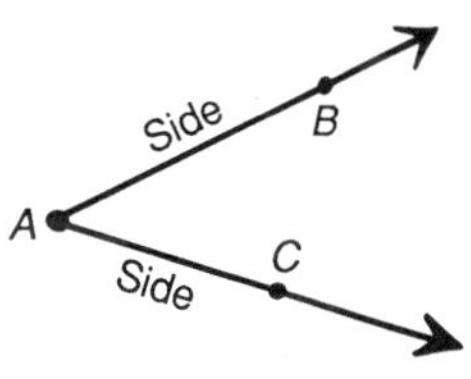

EXAMPLE 8.2.2 How many different angles can be located in the following figure? Name them.

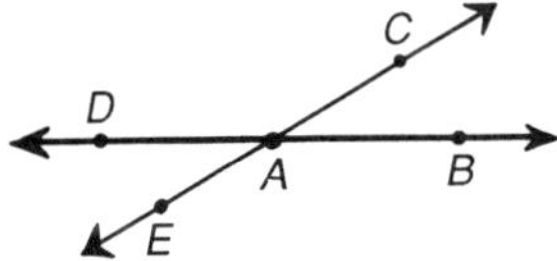

Solution

$\angle DAC$, $\angle DAB$ (straight line), $\angle DAE$, $\angle DAD$

$\angle CAB$, $\angle CAE$ (straight line), $\angle CAC$

$\angle BAE$, $\angle BAB$

$\angle EAE$

There are ten different angles in the figure.

Two rays can be thought of as the two hands of a clock. If the two rays lie on top of each other or coincide at 3, we say they have undergone no rotation, and have an angle measurement of 0° (zero degrees). Other instances of this are $\angle DAD$, $\angle CAC$, $\angle BAB$, and $\angle EAE$ in example 8.2.2 above.

If one hand moves one-fourth of the way around the clock face, then it is at **right angles** to the other hand. This corresponds to a 90° revolution.

If the same hand continues moving until it reaches half of the distance around, then it creates a straight line with the hand that has not moved, and forms a 180° angle.

When the hand moves three-quarters of the way around, it forms an angle of 270°. By the time the hand has moved all the way around, it coincides again with the hand that has not moved. We say that the hand has made a 360° revolution. You may note that a 360° revolution corresponds exactly with the 0° revolution.

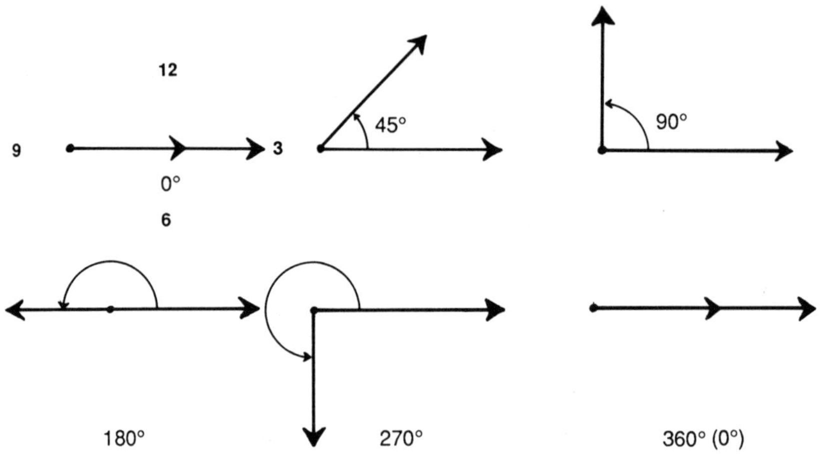

If an angle is less than 90°, it is called an **acute angle.** If the angle is 90°, it is called a **right angle**. An angle that is greater than 90° (and less than 180°) is called an **obtuse angle**. Examples of each appear below.

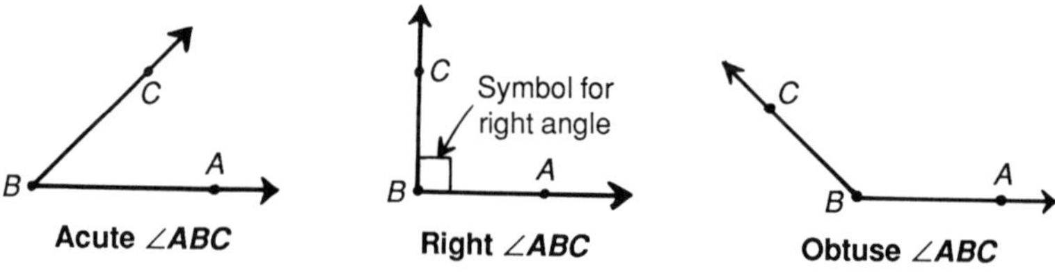

EXAMPLE 8.2.3

Label each angle below as an obtuse, acute, or right angle.

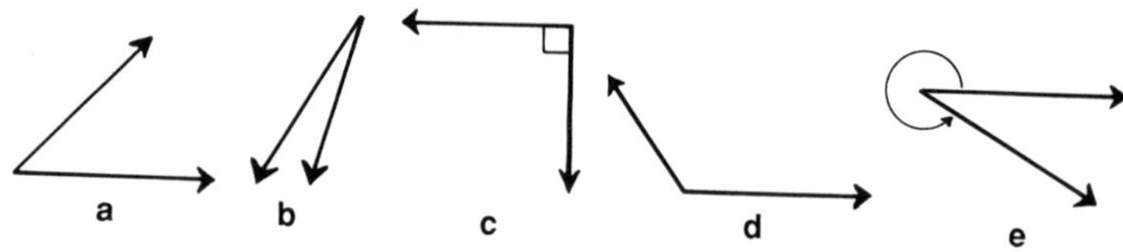

Solution

Comments

a.

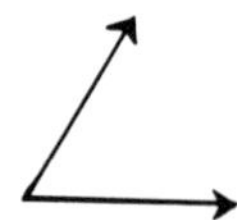

a. This is an acute angle (less than 90°).

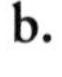

b.

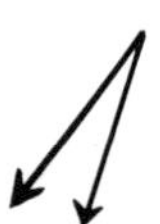

b. This is an acute angle.

c.

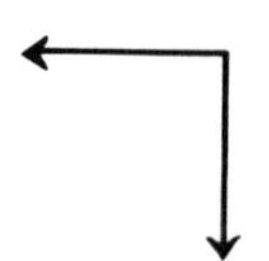

c. This is a right angle (notice right angle symbol).

d.

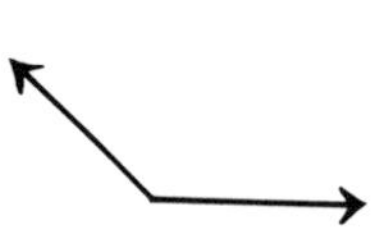

d. This is an obtuse angle (greater than 90° but less than 180°).

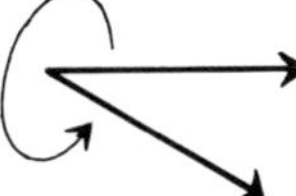

e. The angle indicated by the rotation arrow is more than 270° (three-fourths of a rotation). This angle can be more readily identified by the inside angle measure (denoted by the two lines). This inside angle is acute.

Recall that when two lines cross at one point, we say the lines intersect. If the two lines intersect and form a 90° angle, then the lines are **perpendicular**:

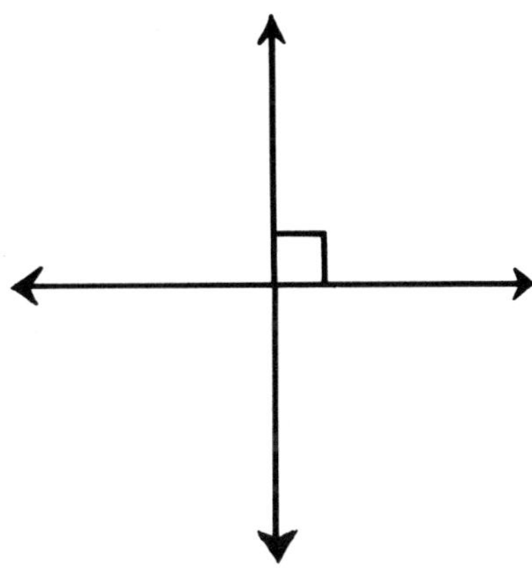

Two angles whose measures add up to 90° are **complementary angles**:

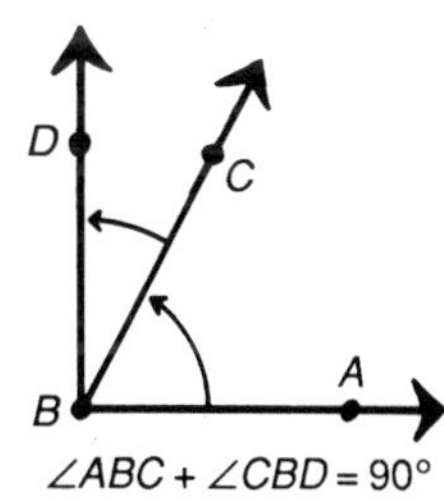

$\angle ABC + \angle CBD = 90°$

Two angles whose measures add up to 180° are **supplementary angles**:

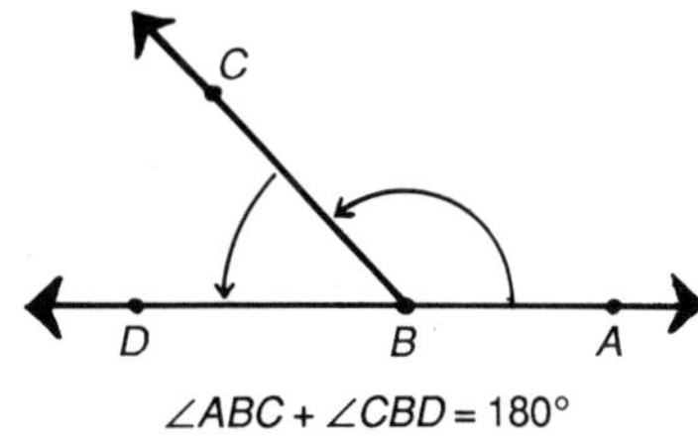

$\angle ABC + \angle CBD = 180°$

EXAMPLE 8.2.4 Name the complementary angles and supplementary angles in the following figures.

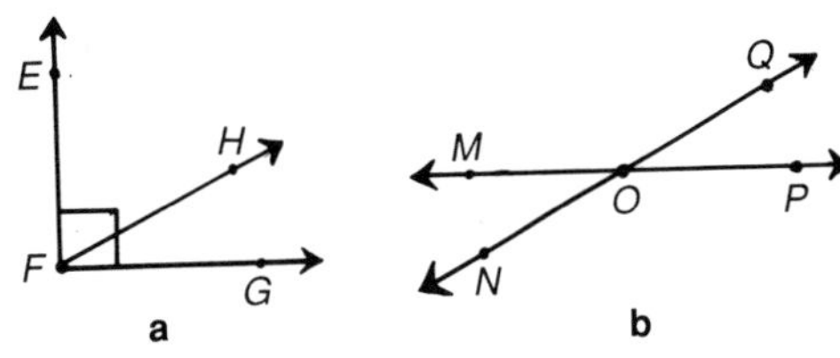

Solution

a.

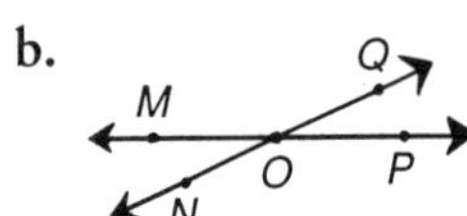

Comments

a. There are two complementary angles: $\angle EFH$ and $\angle HFG$.

Solution

b.

Q
M
O P
N

Comments

b. There are **no** complementary angles in the figure. There are four pairs of supplementary angles, however:

1. $\angle MOQ$ and $\angle QOP$
2. $\angle QOP$ and $\angle PON$
3. $\angle PON$ and $\angle NOM$
4. $\angle NOM$ and $\angle MOQ$

Measuring Angles

If we need to know the precise measurement of a given angle, we can use an instrument called a **protractor**. To use a protractor to measure an angle, follow these steps:

1. Position the vertex of the angle under the hole in the center of the protractor.
2. The 0° reading on the protractor should be on one side of the angle.
3. The other side of the angle should pass through the measurement scale inscribed on the protractor. Read this scale to the nearest degree.

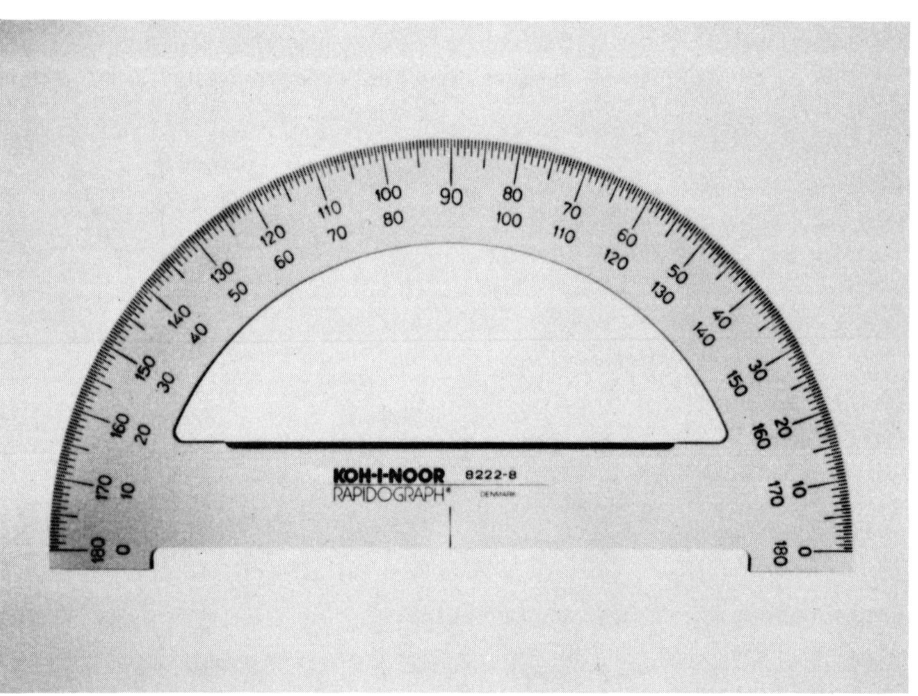

EXAMPLE 8.2.5

Measure the angle below using a protractor.

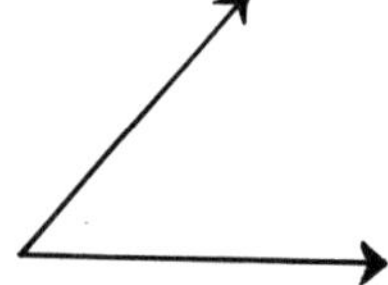

Solution

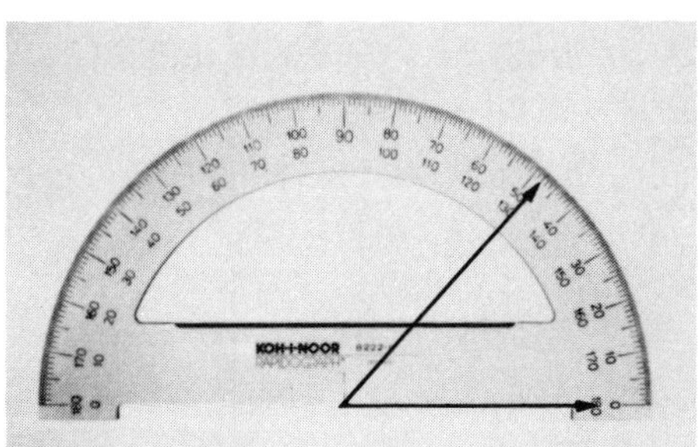

Comments

Line up the vertex with the hole.
The lower side should pass through 0°.
Read the point where the other side passes through scale.

The angle measures 48°.

PROBLEM SET 1

1. Name the line segments that form the sides of the figure *MNOP* in the figure below:

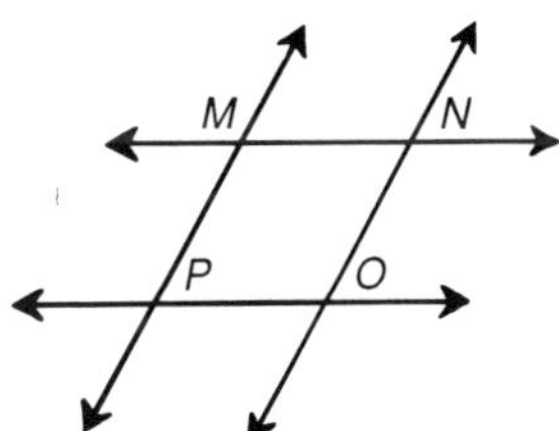

2. Which line segment in the drawing in number 1 is parallel to line segment $\overline{MP}$?
3. Which two line segments intersect at point *N*?
4. Two parallel lines are shown in the figure below with a line intersecting them:

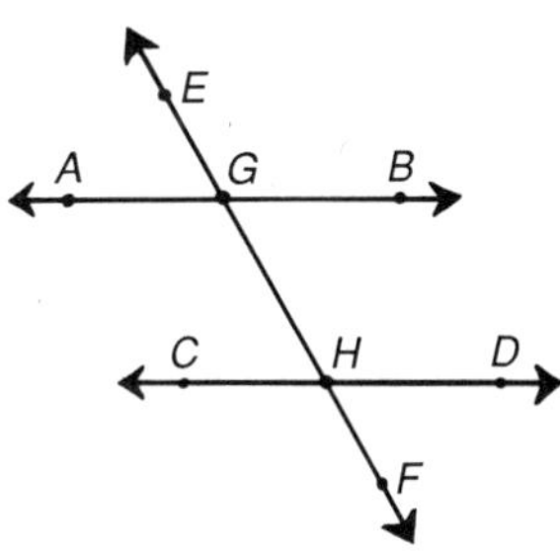

   a. Name the angle that is supplementary to $\angle EGB$.
   b. Name the angle that is supplementary to $\angle CHF$.
   c. Which two lines are parallel?
   d. Name five line segments found in the figure.
   e. At what points do $\overline{AB}$ and $\overline{CD}$ intersect with $\overline{EF}$?

5. Using the figure drawn below, answer the following questions.

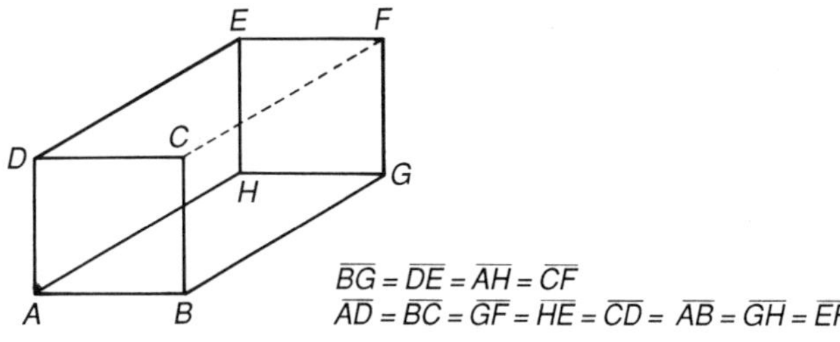

a. Which plane appears to be parallel to plane $ABGH$?
b. Which planes intersect at edge $\overline{AD}$?
c. Which edges form line segments parallel to $\overline{AD}$? (Assume each pair of lines meet at a right angle.)

6. Name all of the angles in the figure below.

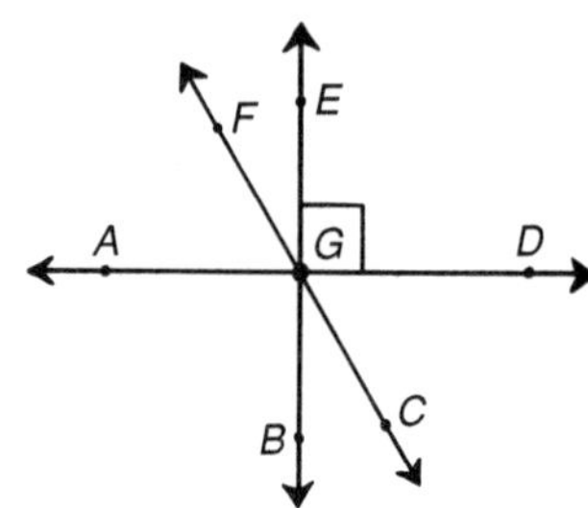

7. Name two pairs of angles found in the figure in problem 6 that are complementary.
8. Using a protractor, measure the following angles to the nearest degree:

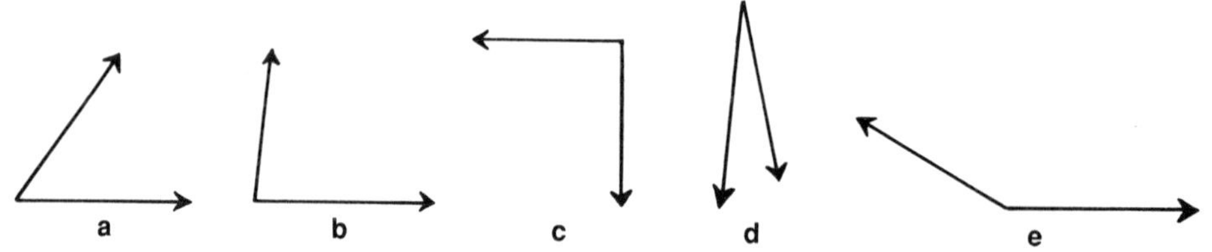

9. Using a protractor, draw angles that have the following measures:
   a. 22° b. 30° c. 60° d. 90° e. 124°
10. Using a protractor, draw angles supplementary to the following:
    a. 48° b. 118° c. 90°
11. Label each angle in problem 8 as either acute, obtuse, or a right angle.

Answers to odd-numbered problems appear on page 236.

8.3 PLANE FIGURES

In this section, we study the area and perimeters of three types of plane figures, the triangle, the parallelogram (including square and rectangle), and the circle.

We begin our study with the simplest plane figure, the triangle.

The Triangle

The triangle is a figure determined by three distinct points connected by three line segments that are *not* in a straight line. There are two ways to classify triangles: by the angles, and by the sides.

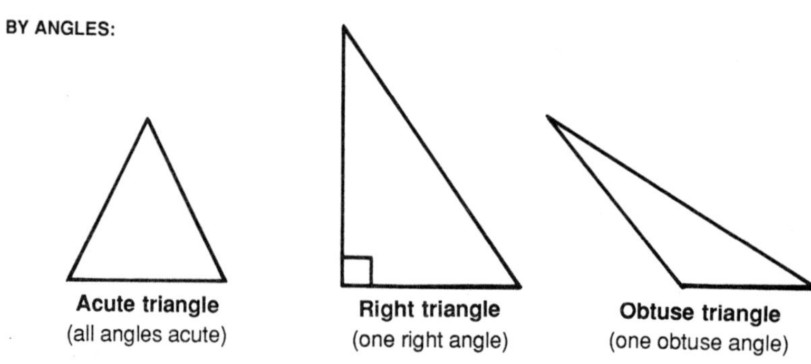

BY SIDES:

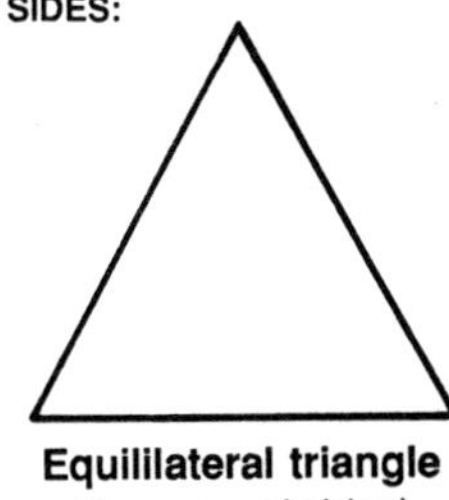

Equililateral triangle
(three equal sides)

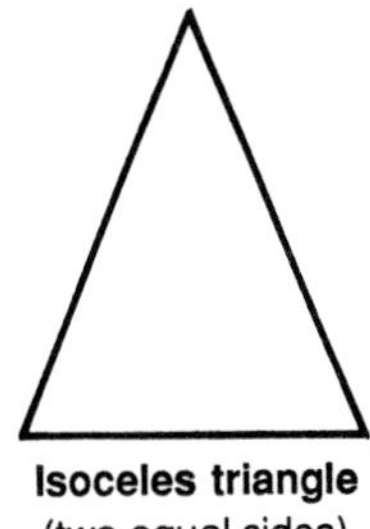

Isoceles triangle
(two equal sides)

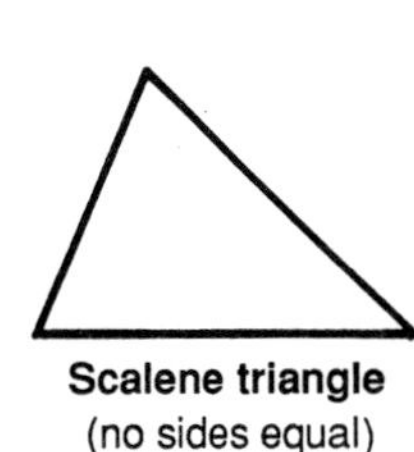

Scalene triangle
(no sides equal)

The sum of the angles of any triangle is always 180°.

EXAMPLE 8.3.1

Find the missing angle of the triangle below.

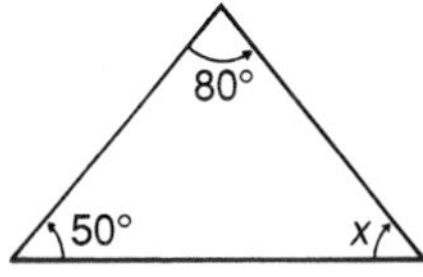

Solution	Comments
$\angle 1 + \angle 2 + \angle 3 = 180°$ $50° + 80° + x = 180°$ $130° + x = 180°$ $x = 180° - 130°$ $x = 50°$	Since all angles must equal to 180°, set up a single algebraic equation to solve for the unknown angle. The missing angle is 50°. Since two of the angles are equal, it is an **isoceles** triangle.

Perimeters of Triangles. To find the **perimeter** of a triangle, simply add the lengths of the three sides together:

$$P = \text{side 1} + \text{side 2} + \text{side 3}$$

EXAMPLE 8.3.2

Given a scalene triangle with $a = 12$ cm, $b = 15$ cm, and $c = 20$ cm, find its perimeter.

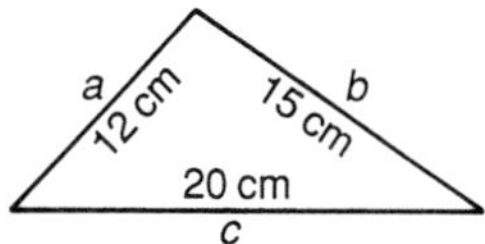

Solution	Comments
$P = a + b + c$	Definition of perimeter.
$P = 12\text{ cm} + 15\text{ cm} + 20\text{ cm}$ $P = 47\text{ cm}$	Substitute the given values into the perimeter formula and evaluate.

If the triangle is a right triangle, and two sides of the triangle are known and one is unknown, we can find the length of the third side by using the **pythagorean theorem.** This theorem states that the square of the long side opposite the right angle (**hypotenuse**) is equal to the sum of the squares of the other two sides:

$$c^2 = a^2 + b^2$$

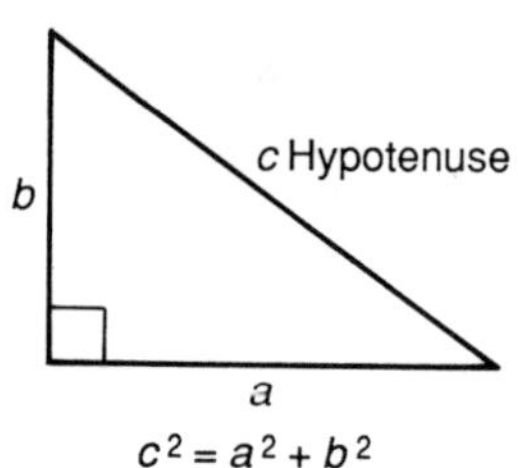

EXAMPLE 8.3.3

Find the perimeter of the triangle below:

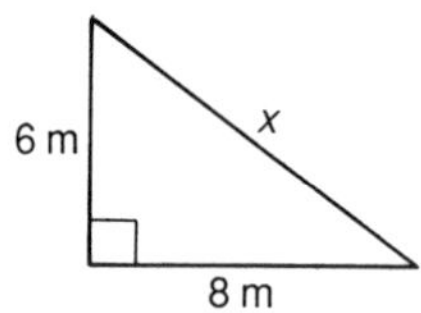

Solution	Comments
$x^2 = (6\text{ m})^2 + (8\text{ m})^2$ $x^2 = 36\text{ m}^2 + 64\text{ m}^2$ $x^2 = 100\text{ m}^2$ $x = 10\text{ m}$	First find the length of the unknown side. Use the Pythagorean theorem. You may use the [√] key on a calculator to find the $\sqrt{c^2}$. Enter the number, press the [√] key. The length of the unknown side is 10 m.
$P = \text{side 1} + \text{side 2} + \text{side 3}$ $P = 6\text{ m} + 8\text{ m} + 10\text{ m}$	Find the perimeter by adding the three sides.
$P = 24\text{ m}$	The perimeter is 24 m.

The Pythagorean theorem may be used to find the length of any unknown side of a right triangle. Simply solve the equation for the unknown side.

EXAMPLE 8.3.4

Find the perimeter of the triangle below.

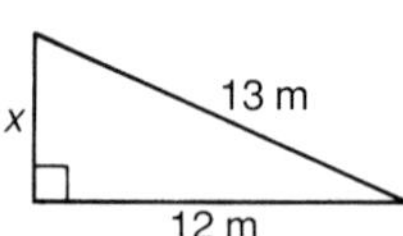

Solution	Comments
$a^2 + b^2 = c^2$	Definition of the Pythagorean theorem.
$(x)^2 + (12\text{ m})^2 = (13\text{ m})^2$ $x^2 = (13\text{ m})^2 - (12\text{ m})^2$	Substitute the known values into the equation. Solve for the unknown side.
$x^2 = 169\text{ m}^2 - 144\text{ m}^2$ $x^2 = 25\text{ m}^2$ $x = \sqrt{25\text{ m}^2} = 5\text{ m}$	Take the square root of both sides of the equation to solve for x.
$P = 5\text{ m} + 12\text{ m} + 13\text{ m}$ $= 30\text{ m}$	Substitute the lengths of all three sides into the perimeter formula.

Area of a Triangle. The area of any triangle is found by multiplying one half the length of the base times the height (or altitude):

$$A = \tfrac{1}{2}bh \qquad b = \text{base},\ h = \text{height}$$

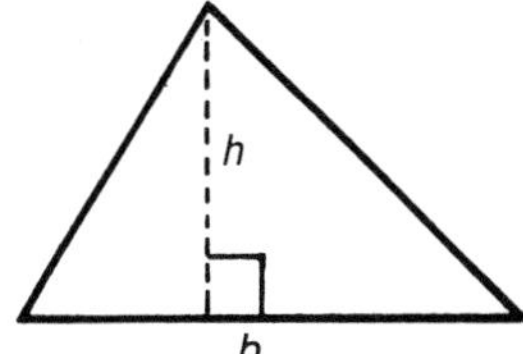

The height or altitude of a triangle is the perpendicular line from any vertex to the opposite side.

EXAMPLE 8.3.5

Find the area of the triangle below:

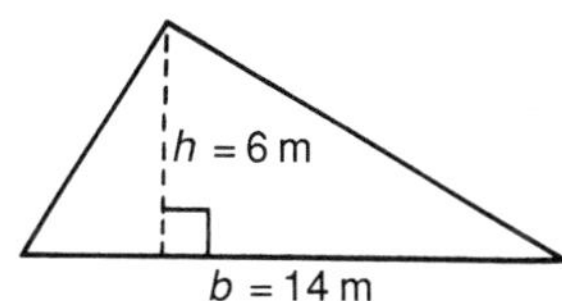

Solution	Comments
$A = \frac{1}{2}bh$	Substitute the values given for b and h into the formula $A = \frac{1}{2}bh$.
$A = \frac{1}{2}\,(14\text{ m})\,(6\text{ m})$ $A = \frac{1}{2}\,(84\text{ m}^2)$	You may multiply the numbers in any order.
$A = 42\text{ m}^2$	Note that the units for area are m^2 (square meters). The units for area are always the square of whatever unit we are using.

EXAMPLE 8.3.6

Find the height of a triangle that has an area of 62.3 ft^2 and a base of length 17.4 ft.

Solution	Comments
$A = \frac{1}{2}bh$ $62.3\text{ ft}^2 = \frac{1}{2}(17.4\text{ ft})h$	Substitute $A = 62.3\text{ ft}^2$ and $b = 17.4$ ft into the formula $A = \frac{1}{2}bh$. Solve for h.
$\frac{(2)(62.3\text{ ft}^2)}{17.4\text{ ft}} = h$	Multiply both sides by 2 and divide both sides by 17.4 ft. Notice that $\text{ft}^2 \div \text{ft} = \text{ft}$.
$7.16\text{ ft} = h$	The height of the triangle is 7.16 ft.

Parallelograms

A **parallelogram** is a four-sided figure with opposite sides equal and parallel. Three special parallelograms are the **square** (all four sides equal with one right angle), the **rectangle** (opposite sides equal with one right angle), and the **rhombus** (all four sides equal with opposite sides parallel).

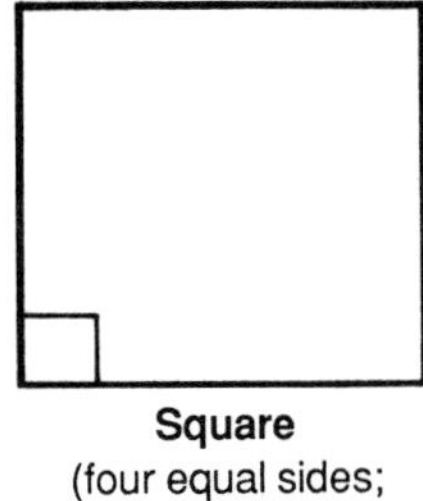

Square
(four equal sides; one right angle)

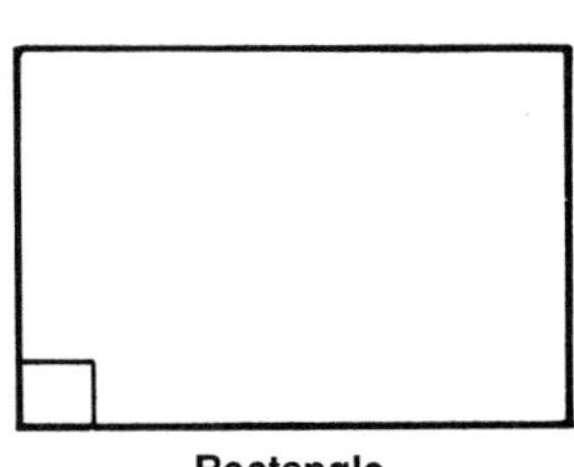

Rectangle
(opposite sides equal; one right angle)

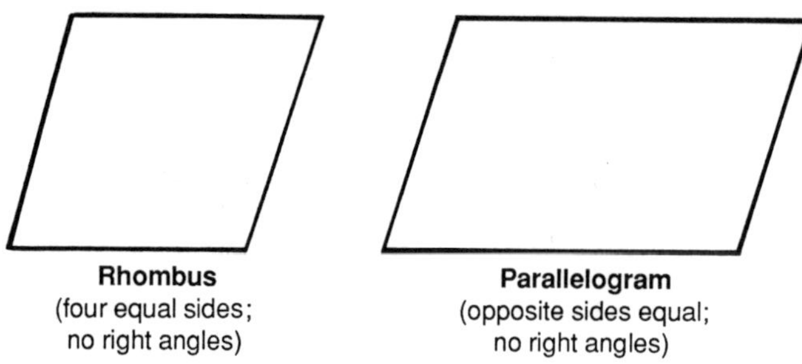

Rhombus
(four equal sides;
no right angles)

Parallelogram
(opposite sides equal;
no right angles)

Perimeter of a Parallelogram. To find the perimeter of any parallelogram, add the measurements of the four sides.

EXAMPLE 8.3.7

Find the perimeters of the following figures.

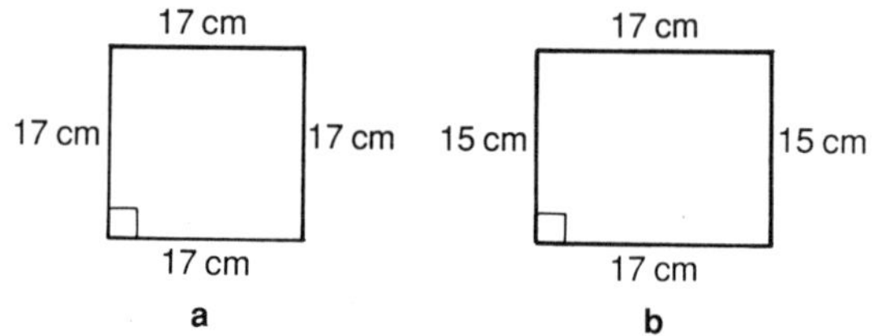

Solution

a.

17 cm

17 cm 17 cm

17 cm

$P = 4(17 \text{ cm})$
$P = 68 \text{ cm}$

b.

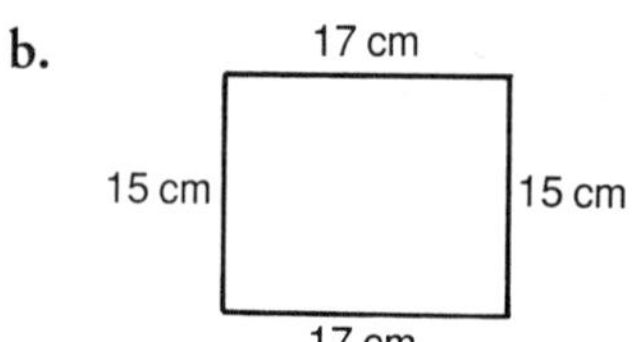

$P = 17 \text{ m} + 15 \text{ m} + 17 \text{ m} + 15 \text{ m}$
$P = 64 \text{ m}$

Comments

a. Since the figure is a square, all four sides must be of equal length. Either add 17 cm four times, or multiply by four. This gives us a formula for the perimeter of a square: $P = 4S$ where S represents the measurement of a side.

b. A rectangle has opposite sides equal. Therefore, we can double the opposite sides and add. This gives us a formula for the perimeter of a rectangle: $P = 2L + 2W$, where L and W represent length and width, respectively.

Areas of Parallelograms. The areas of a square and rectangle can be found by multiplying the length times the width.

Area of a Rectangle:

$$A = L \cdot W$$

Area of a Square:

$A = L \cdot W$; but since $L = W$, let
$S = L = W$, so
$A = S \cdot S$
$A = S^2$

The area of a parallelogram that is not a square or rectangle can be found by multiplying the base times the height where the height is the perpendicular distance from a vertex to the base:

$$A = bh \text{ (parallelogram not a square or rectangle)}$$

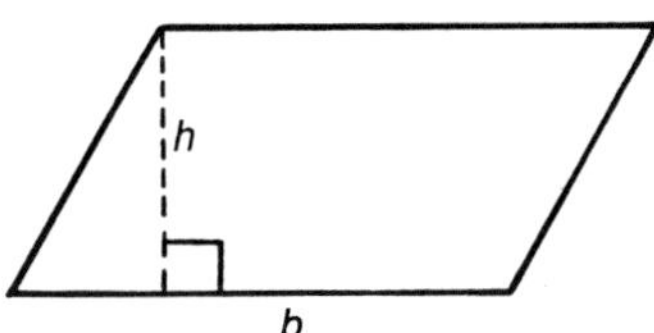

EXAMPLE 8.3.8 Find the areas of the following figures:

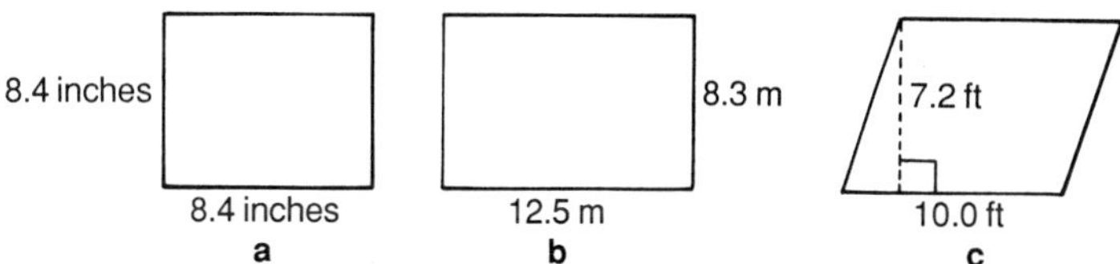

Solution	**Comments**
a. $A = (8.4 \text{ inches})^2$ $A = 71 \text{ inches}^2$	a. Use the formula $A = S^2$. $S = 8.4$ inches
b. $A = (12.5)\ (8.3 \text{ m})$ $A = 1\underline{0}4 \text{ m}^2$ $A = 1\bar{0}0 \text{ m}^2$	b. Use the formula $A = L \cdot W$: $L = 12.5$ m and $W = 8.3$ m. Round off answer to 2 significant digits.
c. $A = (10.0 \text{ ft})\ (7.2 \text{ ft})$ $A = 72 \text{ ft}^2$	c. Use the formula $A = bh$: $b = 10.0$ ft and $h = 7.2$ ft.

EXAMPLE 8.3.9 A table top has the following design:

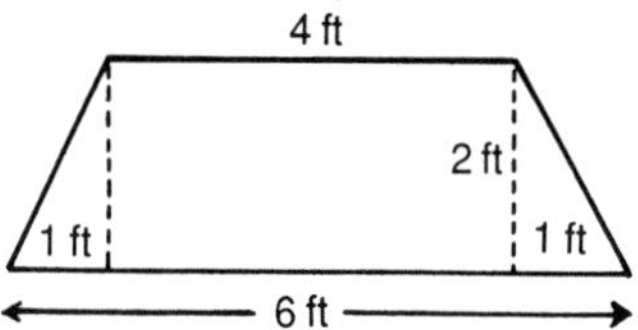

You wish to stain the table top, and you have 1 pt of stain. The label says that 1 pt will cover 56 ft^2. How many table tops can you stain with one pint of the stain? (Assume all measurements given are *exact*.)

Solution	**Comments**
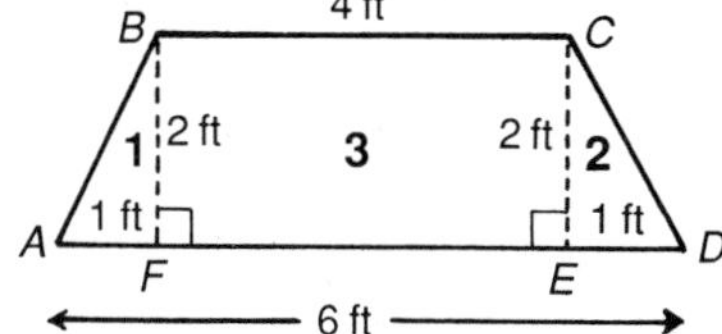	First, divide the figure into two triangles and one rectangle. Drop lines from points B and C perpendicular to F and E, respectively. This gives a rectangle and two right triangles of equal size.
$A = \frac{1}{2}bh$ $A = \frac{1}{2}(1 \text{ ft})\ (2 \text{ ft})$ $A = \frac{1}{2}(2 \text{ ft}^2)$ $A = 1 \text{ ft}^2$	Triangles 1 and 2 have the same dimensions: $b = 1$ ft, $h = 2$ ft. Find the areas of the two triangles.

Solution	Comments
Area of triangle 1 + area of triangle 2 = total area of triangles = 1 ft^2 + 1 ft^2 = 2 ft^2	The total area of the two triangles is 2 ft^2.
$A = L \cdot W$ $A = 4 \text{ ft} \cdot 2 \text{ ft}$ $A = 8 \text{ ft}^2$	Find the area of the middle rectangle: $L = 4$ ft, $W = 2$ ft. The area of the rectangle is 8 ft^2.
Total area $= 8 \text{ ft}^2 + 2 \text{ ft}^2 = 10 \text{ ft}^2$	Now, find the total area of the figure by adding the area of the two triangles to the area of the rectangle.
$\frac{1 \text{ table}}{10 \cancel{\text{ft}^2}} \cdot \frac{56 \cancel{\text{ft}^2}}{1 \text{ pt}}$ $= 5.6$ tables/pt	Use dimensional analysis to find the number of table tops that can be stained with one pint of stain. Recall: 1 pt = 56 ft^2. Let square feet cancel out. You are left with the units tables/per pint of stain.

The Circle

A curve such that all points on the curve have the same distance (r) from a given point (the *center*) is said to be a **circle.** This distance r is called the **radius** of the circle. The distance around the circle is called the **circumference.**

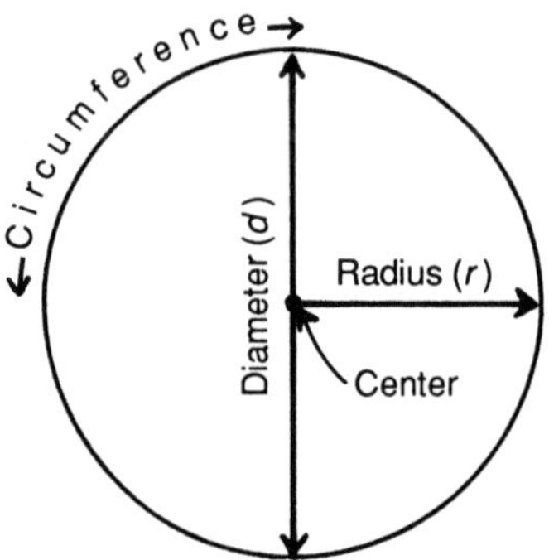

The circumference is related to the radius of the circle by the following formula:

$$C = 2\pi r, \qquad \text{where } \pi \text{ (pi) is a constant}$$

Since $2r$ (twice the radius) is the distance across the circle through the center (called the **diameter,** d), the formula can be written as

$$C = \pi d$$

Pi can be found by rearranging the formula and solving for it:

$$\frac{C}{d} = \pi$$

EXAMPLE 8.3.10

Find π if the circumference of a circular table top is approximately 12.75 ft and the diameter of the table is 4.06 ft.

Solution	Comments
$C = \pi d$ $\frac{C}{d} = \pi$	Substitute $C = 12.75$ ft and $d = 4.06$ ft into the circumference formula.

$\frac{12.75 \text{ ft}}{4.06 \text{ ft}} = \pi$ — Notice that the units cancel out.

$3.14 = \pi$ — Round off your answer.

Pi is a constant representing the ratio of the circumference of any circle to its diameter. It is an irrational number and cannot be expressed exactly as a decimal because it never terminates or repeats. It is frequently approximated by the rational number 3.14 and sometimes by the fraction $\frac{22}{7}$.

In order to obtain a value of π to more than two decimal places, the circumference and diameter must be measured more precisely. The value of π to five decimal places is

$$3.14159$$

For our purposes, we can round off after two decimal places, or let $\pi = 3.14$.

EXAMPLE 8.3.11

Find the circumference of a circle if the radius of the circle is 14.7 mm.

Solution	Comments
$d = 2r$	The diameter is twice the radius.
$d = 2(14.7)$ mm	
$d = 29.4$ mm	
$C = (3.14)(29.4)$ mm	Substitute $d = 29.4$ mm into the equation $C = \pi d$.
$C = 92.3$ mm	

Area of a Circle. To find the surface area of a circle on a plane use the formula

$$A = \pi r^2$$

where A is the area and r is the radius.

EXAMPLE 8.3.12

Find the surface area of a sheet of circular filter paper with a diameter of 11.0 cm. What happens to the area if the radius is doubled?

Solution	Comments
$r = \frac{d}{2}$	The radius is one half of the diameter.
$r = \frac{11.0}{2} = 5.50$ cm	
$A = \pi r^2$ $A = (3.14)(5.50 \text{ cm})^2$ $A = (3.14)(30.2 \text{ cm}^2)$	Substitute into the formula. Remember: Take care of exponents first.
$A = 95.0 \text{ cm}^2$	The area of the original circle is 95.0 cm^2.
$A = 3.14(11.0 \text{ cm})^2$ $A = (3.14)(121 \text{ cm}^2)$	To find the area if the radius doubles substitute 11.0 cm into the area formula.
$A = 380 \text{ cm}^2$	The area of the new circle is 380 cm^2.
$\frac{380 \text{ cm}^2}{95.0 \text{ cm}^2} = 4$	Compare the new area with the original area.
	The area is increased fourfold if the radius is doubled.

PROBLEM SET 2

1. Name each figure below. If it is a triangle, specify which type of triangle.

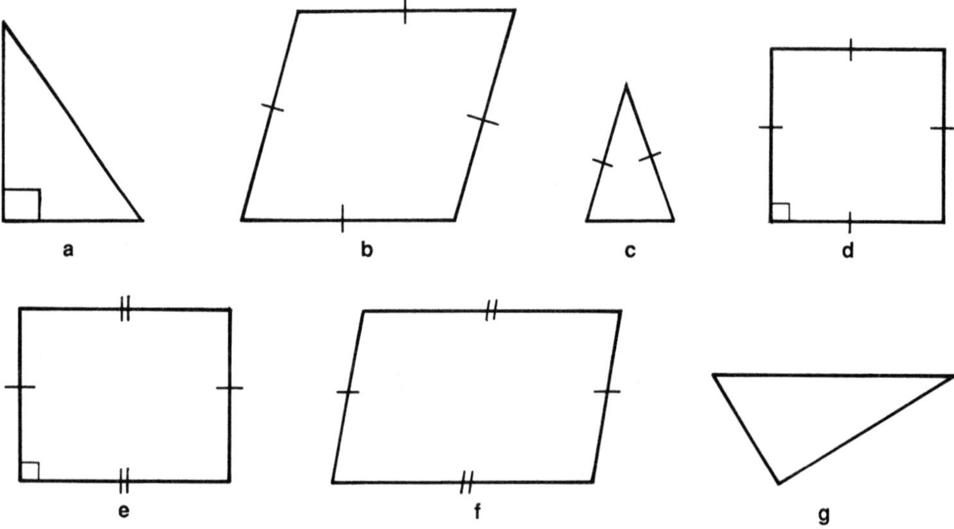

2. Find the perimeters of the following figures. (They may not be drawn to scale.)

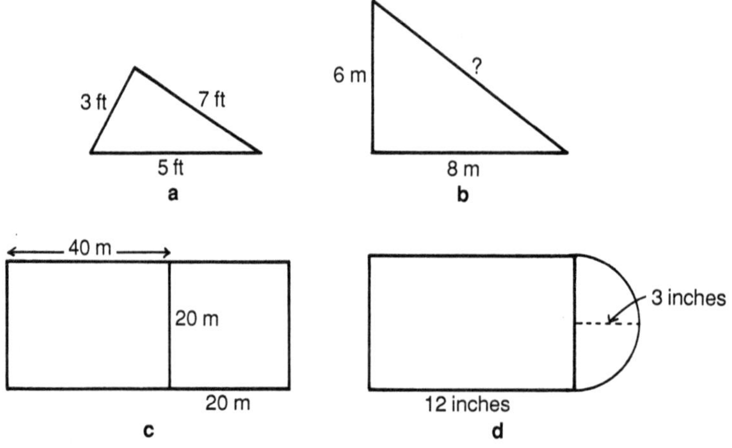

3. Find the area of each figure below. Let $\pi = 3.14$. (For **k**, find the area of the shaded region.)

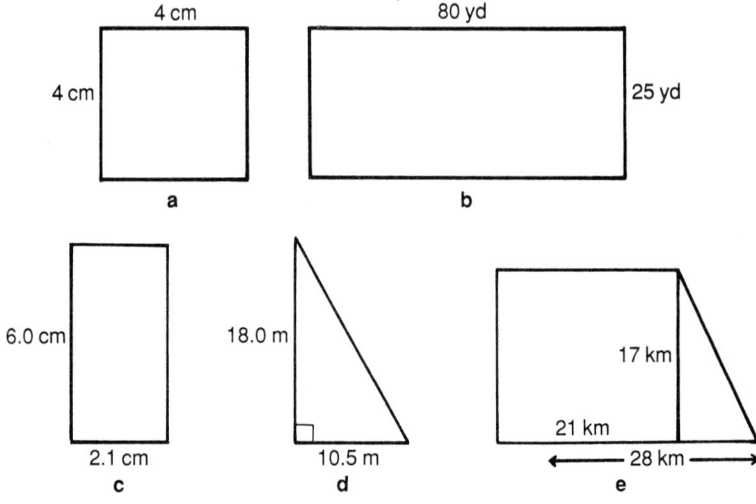

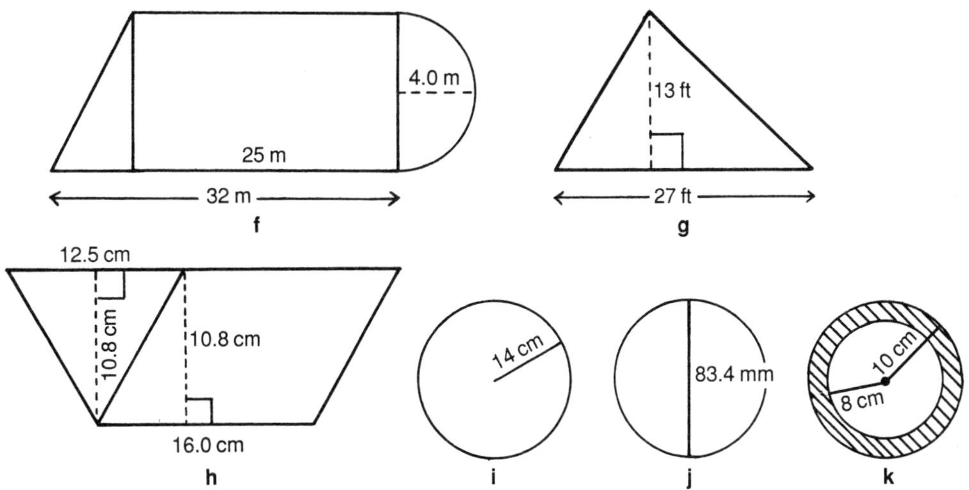

4. A wall has the dimensions 23.4 ft by 35.6 ft. If 1 gal of paint can cover 450 ft^2, how many gallons will it take to give the wall two coats?

5. A gardener has a plot of half-runner beams with the dimensions 55 ft by 105 ft. If a fertilizer is applied at the rate of 10 lb per 50 ft^2, how much fertilizer should the gardener apply to the plot?

6. A laboratory needs a new carpet. The floor measures 25 ft, 4 inches by 32 ft, 8 inches. A tough indoor–outdoor carpet sells for \$8.98 per square yard installed. How much will it cost to carpet the laboratory?

7. A painter uses $8\frac{1}{2}$ gal of paint to cover an entire suite of offices. If the paint label states that 1 gal of paint covers 425 ft^2, how many square feet of surface did the painter cover?

8. Normal air pressure at sea level is approximately 14.7 lb/$inch^2$. A man 72 inches tall weighing 180 lb has a skin surface area of approximately 3100 $inch^2$. What is the air pressure exerted upon the man's skin?

9. Number 1 filter paper is 11.0 cm in diameter. Number 42 filter paper is 7.0 cm in diameter. How much more area does number 1 filter paper have than number 42?

10. The instructions of a bottle of developing replenisher state that "1 gal of replenisher should be added for every fifty 14 by 17 inch x-ray films or equivalent area developed." How many 4 by 4 inch films can be developed with 1 gal of replenisher?

11. Thirty-five millimeter film is in wide use today by both professional and amateur photographers. The distance from one side of the negative to the other is 36 mm.

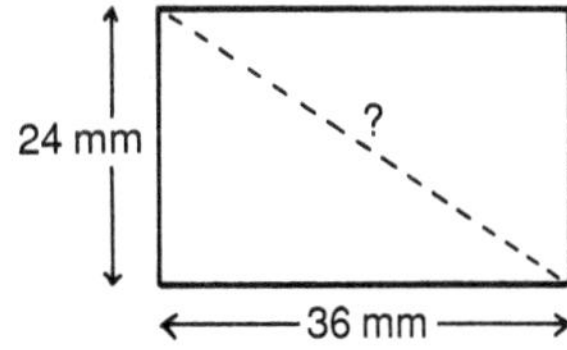

 a. If the negative is 24 mm wide, find the area of the negative.
 b. Find the length of the diagonal from one corner of the negative to the opposite corner.

Answers to odd-numbered problems appear on page 236.

8.4 SOLID FIGURES

Solid figures with flat surfaces are called **polyhedra**. In this section we will study the surface area and volume formulas for two such polyhedra, the prism and the pyramid.

We will also study surface area and volume formulas for such curved figures as the sphere, cylinder, and the cone.

Surface Area. A solid figure is enclosed by a surface, which may be a series of flat planes such as a polyhedron, or by a curved surface, as in a sphere. The area of this surface is called the **surface area**. If we wanted to know how much paint we needed to cover the surface of a cylinder, we would need to know the surface area.

Volume. The **volume** of a solid figure is the amount of space enclosed within the solid figure. If we needed to know the amount of space within a cylindrical oxygen tank, we would have to calculate the volume of the tank.

The Prism

There are various forms of the prism. A **prism** is a polyhedron with two sides of the same size in parallel planes, with the remaining sides in the shape of a parallelogram. We will consider prisms with either square or rectangular bases.

The simplest prism is the **cube**, which has six equal sides, called **faces**. The sides of the faces are called **edges**. The corners of the cube are called the **vertices**.

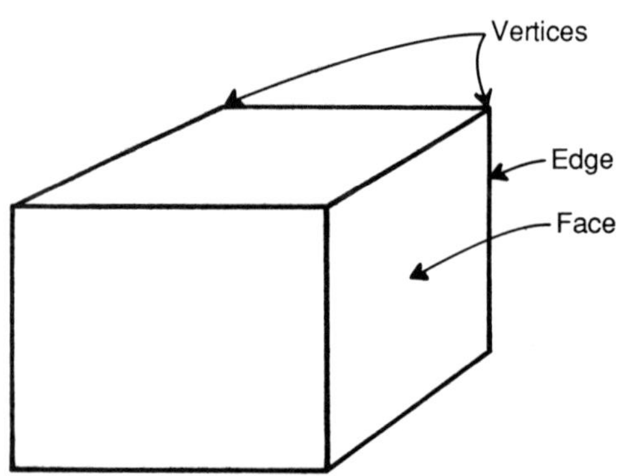

Surface Area. To find the surface area of the cube, find the area of each face and multiply it by 6. We may write the formula

$$A = L \cdot W \quad \text{or} \quad A = S^2 \quad \text{since length} = \text{width}$$

and multiply the result by 6:

$$A = 6S^2$$

The result will have the unit associated with each dimension squared.

Volume. To find the volume of any prism with square or rectangular bases, use the formula

$$V = L \cdot W \cdot H$$

where L is the length, W is the width, and H is the height. You must remember that the units of all three dimensions must be the same, and that the result will have the unit cubed.

EXAMPLE 8.4.1

Find the surface area and the volume of a sugar cube 0.35 inch on a side.

Solution	**Comments**
$A = S^2$ $A = (0.35 \text{ inch})^2$ $A = 0.12 \text{ inch}^2$ Total surface area $= (6)(0.12 \text{ inch}^2)$ $= 0.72 \text{ inch}^2$	To find the surface area, find the area of one side, and multiply by 6.

$V = L \cdot W \cdot H$ $V = (0.35 \text{ inch})(0.35 \text{ inch})(0.35 \text{ inch})$	To find the volume, substitute $L = 0.35$ inch $W = 0.35$ inch and $H = 0.35$ inch.
$V = 0.043 \text{ inch}^3$	The unit inch^3 is called cubic inches.

The Rectangular Box

Another common prism is the rectangular box, in which the three sets of opposite sides are equal.

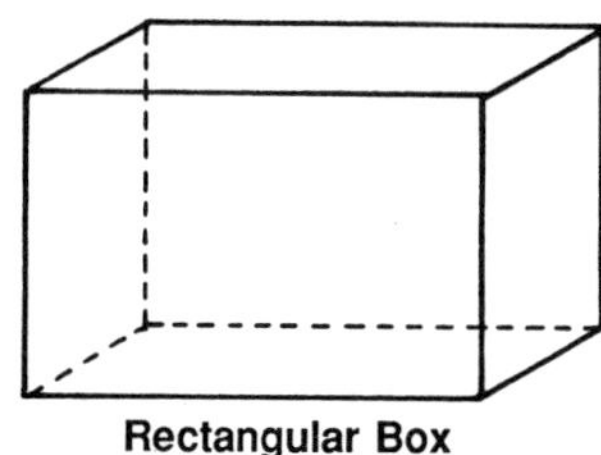

Rectangular Box

A brick, a room, and a gold ingot may have the shape of a rectangular box.

Surface Area. The surface area of a rectangular box is calculated by determining the area of each different size face and multiplying by 2, since the opposite face is of equal area. The areas of these pairs of faces are then added together to obtain the total surface area:

$$A = 2A_1 + 2A_2 + 2A_3$$
$$A = 2(L_1 W_1) + 2(L_2 W_2) + 2(L_3 W_3)$$

where A_1, L_1, and W_1 are the area, length, and width of the first pair of faces, A_2, L_2, and W_2 are the area, length, and width of the second pair of faces, respectively, and A_3, L_3, and W_3 are the area, length, and width of the third pair of faces.

Volume. The volume of a rectangular box is found by the formula

$$V = L \cdot W \cdot H$$

where L is the length, W is the width, and H is the height.

EXAMPLE 8.4.2

Find the total surface area and volume of a rectangular box with the following dimensions: $L = 18.7$ cm; $W = 7.4$ cm; and $H = 2.6$ cm.

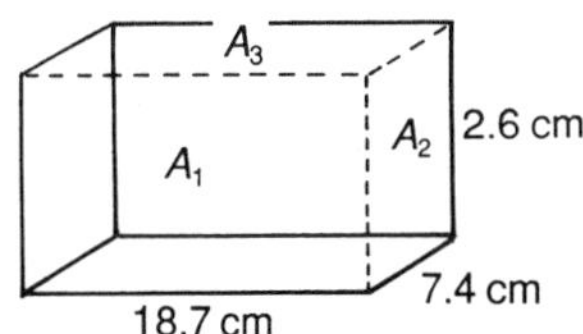

Solution	**Comments**
$A_1 = L_1 \cdot W_1$ $A_1 = (18.7 \text{ cm})\ (2.6 \text{ cm})$ $A_1 = 49 \text{ cm}^2$ $2A_1 = 98 \text{ cm}^2$	Find the area of the side A_1 rectangles: $L_1 = 18.7$ cm, and $W_1 = 2.6$ cm. Multiply by 2 since there are two sides with this area.
$A_2 = (7.4 \text{ cm})\ (2.6 \text{ cm})$ $A_2 = 19 \text{ cm}^2$ $2A_2 = 38 \text{ cm}^2$	Find the area of the side A_2 rectangles: $L_2 = 7.4$ cm and $W_2 = 7.6$ cm. Multiply by 2.
$A_3 = (18.7 \text{ cm})\ (7.4 \text{ cm})$ $A_3 = 140 \text{ cm}^2$ $2A_3 = 280 \text{ cm}^2$	Find the area of the side A_3 rectangles: $L_3 = 18.7$ cm and $W_3 = 7.4$ cm. Multiply by 2.

$A = 2A_1 + 2A_2 + 2A_3$ $A = 98 \text{ cm}^2 + 38 \text{ cm}^2 + 280 \text{ cm}^2$	Find the total surface area by adding the areas of the sides.
$A = 416 \text{ cm}^2$ $V = L \cdot W \cdot H$	The total surface area is $4.2 \cdot 10^2 \text{ cm}^2$ (two significant digits).
$V = 18.7 \text{ cm} \cdot 7.4 \text{ cm} \cdot 2.6 \text{ cm}$	Find the volume by substituting $L = 18.7$ cm, $W = 7.4$ cm, and $H = 2.6$ cm into the volume formula.
$V = 360 \text{ cm}^3$	The volume is $3.6 \cdot 10^2 \text{ cm}^3$ (two significant digits).

The Pyramid

A **pyramid** is a figure with a base and as many triangular sides as the base has sides. Pictured below are the two most common pyramids: the triangular pyramid and the rectangular pyramid.

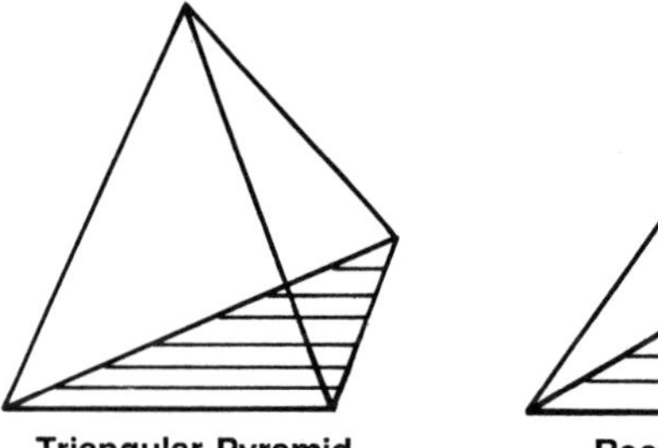

Triangular Pyramid

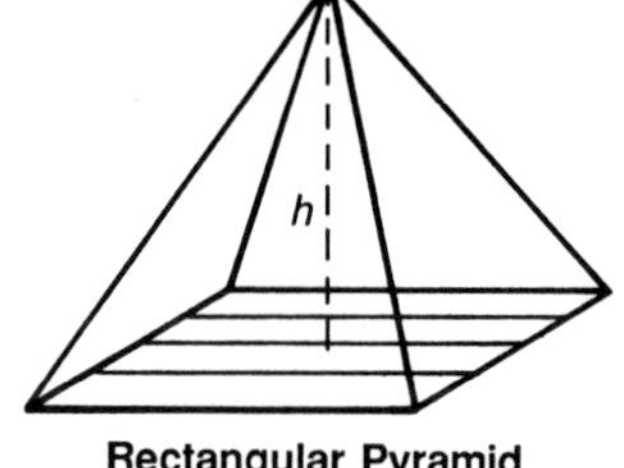

Rectangular Pyramid

The **altitude** denoted by h is the perpendicular distance from the **apex** to a point on the base.

Volume. The formula for the volume of a pyramid is

$$V = \tfrac{1}{3}Bh$$

where B is the area of the base and h is the altitude.

EXAMPLE 8.4.3

Find the volume of the pyramid below.

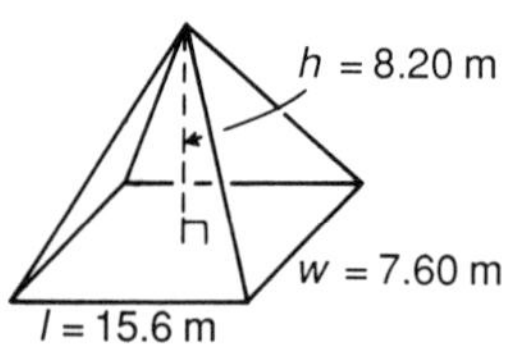

Solution	**Comments**
$V = \tfrac{1}{3}Bh$ $B = L \cdot W$ $B = (15.6 \text{ m})\ (7.60 \text{ m})$ $B = 119 \text{ m}^2$	Write the formula for volume. B in this case is the area of the rectangular base, $L = 15.6$ m, and $W = 7.60$ m.
$V = \tfrac{1}{3}(119 \text{ m}^2)\ (8.20 \text{ m})$ $V = \tfrac{1}{3}(976 \text{ m}^3)$ $V = 325 \text{ m}^3$	Substitute $B = 119 \text{ m}^2$ and $h = 8.20$ m into the volume formula.

The Sphere

A **sphere** is a three-dimensional figure where all points on the surface are equidistant from the center. The **radius** of the sphere is the distance from the center to a point on the surface. The **diameter** extends from a point on the surface through the center to a point on the opposite surface.

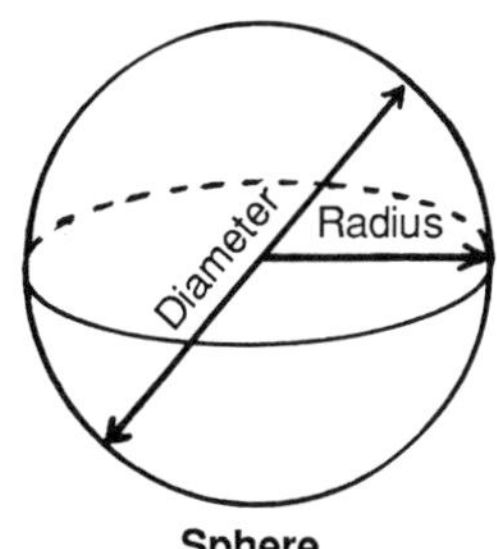

Sphere

Surface Area. The surface area (S) of a sphere is found by using the formula

$$S = 4\pi r^2$$

Volume. The volume of a sphere is found by the formula

$$V = \tfrac{4}{3}\pi r^3.$$

The atom can be thought of as a sphere, with the center of the nucleus as the center of the sphere. The distance from the center of the nucleus to the outermost electron is the radius of the sphere. With this in mind, study the following examples.

EXAMPLE 8.4.4

Find the surface area and volume of a chromium atom that has a diameter of $2.36 \cdot 10^{-10}$ m.

Solution	**Comments**
$d = 2r$	Using the diameter, find the radius.
$\frac{d}{2} = r$	
$\frac{2.36 \cdot 10^{-10}}{2} \text{ m} = r$	
$1.18 \cdot 10^{-10} \text{ m} = r$	
$S = 4\pi r^2$	To find the surface area, substitute $r = 1.18 \cdot 10^{-10}$ m into the formula.
$= 4(3.14)\ (1.18 \cdot 10^{-10} \text{ m})^2$	Square the radius first.
$= 4(3.14)\ (1.39 \cdot 10^{-20} \text{ m}^2)$	
$= 17.5 \cdot 10^{-20} \text{ m}^2$	
$= 1.75 \cdot 10^{-19} \text{ m}^2$	The surface area is $1.75 \cdot 10^{-19}$ m^2.
$V = \frac{4}{3}\pi r^3$	To find the volume of the atom, substitute
$= \frac{4}{3}(3.14)\ (1.18 \cdot 10^{-10} \text{ m})^3$	$r = 1.18 \cdot 10^{-10}$ m into the formula.
$= \frac{4}{3}(3.14)\ (1.64 \cdot 10^{-30} \text{ m}^3)$	Cube the radius first.
$= \frac{20.6}{3} \cdot 10^{-30} \text{ m}^3$	
$= 6.87 \cdot 10^{-30} \text{ m}^3$	The volume of the chrominum atom is $6.87 \cdot 10^{-30}$ m^3.

EXAMPLE 8.4.5

How much more volume will a cesium atom have if its radius is twice that of the chromium atom?

Solution		**Comments**
Cr atom	*Cs atom*	A simple way to find the change in volume is to let the chromium radius equal r and the cesium equal $2r$.
$V = \frac{4}{3}\pi r^3$	$V = \frac{4}{3}\pi(2r)^3$	

$V = Kr^3$	$V = K(2r)^3$	Let the letter K equal $\frac{4}{3}\pi$ in both equations. $\frac{4}{3}\pi$ is a constant.
$V = Kr^3$	$V = K(8r^3)$	Cube the radius of the cesium atom $(2r)$.
$V = Kr^3$	$V = 8Kr^3$	Compare the volumes. The volume of the cesium atom is 8 times larger than the volume of the chromium atom.

The Cylinder

The **cylinder** is a very common geometric figure encountered in the laboratory. A **right circular cylinder** is a solid figure formed by enclosing with perpendicular line segments the space between two circles with equal radii in parallel planes.

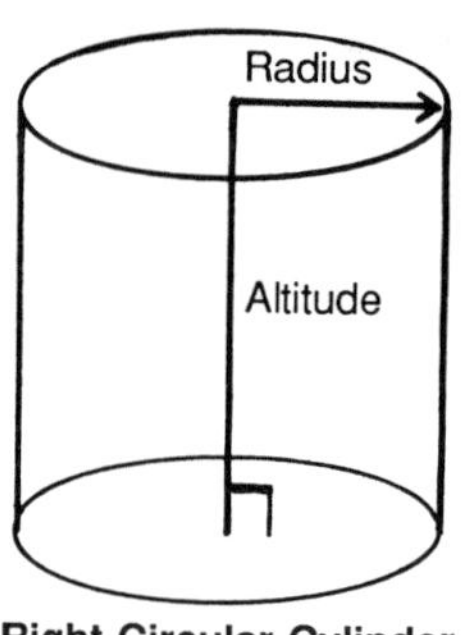

Right Circular Cylinder

Surface Area. We can find the surface area of a right circular cylinder by finding twice the area of the top or bottom (both circles) and adding it to the area of the circular side. If a soda can, which is a right circular cylinder, is torn apart and flattened, it will have the shape shown below. The sides form a rectangle, and the top and bottom form two circles.

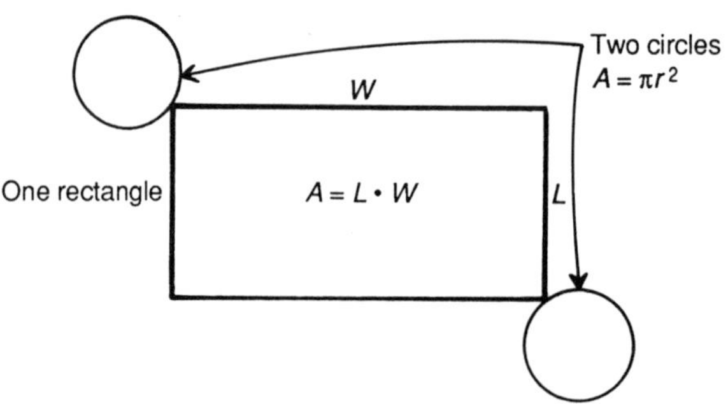

The total surface area then becomes

$$S = 2(\pi r^2) + L \cdot W$$

but since the length of the rectangle is the circumference of the top and bottom circles, and the width of the rectangle is equal to the altitude of the cylinder, the formula becomes

$$S = 2\pi r^2 + 2\pi rh$$

or

$$S = 2\pi r(r + h)$$

Volume. The volume of a right circular cylinder is given by the formula

$$V = \pi r^2 h$$

EXAMPLE 8.4.6

A soda can has the following dimensions:

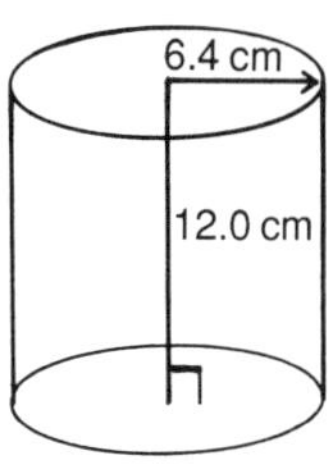

Find the surface area and volume of the can.

Solution	**Comments**
$S = 2\pi r(r + h)$ $S = 2(3.14)(6.4 \text{ cm})(6.4 \text{ cm} + 12.0 \text{ cm})$ $S = 2(3.14)(6.4 \text{ cm})(18.4 \text{ cm})$ $S = 740 \text{ cm}^2$	Substitute $\pi = 3.14$, $r = 6.4$ cm, and $h = 12.0$ cm into the formula for surface area. Add inside the parenthesis first.
$V = \pi r^2 h$ $V = (3.14)(6.4 \text{ cm})^2(12.0 \text{ cm})$	Substitute the appropriate values the volume formula. Square the radius first.
$V \approx 1543 \text{ cm}^3$ $= 1.5 \cdot 10^3 \text{ cm}^3$	Round off your answer to two significant digits.

The Right Circular Cone

The **right circular cone** has a circular base with line segments connecting the circumference of the base to a point located directly above the center of the base.

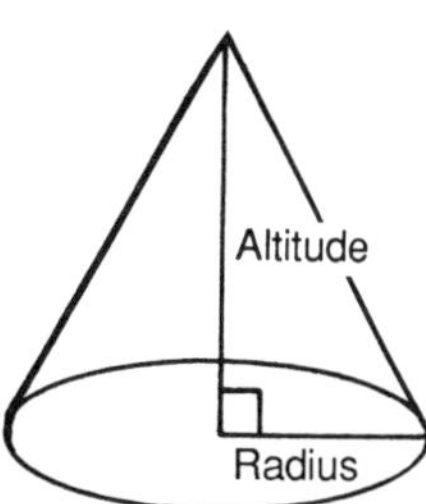

Right Circular Cone

Volume. The formula for the volume of the cone is the same as for the pyramid:

$$V = \tfrac{1}{3}Bh$$

where B is the area of the base and h is the perpendicular distance from the **apex** to the center of the circular base.

Since the base is a circle, the formula can be rewritten as

$$V = \tfrac{1}{3}\pi r^2 h$$

The right circular cone has many interesting geometric properties. If various pieces of the right circular cone are cut off and looked at in cross section, some basic geometric figures are found, as is shown in the figure below.

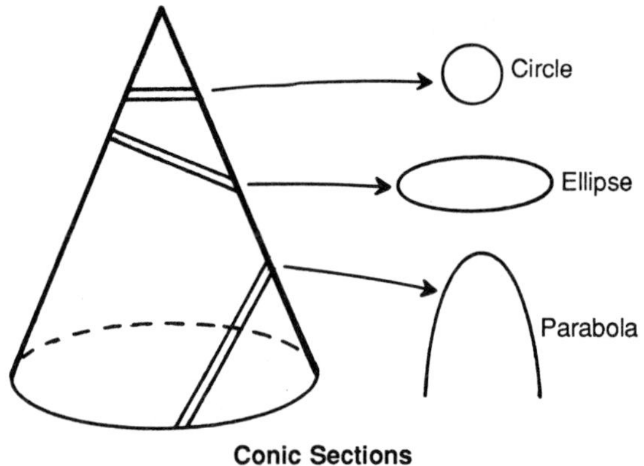

Conic Sections

EXAMPLE 8.4.7

Find the volume of a right circular cone with a radius of $4.00 \cdot 10^{-2}$ m and an altitude of $8.72 \cdot 10^{-1}$ m.

Solution	Comments
$V = \frac{1}{3}\pi r^2 h$	Write down the formula for the volume of the cone.
$V = \frac{1}{3}(3.14)(4.00 \cdot 10^{-2} \text{ m})^2 \cdot (8.72 \cdot 10^{-1} \text{ m})$	Substitute $r = 4.00 \cdot 10^{-2}$ m and $h = 8.72 \cdot 10^{-1}$ m into the formula.
$V = \frac{1}{3}(3.14)(16.0 \cdot 10^{-4} \text{ m}^2) \cdot (8.72 \cdot 10^{-1} \text{ m})$	Square the radius first.
$V = \dfrac{438 \cdot 10^{-5} \text{ m}^3}{3}$	
$V = 146 \cdot 10^{-5} \text{ m}^3 = 1.46 \cdot 10^{-3} \text{ m}^3$	The volume of the cone is $1.46 \cdot 10^{-3}$ m^3.

PROBLEM SET 3

1. Find the surface area of the solid figures pictured below.

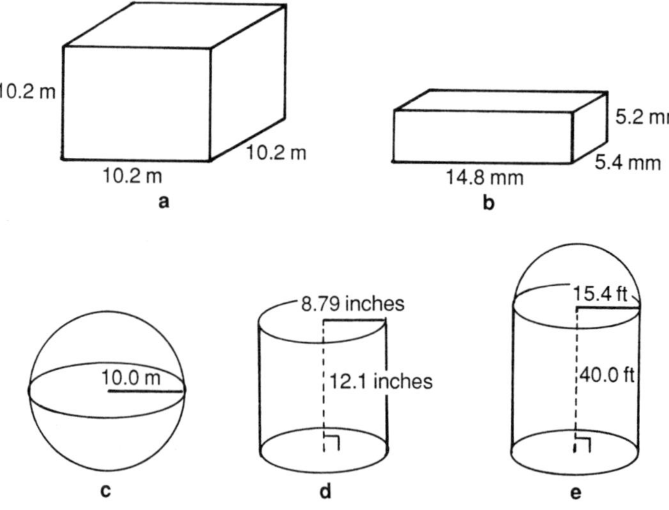

2. Find the volume of each figure pictured above.
3. Find the volume of the rectangular pyramid below.

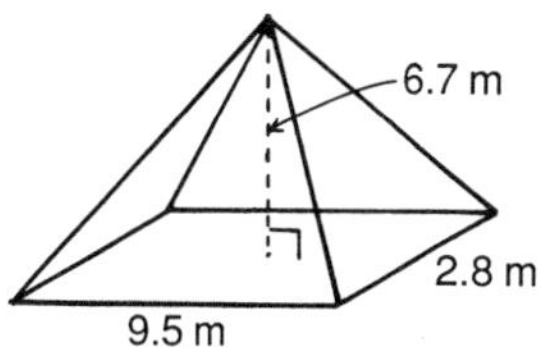

6.7 m
2.8 m
9.5 m

4. The Great Pyramid of Eqypt is a square pyramid with a base of 227 m and an altitude of 137 m. What is its volume?

5. Calculate the volume of an ice cream cone if it has a radius of 1.0 inch and a height of 6.0 inches.

6. A typical cloud droplet, which is small enough to float in the air, has an essentially spherical shape. The radius of a cloud droplet is approximately 0.0005 cm. Find its volume.

7. A typical raindrop, which is also spherical, has a radius of 0.005 cm. What is its volume?

8. Using the results of numbers 6 and 7, determine the number of cloud droplets needed to form one raindrop.

9. Assume that a basketball has a radius of 5.0 inches. Ignoring the thickness of the walls of the basketball, determine how many pounds of pressure would be exerted against the walls of the basketball if it were inflated to 30 lb/inch^2?

10. Find the volume of a metal block whose dimensions are 4.5 cm · 12.54 cm · 1.25 cm. What is the volume of the metal block in cubic meters?

11. Assume all containers listed below are cylinders. Find their volumes.
    a. A beaker: d = 5.7 cm, h = 8.1 cm
    b. A beaker: d = 7.1 cm, h = 8.7 cm
    c. A test tube: d = 16 mm, h = 125 mm
    d. A culture tube: d = 72 mm, h = 175 mm
    e. A buret: d = 1.3 mm, h = 65 mm

12. One mole of any gas at conditions of standard temperature and pressure (STP) will occupy the same volume as a cube 28.2 cm on an edge. Find this volume in liters.

13. If a cylindrical container with a radius of 12.3 cm and an altitude of 28.7 cm is filled with pure water, approximately how many kilograms of water are contained in the container? (1 cm^3 of water $\approx$ 1 g.)

14. What would be the density of the sun if its mass ($2 \cdot 10^{30}$ kg) were compressed to 1.5 km in diameter?

15. An ingot of pure gold has the dimensions 20.0 cm · 3.0 cm · 7.5 cm. What is the mass of the ingot if its density is 19.32 g/cm^3?

16. What is the radius of a metal ball with a mass of $4.00 \cdot 10^3$ g if the metal is
    a. iron
    b. aluminum
    c. lead?
    (*Hint*: First, look up the density of each metal in a chemistry textbook, then use the density formula to determine the volume of the ball.) Use a calculator with a exponential functions.

17. A typical atom has a radius of approximately $5 \cdot 10^{-11}$ m. This is essentially the distance from the center of the nucleus to the outermost electron. The nucleus has

a radius of $1 \cdot 10^{-14}$ m. Now, imagine that the nucleus was enlarged to the size of a basketball, with a radius of $1.27 \cdot 10^{-1}$ m. How far away would the outermost electron be?

18. The atomic radius of iron is $1.17 \cdot 10^{-10}$ m. Assuming the atom to be a sphere, how many iron atoms, ignoring empty space, could be fitted into a cube of iron 1.00 cm on an edge?

Answers to odd-numbered problems appear on page 237.

CHAPTER REVIEW

(8.2)

1. Given the drawing below, answer the following questions:

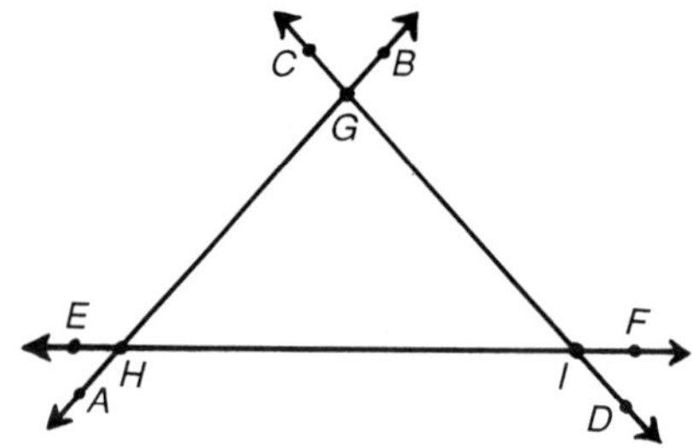

   a. Which lines intersect at point G?
   b. Which angles form the vertices of a triangle?
   c. Name at least two angles that are supplementary.
   d. Name the angles that have point H at the vertex.
   e. Name all the line segments along $\overleftrightarrow{CD}$.
   f. Are any of the lines parallel?

2. Using a protractor, measure the angles below:

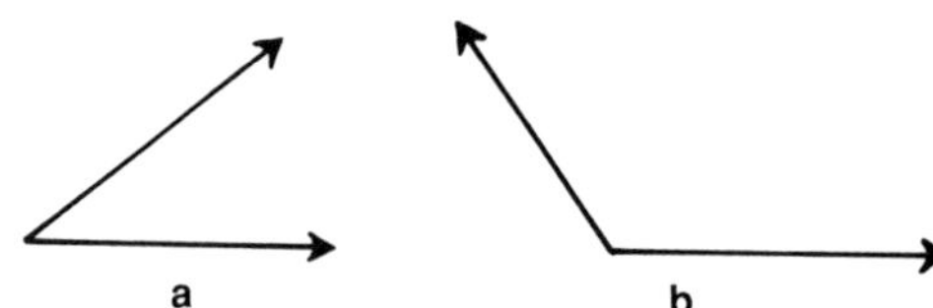

3. Using a protractor, draw angles with the following measures:
   a. 45°
   b. 135°
   c. 390°
   d. Which of the angles above are acute? Obtuse?

(8.3)

4. A wall has the dimensions 18.2 ft · 7.0 ft. There is one window in the wall 3.0 ft wide and 4.5 ft high. How many square feet of surface area does the wall contain?

5. Find the area of a isoceles triangle with a base of 14.0 cm and an altitude of 28.0 cm.

6. Find the perimeter of the triangle in problem 5.

7. Find the area of the following figure:

10.0 cm
10.0 cm
10.0 cm
25.0 cm
20 cm

8. Find the area of the shaded region:

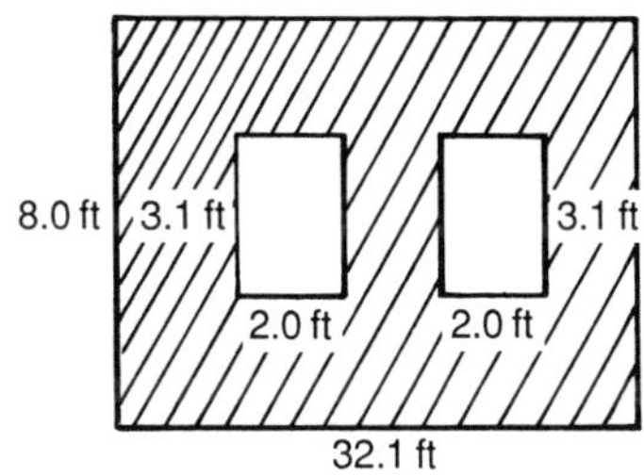

9. To properly develop x-ray film, $2\frac{3}{4}$ oz of replenisher is needed for each 196 inch^2 of film developed. How many $14 \cdot 17$ inch film negatives can be developed from $\frac{1}{2}$ gal of replenisher? (32 oz = 1 quart)

(8.4) 10. Calculate the volumes of the figures below.
   a. A cube: $3.0 \cdot 10^4$ dm on each edge
   b. A sphere: 40.0 cm in diameter
   c. A cylinder: $r = 84.6$ mm, $h = 148.7$ mm
   d. A cone: $r = 3.25$ cm, $h = 12.00$ cm

11. Find the surface area of the figures in problems 10a, 10b, and 10c.

12. How many grams of water can a beaker hold that has a diameter of 12.0 cm and a height of 16.0 cm? 1 g of water $\approx$ 1 cm^3

13. What is the mass in grams of a cloud droplet if its radius is 0.0005 cm? Assume the cloud droplet is a sphere.

14. One atom of aluminum has an atomic radius $1.25 \cdot 10^{-10}$ m. How many of these atoms laid side by side would it take to cross the head of a pin ($d = 1.5$ mm)?

Answers to odd-numbered problems appear on page 237.

chapter 9

Statistics

OBJECTIVES

After studying this chapter, the student should be able to:

1. Find and interpret the mean, median, and mode for a set of numerical data.
2. Find and interpret the range and standard deviation for a set of numerical data.
3. Construct a frequency table and frequency polygon for a set of numerical data.
4. Construct and interpret a grouped frequency distribution and find the mean, median, mode, range, and standard deviation for this grouped data.
5. Construct a graphical presentation of grouped data.

9.1 INTRODUCTION

The purpose of this chapter is to help the student deal effectively with numerical information. Although you will not be a complete statistician after studying this chapter, you should be able to organize and correctly interpret numerical data collected by yourself or others. **Numerical data** are a set of numerical values obtained either by experiment or other sources.

9.2 DEFINITION

Statistics is the organization and interpretation of numerical information or data. It is essential that data be organized correctly, and interpreted in a manner that will allow intelligent decisions to be made on the basis of this information.

9.3 MEASURES OF CENTRAL TENDENCY: MEAN, MEDIAN, AND MODE

For any set of numerical data, the student will want to find three measures—the mean, median, and mode. These values are called measures of **central tendency.**

Mean

The **mean** of a set of numerical data is the result obtained by finding the sum of all numerical entries and dividing that sum by the total number of entries. It is indicated by the symbol $\bar{x}$ and is given by the formula

$$\bar{x} = \frac{\sum x}{n}$$

x is the variable representing each of the values in the data. Σ is the Greek letter "sigma" and means "the sum of" the xs in the formula; n is the total number of values in the data.

In rounding off the answer, always carry one more decimal place than occurs in the data. For instance, in example 9.3.1, each item of data is measured to the nearest tenth, so the mean is rounded to the nearest one hundredth.

EXAMPLE 9.3.1

Find the mean of the following set of numbers: 10.2, 3.6, 7.4, 8.1, 12.0.

Solution

$$\frac{10.2 + 3.6 + 7.4 + 8.1 + 12.0}{5}$$

$$\bar{x} = \frac{41.3}{5} = 8.26$$

Comments

Find the sum of all five entries and divide by the total number of entries, which is five.

EXAMPLE 9.3.2

Find the mean weight of ten fourth graders whose weights (in kilograms) are given below:

45	60	62
42	54	48
40	70	
68	64	

Solution

45 kg
42 kg
40 kg
68 kg
60 kg
54 kg
70 kg
64 kg
62 kg
+ 48 kg
553 kg

$$\bar{x} = \frac{553 \text{ kg}}{10} = 55.3 \text{ kg}$$

Comments

Find the sum of all the weights and divide it by ten, the number of weights involved ($n = 10$).

If one pictures numerical entries as weights suspended from a horizontal bar, the mean would be the "balance point". To explain further, suppose that, in the above example, we could suspend the weights from a bar which is marked off uniformly by units ranging from 40 to 70, as in the figure below.

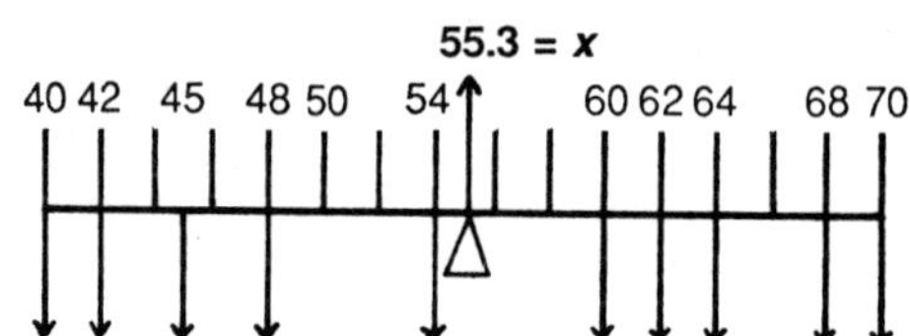

If we think of this bar with the suspended weights as a "seesaw", it would be balanced if we placed another bar under it at the exact point 55.3. Therefore, one can think of the mean as the point where the numerical values are "balanced."

Median

To find the **median**, proceed with the following steps:

1. Arrange the numerical entries in order from smallest to largest.

2a. If there are an odd number of entries, the median will be the middle number.

To illustrate, consider the five entries in example 9.3.1. If they are arranged from smallest to largest, the middle number, 8.1, is the median of these entries:

3.6, 7.4, <u>8.1</u>, 10.2, 12.0

2b. If there are an even number of entries, then the mean of the two middle numbers is the median. To illustrate, consider the ten entries in example 9.3.2. If they are arranged in order, the mean of the two middle numbers, 57, is the median of these entries:

40, 42, 45, 48, <u>54</u>, <u>60</u>, 62, 64, 68, 70

$$\tilde{x} = \frac{54 + 60}{2} = 57$$

The **median** can therefore be defined as the middle number of a set of numerical entries. It is indicated by $\tilde{x}$. Its **position** can be found by the formula

$$P = \frac{n + 1}{2},$$

where P is the position of the median and n is the number of entries.

Suppose that the median income for all allied health professionals in the United States is $24,500 per year. This means that there are exactly as many allied health professionals making less than $24,500 per year as there are making more than $24,500 per year.

EXAMPLE 9.3.3

Find the median income for the following seven respiratory therapists' annual salaries:

$29,500	$28,000
$32,300	$30,500
$34,000	$28,500
$38,000	

Solution

$28,000
$28,500
$29,500
<u>$30,500</u>
$32,300
$34,000
$38,000

$\tilde{x}$ = $30,500

Comments

Arrange the salaries from smallest to largest.

Since there is an odd number (seven) of entries, the middle number is the median income.

EXAMPLE 9.3.4

Find the median height for the following eight hospital outpatients:

70 inches	62 inches	74 inches	58 inches
69 inches	72 inches	66 inches	63 inches

Solution

58 inches
62 inches
63 inches
<u>66</u> inches
<u>69</u> inches
70 inches
72 inches
74 inches

$$\tilde{x} = \frac{66 \text{ inches} + 69 \text{ inches}}{2} = 67.5 \text{ inches}$$

Comments

Arrange the heights from smallest to largest.

Since there are an even number (eight) of entries, the mean of the two middle numbers is the median height.

If there are an even number of entries and the two middle numbers are equal, then this value is the median.

EXAMPLE 9.3.5

Find the median temperature for the following readings:

98.6°F	99.0°F	99.2°F
99.2°F	100.2°F	101.0°F

Solution

98.6°F
99.0°F
99.2°F The two middle
99.2°F temperatures
100.2°F are equal.
101.0°F

$\tilde{x} = 99.2°F$

Comments

Arrange the numbers in order.

Since the two middle values are equal to 99.2°F, this is the median temperature.

Mode. The last measure of central tendency is called the mode. The **mode** is the *single* most frequently occurring value in the data. The word "single" here is important. The mode is *one* value that appears with the greatest frequency.

For example, the mode for the following set of values is 27, since it is the single number with the greatest frequency:

22, 23, 27, 27, 27, 28, 28, 30

If two or more numbers appear with the same frequency and this frequency is greater than all other frequencies, then the data are said to be **bimodal** or **multimodal**.

For example, the following set of numbers is bimodal since 98.6 and 99 both have the same frequency, which is greater than the other frequencies:

98, 98.6, 98.6, 98.6, 99, 99, 99, 99.5, 100, 100.5, 100.5, 102

PROBLEM SET 1

Find the mean, median, and mode (if it exists) for each of the sets of data in problems 1–5.

1. The laboratory expenses per patient per day reported by six private physicians were \$32, \$38, \$40, \$45, \$50, and \$40.
2. The diastolic blood pressures of eight patients were 80, 82, 82, 82, 90, 90, 90, and 92.
3. The heights (to the nearest inch) of ten junior high girls were 60, 62, 63, 66, 63, 64, 68, 70, 58, and 60.
4. The numbers of cases of hepatitis reported by five outpatient clinics were 8, 6, 7, 10, and 10.
5. The weight gains (in kilograms) in 1 month for 12 people were 2.4, 3.1, 3.2, 3.5, 3.5, 4.0, 4.1, 4.2, 4.3, 4.5, 4.5, and 4.5.
6. Which measure of central tendency sometimes does not exist?
7. Can the mean equal the median, the mode, or both? Gives examples.
8. Consider the following list of health professionals' salaries: 14,500, 15,000, 12,000, 13,000, 15,500, 19,000, 92,500, 50,000, 65,000, 80,000, and 75,000. Which measure of central tendency is a more "accurate reflector" of these data? Why?

Answers to odd-numbered problems appear on page 238.

9.4 MEASURES OF DISPERSION: RANGE AND STANDARD DEVIATION

Suppose the mean recovery time for three patients on one medication was 5 days. Suppose that the mean recovery time for three patients on another type of medication was also 5 days.

If we look strictly at the means, we may conclude that each medication is equally effective. However, a closer look at the data reveals that the recovery times were as follows:

Medication A	**Medication B**
Patient *X*—4 days	Patient *P*—1 day
Patient *Y*—5 days	Patient *Q*—5 days
Patient *Z*—6 days	Patient *R*—9 days

Notice that although the mean and median recovery times are the same, there is a wider variation in the recovery time for medication B.

One measure of the variation in a set of data is called the range. The **range** is defined as the difference between the highest and lowest score in a set of data:

$$\text{Range} = H - L$$

where H represents the highest data score and L represents the lowest data score.

Even though the mean recovery times are the same for both medications, the recovery time for medication A ranges over a 2-day period while the recovery time for medication B ranges over a 9-day period. This could possibly indicate a significant difference in the medications that the mean, median, or mode recovery times would not show.

Another measure of variation or spread in the data is given by the standard deviation. The **standard deviation** may be thought of as an indicator of how widely numerical data are dispersed about the mean. In other words, the standard deviation is an indicator of how much each score differs from the mean.

Suppose you and a friend are in two different sections of the same course. On the first test you receive a score of 80 where the class mean is 72 and the standard deviation is 4. Your friend receives an 84. The mean in his class is 80 with a standard deviation of 2. Your score is 2 standard deviations above the mean in your class. (One standard deviation in your class is 4 points.) Your friend's score is also 2 standard deviations above the mean in his class. (One standard deviation in his class is 2 points.) Although his score is higher than yours, you are each competing equally well within your respective classes, assuming the tests were of comparable difficulty.

The standard deviation not only provides vital information about the dispersion or spread of scores, but as shown above, it also provides a way to make meaningful comparisons of different sets of data.

The standard deviation for a sample set of data, indicated by s, is defined as follows:

$$s = \sqrt{\frac{(x_1 - \bar{x})^2 + (x_2 - \bar{x})^2 + \cdots + (x_n - \bar{x})^2}{n - 1}}$$

The formula is interpreted as follows:

Step 1. Subtract the mean from each item of data.
Step 2. Square each of these differences.
Step 3. Add these squares.
Step 4. Divide this sum by the number of entries minus one. This number, in square units, is called the **variance** of the data.
Step 5. Take the square root of this quotient. This is done so that the standard deviation will have the same units as the data. The standard deviation is the square root of the variance calculated in step 4.

Remember to round off your final number to one more decimal place than your data. For example, if your data are reported in whole numbers, round the standard deviation to the nearest tenth.

EXAMPLE 9.4.1

Find the standard deviation for the following set of numbers: 72, 70, 71, 74, 73, 78.

Solution	**Comments**
$\bar{x} = \dfrac{72 + 70 + 71 + 74 + 73 + 78}{6}$ $= 73$	Find the mean.
$(72 - 73)^2 = (-1)^2 = 1$ $(70 - 73)^2 = (-3)^2 = 9$ $(71 - 73)^2 = (-2)^2 = 4$ $(74 - 73)^2 = (1)^2 = 1$ $(73 - 73)^2 = 0^2 = 0$ $(78 - 73)^2 = 5^2 = 25$	Subtract each piece of data from the mean and square the difference.
$= 40$	Find the sum of these squares.
$\dfrac{40}{5} = 8$	Divide this sum by 5, the number of entries minus one.
$s = \sqrt{8} = 2.8$	Take the square root of this quotient. Round off.

A standard deviation of 2.8 indicates that the numerical entries in these data occur close to the mean of 73. That is to say that most of the scores are "packed somewhat tightly" about the mean.

Another set of data could have the same mean, 73, but a higher standard deviation. The scores in this set of data would be more widely dispersed about 73.

Suppose a physician can prescribe the two medications discussed at the beginning of this section. Assuming that all other factors are equal, he would probably prescribe medication A because its effect would be more predictable, that is, there would be less variation in patients' recovery times. One can more fully understand this, however, by examining the standard deviation of recovery times.

As a further example of standard deviation, consider the normal distribution. A set of data is said to be **normally distributed** if approximately 68% of the data lie within *one* standard deviation of the mean, approximately 95% of the data lie within *two* standard deviations of the mean, and approximately 99.7% of the data lie within *three* standard deviations of the mean. The normal distribution is shown graphically below.

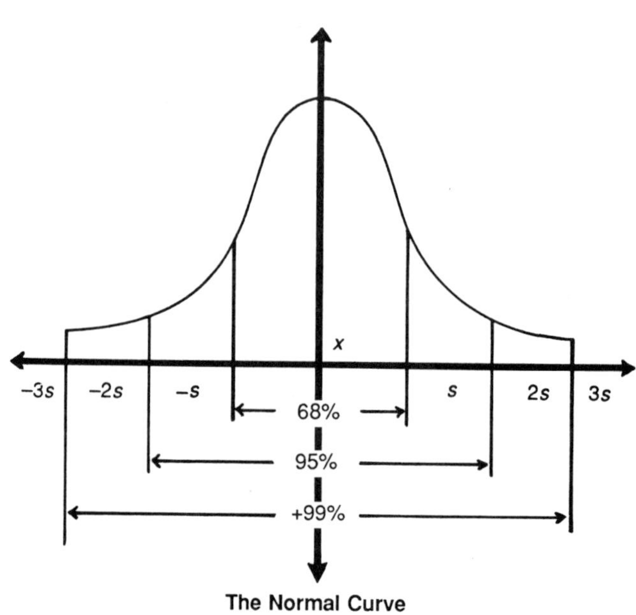

The Normal Curve

Suppose a group of patients with the same disease were divided into two groups. Group 1 takes medication A and group 2 takes medication B. Suppose that the recovery times for patients in group 1 were normally distributed with a mean of 15 days and a standard deviation of 4 days. This means that approximately 99.7% of these patients recovered within 12 days of the mean time of 15 days, since 12 days represent 3 standard deviations, that is, $3 \cdot 4$ days $= 12$ days. Therefore approximately 99.7% of these patients took between 3 $(15 - 12)$ and 27 $(15 + 12)$ days to recover.

If the recovery times for patients in group 2 were normally distributed with the same mean of 15 days, but a different standard deviation of 2 days, then approximately 99.7% of these patients took between 9 $(15 - 6)$ and 21 $(15 + 6)$ days to recover. This is a smaller interval and may indicate that mediation B (group 2) is more reliable. These results are summarized in the following table:

	Mean	Standard Deviation	Recovery Time Intervals (%) 68%	95%	99.7%
Group 1	15 days (d)	4 d	11–19 d	7–23 d	3–27 d
Group 2	15 d	2 d	13–17 d	11–19 d	9–21 d

Even though both groups have the same mean recovery time, the group with the higher standard deviation had recovery times more widely dispersed about the mean.

This example shows that the standard deviation provides essential information concerning the data that the mean, median, and mode do not.

Suppose that we wish to compare an individual in group 1 with an individual in group 2 relative to how well each is responding to his medication. This is done by using the **z score** or **standard score** (z), which is defined as follows:

$$z = \frac{x - \overline{x}}{s}$$

where x is a selected item of data, $\overline{x}$ is the mean of the data, and s is the standard deviation.

This formula will indicate how many standard deviations a particular value of the data is above or below the mean. A negative z score will indicate that a score is that many standard deviations below the mean, and a positive z score indicates that a score is that many standard deviations above the mean.

EXAMPLE 9.4.2

Using the data in the table above, find the z scores for **a.** a patient in group 1 who had a recovery time of 17 days, and **b.** a patient in group 2 who also had a recovery time of 17 days.

Solution

a. $z = \dfrac{x - \overline{x}}{s}$

$z = \dfrac{17 - 15}{4}$

$z = \dfrac{2}{4} = \dfrac{1}{2} = 0.5$

b. $z = \dfrac{17 - 15}{2}$

$z = \dfrac{2}{2} = 1$

Comments

a. For a patient in group 1, $x = 17$, $\overline{x} = 15$, and $s = 4$.

This patient's recovery time is 0.5 standard deviations above the mean of the group.

b. For a patient in group 2, $x = 17$, $\overline{x} = 15$, and $s = 2$.

This patient's recovery time is 1 standard deviation above the mean of the group.

The higher z score for the patient in group 2 indicates that, relative to the group, the patient is taking longer to respond to medication than the patient in group 1 is responding relative to that group.

The z score is a means of comparing individual scores in different data groups relative to their standing within those respective groups.

There are many uses of the standard deviation that are beyond the scope of this text. Our purpose here is to point out that the mean, median, and mode do not offer a complete picture of numerical data, and to offer a brief introduction to the concepts of standard deviation, variance, and normality.

PROBLEM SET 2

1–5. Find the standard deviation for the numerical data given in problems 1–5 in problem set 1.

6. Give an example of two sets of data where the means are the same, but the standard deviations are different. What are the implications of these different standard deviations?

7. Which is more "deviant"—a score of 70 where the mean is 60 and the standard deviation is 10 or a score of 75 where the mean is 66 and the standard deviation is 2? (*Hint*: use z scores.)

8. Who has a lower relative pulse rate—a patient with a pulse of 84 from a group with a mean pulse rate of 76 and a standard deviation of 8, or a patient with a pulse of 84 from a group with a mean pulse rate of 72 with a standard deviation of 10.5?

Answers to odd-numbered problems appear on page 238.

9.5 FREQUENCY TABLES AND FREQUENCY POLYGONS

Sometimes certain numerical values occur with frequencies greater than 1. We illustrate this situation with a **frequency table**.

EXAMPLE 9.5.1

Make a frequency table for the following set of data: 5, 5, 6, 7, 7, 8, 8, 8, 9, 10, 11, 11, 12, 12, 14, 15, 15, 15, 15, 15, 20, 20.

Solution

Entry	*Frequency*
5	2
6	1
7	2
8	3
9	1
10	1
11	2
12	2
14	1
15	5
20	2
	22

Comments

Arrange the *different* numbers in order. Under the frequency column, write the number of times it occurs.

The sum of the frequency column should equal the total number of individual entries.

If one wishes to look at the above data graphically, a **frequency polygon** can be constructed as follows: Let the horizontal axis represent the numbers in the data. The vertical axis will represent the frequency with which each entry occurs. For example, as shown in the figure below, if 5 occurs twice, we plot the point (5,2): the first coordinate represents the score and the second coordinate represents its frequency.

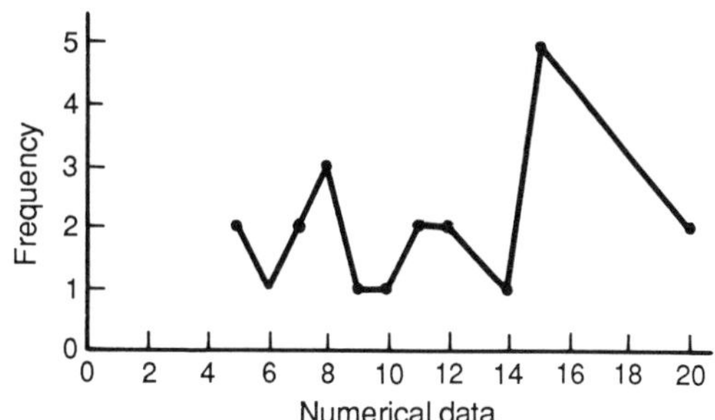

Finally, we connect the plotted points with a series of line segments. With this broken line segment, we can quickly see where the frequencies occur and possibly spot trends in the data.

To review all the ideas expressed so far in this chapter, consider the following example.

EXAMPLE 9.5.2

Given the following weights (in pounds) of twenty 6-year-old children—40, 40, 40, 44, 44, 46, 52, 52, 60, 52, 58, 60, 50, 52, 42, 43, 45, 45, 45, 44—find the mean, median, mode, and standard deviation. Construct a frequency table and a frequency polygon for these data.

Solution

Entries		*Frequencies*		
40	·	3	=	120
42	·	1	=	42
43	·	1	=	43
44	·	2	=	88
45	·	4	=	180
46	·	1	=	46
50	·	1	=	50
52	·	4	=	208
58	·	1	=	58
60	·	2	=	120
		20		960

Comments

Calculations will be easier if the data are first arranged in a frequency table.

$$\bar{x} = \frac{960}{20} = 48$$

To calculate the mean from a frequency table, form a third column containing the product of each entry and its frequency. Find the sum of this column and divide it by the number of entries. (In this case, it is 20.)

$$P = \frac{20 + 1}{2} = 10.5$$

$$\tilde{x} = 45$$

The position of the median is halfway between the 10th and 11th scores. Checking the table, the 10th score from the top is 45 and the 11th score is 45; so the median is 45.

Bimodal

It is bimodal since there are *two* scores tied with the greatest number of frequencies.

$$(40 - 48)^2 \cdot 3 = 192$$
$$(42 - 48)^2 \cdot 1 = 36$$
$$(43 - 48)^2 \cdot 1 = 25$$
$$(44 - 48)^2 \cdot 2 = 32$$
$$(45 - 48)^2 \cdot 4 = 36$$
$$(46 - 48)^2 \cdot 1 = 4$$
$$(50 - 48)^2 \cdot 1 = 4$$
$$(52 - 48)^2 \cdot 1 = 64$$

To calculate the standard deviation, find the difference between each score and the mean, square each difference, and multiply it by the frequency of the score. By using a frequency table, we need to calculate the square of the difference between a score and the mean only once, regardless of how often that particular score occurs.

$(58 - 48)^2 \cdot 1 = 100$
$(60 - 48)^2 \cdot 2 = \underline{8}$
501

We then multiply this value by the frequency with which a particular score occurs.

$$s = \sqrt{\frac{501}{19}} = \sqrt{26.37} = 5.1$$

Find the sum of these products, divide by 10, and take the square root of this quotient. Round off your answer.

The frequency polygon can be constructed as follows: Let the horizontal axis represent the weights and the vertical axis represent the frequency of each weight. Notice that the horizontal scale begins at 40 since there are no weights below this value.

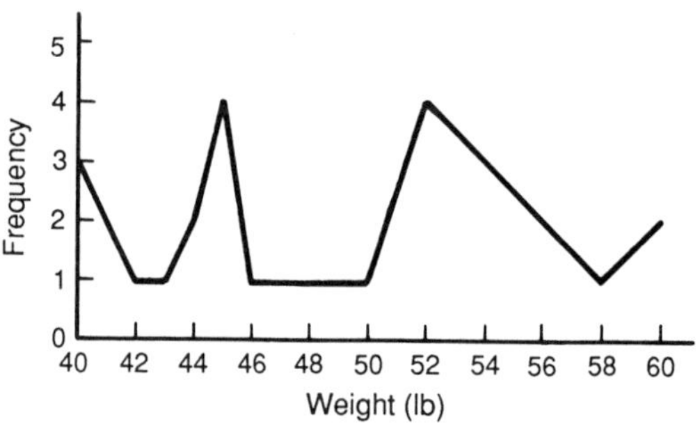

PROBLEM SET 3

1–5. Make a frequency table and construct a frequency polygon for the numerical data in problems 1–5 in problem set 1.

6. Construct a frequency polygon from each of the following frequency tables:

Length of Physical Therapy (days)	Frequency
20	2
24	5
25	4
28	1
30	2

Chloresterol Readings (for Cardiac Patients) (mg/dL)	Frequency
250	5
260	6
282	10
300	4
350	8
380	2

7. Find the mean, median, mode, and standard deviation for the numerical data in both parts of problem 6.

Answers to odd-numbered problems appear on page 238.

9.6 GROUPED FREQUENCY DISTRIBUTION

When there are a large number of values (usually 20 or more) in a sample, it is often more convenient to arrange the scores into a **grouped frequency distribution.** To do this, the researcher places the values in intervals of equal width. The number of intervals, called **classes**, is usually between 4 and 12 and the **class width** should be an odd number.

EXAMPLE 9.6.1

Arrange this data given by the following weights (lb) of 25 male cardiac patients into a grouped frequency distribution:

140	164	173	185	204
146	166	175	185	206
150	168	176	185	210
158	168	180	190	215
160	170	180	196	215

Solution	Comments
Range = 215 − 140 = 75	*Step 1:* Find the range of the data.
$7 \cdot 11 = 77$	*Step 2:* Find a number slightly larger than the range that has two factors somewhat close together, at least one of which should be odd. This number can vary (such as $6 \cdot 13 = 78$, or $9 \cdot 9 = 81$).
140–150 151–161 162–172 173–183 184–194 195–205 206–216	*Step 3:* Arrange data into seven intervals where the difference between the smallest number in one interval and the smallest number in the next interval is equal to 11. These intervals are called classes and this constant difference is called class width.

	Patients
140–150	3
151–161	2
162–172	5
173–183	5
184–194	4
195–205	2
206–216	4

Step 4: Indicate the frequency (how many patients) in each class.

Note that we could have also arranged the data into 11 classes with a class width of 7, or 6 classes with a class width of 13, or 9 classes with a class width of 9. It is up to the student to determine the class size and width within the guidelines of step 2. We further recommend that there be between 4 and 12 classes, and that the class width should always be odd.

The smallest and largest numbers in each class are called the **class limits**, for example 140 and 150 are the lower and upper limits, respectively, of the first class in example 9.6.1. If the class limits are added and divided by two, the **class mark** is obtained: The class mark is, therefore, the mean of the class limits.

$$\text{Class mark } (X) = \frac{\text{Lower limit} + \text{upper limit}}{2}$$

This number, indicated by X, is used extensively to find the mean and standard deviation of a grouped frequency distribution. The class mark will represent every number in a class.

EXAMPLE 9.6.2

Find the class limits and class mark for the class 140–150 in example 9.6.1.

Solution	Comments
Lower class limit = 140 Upper class limit = 150	Definition of class limits.

$$X = \frac{140 + 150}{2} = 145$$

Definition of class mark.

There were three weights (140, 146, 150) in the table in example 9.6.2 that fell into the first class (140–150). They will now be equal to the class mark, 145.

To find the mean and standard deviation of a grouped frequency distribution, we use the following formulas:

Mean of a grouped frequency distribution:

$$\bar{x} = \frac{\sum Xf}{\sum f}$$

where $\sum Xf$ is the sum of the products of each class mark and its frequency and $\sum f$ is the sum of the frequencies. $\sum f$ should be equal to the total number of original values (25 weights).

Standard deviation of a grouped frequency distribution:

$$s = \sqrt{\frac{\sum X^2 f - \frac{(\sum Xf)^2}{n}}{n - 1}}$$

where $\sum X^2 f$ is the sum of the products of the squares of the class marks and their frequency, $(\sum Xf)^2$ is the square of the sum of the products of the class marks and their frequencies, and n is the sum of the frequencies, $\sum f$.

The table in example 9.6.3 is an extension of the table in example 9.6.1 and consists of information that will be necessary to calculate the mean and standard deviation of the grouped frequency distribution.

EXAMPLE 9.6.3

Find the mean of the grouped frequency distribution in the following table:

x	f	X	Xf	X^2	X^2f
140–150	3	145	435	21,025	63,075
151–161	2	156	312	24,336	48,672
162–172	5	167	835	27,889	139,445
163–173	5	178	890	31,684	158,420
184–194	4	189	756	35,721	142,884
195–205	2	200	400	40,000	80,000
206–216	4	211	844	44,521	178,084
	$\sum f = 25$	$\sum X = 1246$	$\sum Xf = 4472$	$\sum X^2 = 225{,}176$	$\sum X^2 f = 810{,}580$

Solution

$$\bar{x} = \frac{\sum Xf}{\sum f}$$

$$\bar{x} = \frac{4472}{25}$$

$$\bar{x} = 178.9 \text{ lb}$$

Comments

Definition of mean of grouped frequency distribution.

Substitute values from the table into formula and calculate.

This is the mean weight of grouped frequency distribution for the 25 male cardiac patients given in the table above.

EXAMPLE 9.6.4

Find the standard deviation of the grouped frequency distribution in the table in example 9.6.3.

Solution	Comments
$$s = \sqrt{\frac{\sum X^2 f - \frac{(\sum Xf)^2}{n}}{n - 1}}$$	Definition of standard deviation of grouped frequency distribution.
$$s = \sqrt{\frac{810{,}580 - \frac{(4472)^2}{25}}{25 - 1}}$$	Substitute values from the table in example 9.6.3 and calculate.
$$s = \sqrt{\frac{810{,}580 - \frac{19{,}998{,}784}{25}}{24}}$$	
$$s = \sqrt{\frac{810{,}580 - 799{,}951}{24}}$$	
$s = 21$	This is the standard deviation of the grouped frequency distribution for the 25 male cardiac given in the table in example 9.6.3.

EXAMPLE 9.6.5

Find the median and the mode of the weights of the 25 cardiac patients in the table in example 9.6.1.

Solution	Comments
$$P = \frac{n + 1}{2}$$	Definition of the position of the median.
$$P = \frac{25 + 1}{2}$$	There are 25 weights. Substitute into position formula.
$P = 13$ $\tilde{x} = 176$ lb	The median weight is the 13th weight counting from the smallest in the table in example 9.6.1 (i.e., beginning with 140 lb).
mode = 185 lb	The weight that occurs most frequently is 185 lb.

PROBLEM SET 4

1. A control group of college females had the following set of diastolic blood pressure readings:

62	72	76	86	99
64	74	78	88	99
66	74	78	88	100
66	76	78	88	102
68	76	80	90	104
70	76	82	94	106

a. Arrange these data into a grouped frequency distribution and find its

b. Mean

c. Mode

d. Range

e. Standard deviation

2. A control group of ironworkers had the following set of cholesterol levels:

173	258	175	172	306
262	280	176	370	300
150	225	280	315	290
120	220	296	345	185
122	220	310	242	170
122	226	330	222	176
126	230	342	234	162
315	186	316	188	310
128	183	154	138	144
130	160	154	210	328

a. Arrange these data into a grouped frequency distribution and find its:

b. Mean

c. Median

d. Mode

e. Range

f. Standard deviation

(*Hint*: First arrange data in numerical order.)

Answers to odd-numbered problems appear on page 239.

9.7 CONSTRUCTING FREQUENCY HISTOGRAMS

We can graphically depict the data from the grouped frequency distribution given in Section 9.6. To do this, we utilize the **class boundaries**, which are the class limits extended by one half of a unit. For example, the class boundaries for the first class of weights depicted in example 9.6.1 (140–150 lb) would be 139.5 and 150.5.

The graph of a grouped frequency distribution is called a **histogram** or **bar graph.** It consists of rectangles whose sides coincide with the class boundaries. We let the horizontal axis represent the weights. Along this axis, we mark off the class boundaries. The vertical axis represents the frequencies of each class. The frequency of each class is represented by a rectangle with a width equal to the class width and a height equal to the frequency of that particular class.

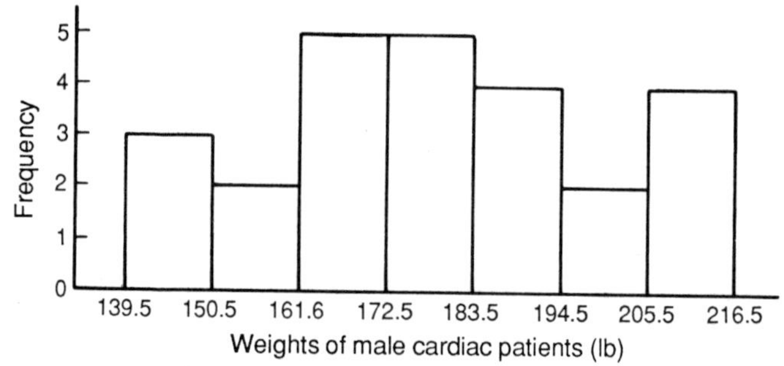

Be sure to label the graph and each axis so that the reader can obtain accurate information at a glance.

PROBLEM SET 5

1. Construct a frequency histogram for the data in problem 1 of problem set 4.
2. Construct a frequency histogram for the data in problem 2 of problem set 4.

Answers to odd-numbered problems appear on page 239.

CHAPTER REVIEW

1. The number of blood tests processed at several rural clinics during a 2-day period were as follows:

   1, 3, 4, 4, 6, 6, 7, 7, 7, 9, 9, 9, 3, 2, 1, 1, 6, 4, 4, 5, 5, 3, 3, 2, 2, 2, 8, 10, 6, 6

   Find the following measures or perform the indicated tasks:

(9.3)
   a. Mean
   b. Median
   c. Mode

(9.4)
   d. Standard deviation

(9.5)
   e. Construct a frequency table.
   f. Construct a frequency polygon.

2. The radiation (in rads) per year for 1000 radiation technologists is given below:

Rads	Frequency
20	250
25	100
26	350
28	180
30	120

(9.3)
   a. Mean
   b. Median
   c. Mode

(9.4)
   d. Standard deviation (*Hint*: Treat as a grouped frequency distribution where the rad numbers are class marks.)

(9.5)
   e. Construct a frequency polygon.

3. Given the following frequency polygon on page 178, find the following measures:

(9.3)
   a. Mean
   b. Median
   c. Mode

(9.4)
   d. Standard deviation

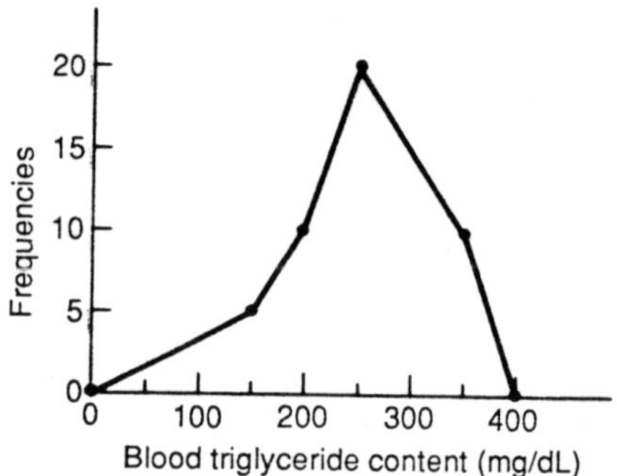

(9.4) 4. Who has a lower relative systolic blood pressure reading: a patient with a reading of 150 from a group with a mean of 140 and a standard deviation of 10, or a patient with a reading of 146 from a group with a mean of 132 and a standard deviation of 6? Compare z scores. Explain your conclusion.

(9.5) 5. Arrange the following set of 50 resting pulse rates of a group of male office workers into a grouped frequency distribution:

49	52	59	63	68	70	76	78	84	89
49	54	59	63	68	70	76	80	84	90
50	54	60	64	68	72	77	81	86	92
50	56	61	66	68	72	77	82	87	94
51	57	62	66	70	72	78	82	89	98

6. For the grouped frequency distribution in problem 5, find the **a.** mean **b.** median **c.** mode **d.** range **e.** standard deviation.

7. Use the information found in problems 5 and 6 above to construct a frequency histogram for the data given in problem 5.

Answers to odd-numbered problems appear on pages 240-241.

chapter **10**

Drawing and Interpreting Graphs

OBJECTIVES

After studying this chapter, the student should be able to:

1. Plot points on the rectangular coordinate system.
2. Graph a linear equation.
3. Given a data table, graph the data in the appropriate format.
4. Draw circle and bar graphs from data provided.
5. Interpret circle graphs, bar graphs, and rectangular coordinate graphs, and draw conclusions from them.

10.1 INTRODUCTION

Often, patterns or trends that occur in a set of raw data are obscured by the sheer volume of the data. The best way to present these patterns or trends is through the use of graphs. In this chapter, we learn to construct and interpret several types of graphs. We begin our discussion with the rectangular coordinate system.

10.2 THE RECTANGULAR COORDINATE SYSTEM

The French mathematician René Descartes is credited with developing a system of graphing points on a plane that is called the **rectangular coordinate system** or **Cartesian coordinate system.** This system utilizes a standard number line as its basic feature:

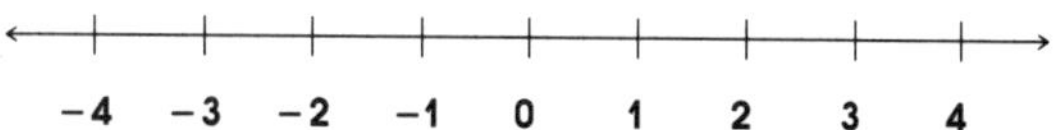

Imagine another number line superimposed at a right angle on the number line shown above, and intersecting it at the point 0. The two number lines thus formed are the basis of the rectangular coordinate system:

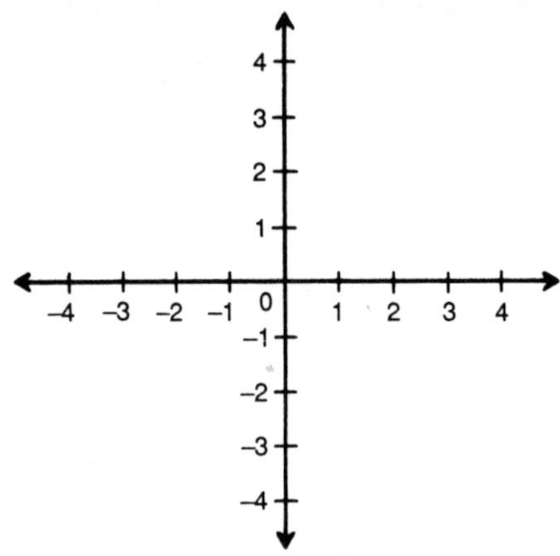

The plane shown above is divided into four **quadrants.** They are numbered with Roman numerals in a counterclockwise direction:

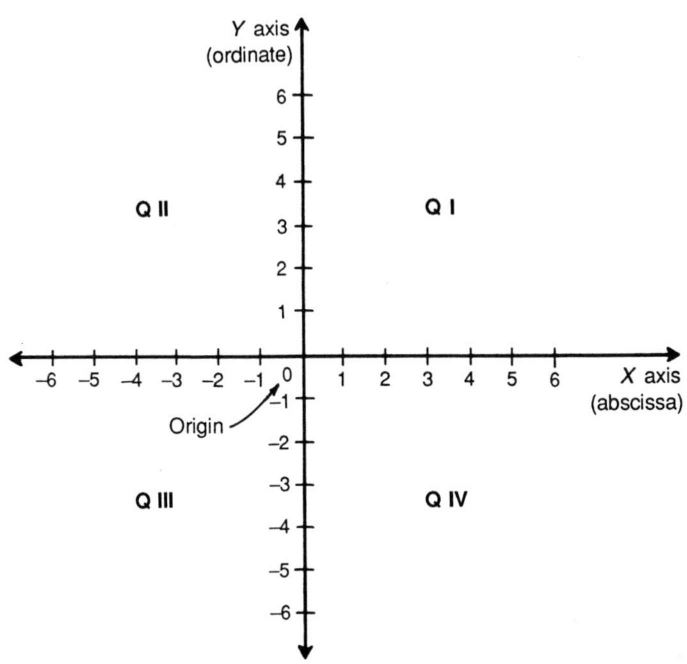

The horizontal number line is called the X axis, or the **abscissa,** and the vertical number line is called the Y axis, or the **ordinate.** The point where the two axes intersect is called the **origin.**

Any point on this plane can be located by the use of an **ordered pair,** which describes the distance of the point to the left or right of the origin on the X axis and then up or down from the origin on the Y axis. The X coordinate is always written first, and the Y coordinate is always written second. The two coordinates are always separated by a comma and placed inside a set of parentheses. The ordered pair (3,2) means that you move 3 units to the right of the origin on the X axis, and 2 units up from the origin on the Y axis:

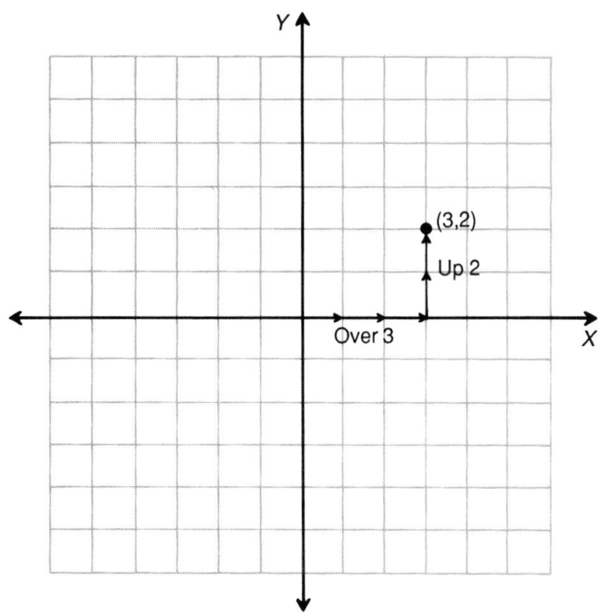

EXAMPLE 10.2.1

Locate the following points on the rectangular coordinate system plane: (4,1); $(-2,3)$; $(-4,-1)$; $(5,-2)$.

Solution

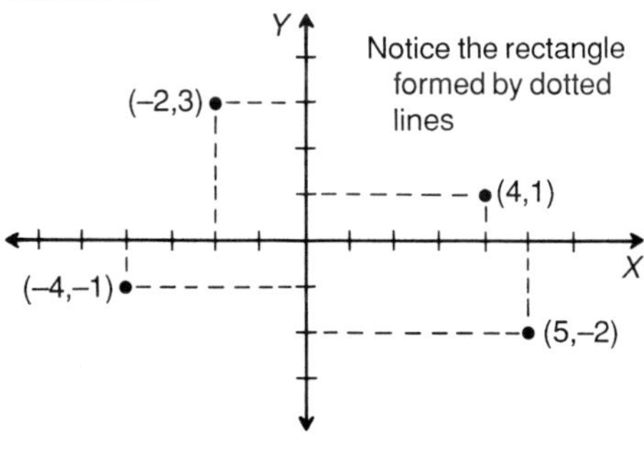

Comments

Since all ordered pairs are in the form (X,Y), locate the X position first, then go up for positive values of the Y coordinate or down for negative values of the Y coordinate.

Note that the point (0,0) is at the origin. Also notice that lines drawn to the point from the respective coordinates make a rectangle with respect to the X and Y axes—hence the term rectangular coordinate system.

EXAMPLE 10.2.2

Find the ordered pairs that correspond to the points on the graph:

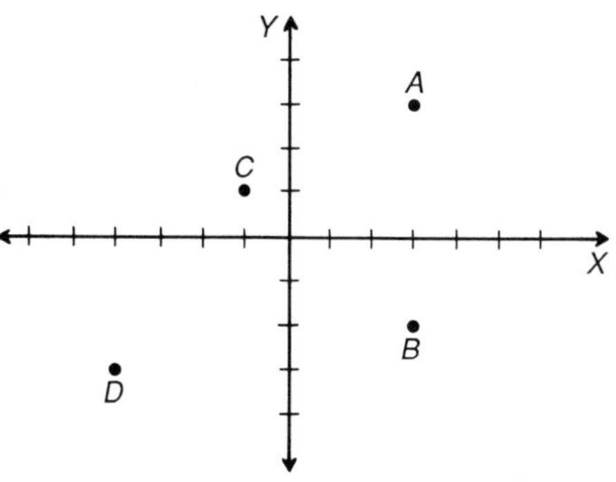

Solution

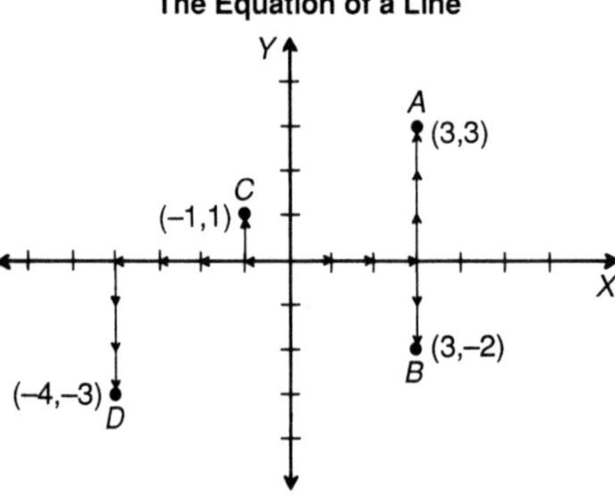

Comments

All points are in the form (X,Y).

Point A: X axis—right 3
Y axis—up 3
(3,3)

Point B: X axis—right 3
Y axis—down 2 (-2)
$(3,-2)$

Point C: X axis—left 1 (-1)
Y axis—up 1
$(-1,1)$

Point D: X axis—left 4 (-4)
Y axis—down 3, (-3)
$(-4,-3)$

The Equation of a Line

If we have an equation in one variable, the equation can have one solution. For example, the equation

$$2x + 4 = 16$$

has the solution

$$x = 6$$

An equation may have two variables, such as the equation

$$y = 2x - 1$$

We cannot solve this equation in the same manner as we solve an equation with only one variable. To solve the equation, we first choose a value for x, and then solve the equation for y. If we let x equal 2, then

$$y = 2x - 1$$

becomes

$$y = 2(2) - 1$$
$$y = 4 - 1$$
$$y = 3$$

The equation has a value for y that corresponds to the value for x. We may write this solution as an ordered pair (x,y). The ordered pair (2,3), then, is a solution to the equation

$$y = 2x - 1$$

There can be an infinite number of solutions to an equation in two variables.

EXAMPLE 10.2.3

Find the ordered pairs that are the solutions of the equation $y = 2x - 1$. Let $x = 0$, 3, and -3.

Solution

$y = 2(0) - 1$
$y = 0 - 1$
$y = -1$

$y = 2(3) - 1$
$y = 6 - 1$
$y = 5$

Comments

Let $x = 0$, and then solve for y. This gives an ordered pair, which is one solution.

Repeat this process for $x = 3$ and $x = -3$.

$$\begin{aligned} y &= 2(-3) - 1 \\ &= -6 - 1 \\ &= -7 \end{aligned}$$

x	y
0	−1
3	5
−3	−7

Make a table for the values of x and y. Let x be the left-hand column and y be the right-hand column.

The solutions are $(0,-1)$, $(3,5)$, and $(-3,-7)$, and $(2,3)$ from the first solution.

Write the solutions as ordered pairs.

Let us see what happens when these ordered pairs are graphed on the rectangular coordinate system:

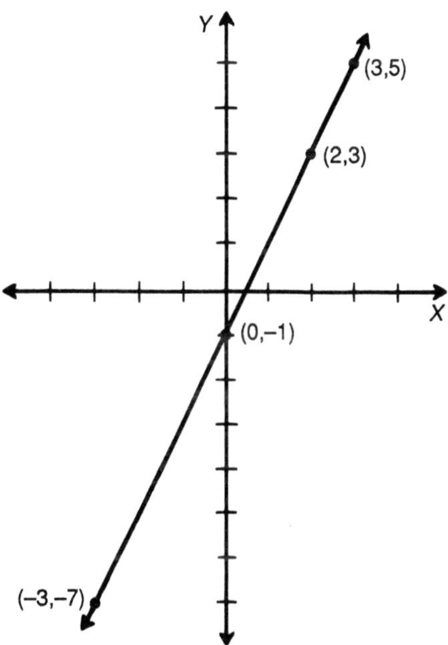

All of the points lie in a straight line. We call the equation $y = 2x - 1$ a **linear equation** because all of the ordered pairs that are solutions to the equation (there are an infinite number) lie in a straight line. The equation $y = 2x - 1$ may be rewritten, by subtracting $2x$ from both sides, as:

$$-2x + y = -1$$

Equations that can be put in the same form as $-2x + y = -1$ are called **linear equations.** These equations may be represented by the general form

$$ax + by = c$$

where a, b, and c are real numbers.

EXAMPLE 10.2.4 Draw a graph of the equation $3x - 2y = 6$. Let $x = 0$, 2, and -3.

Solution

$$\begin{aligned} 3x - 2y &= 6 \\ -2y &= -3x + 6 \\ \frac{-2y}{-2} &= \frac{-3x}{2} + \frac{6}{2} \end{aligned}$$

Comments

You may rewrite the equation by solving for y. This step, while not necessary, may make your work easier.

$$y = -\frac{3}{2}x + 3$$

$$y = -\frac{3}{2}(0) + 3$$

Solve for y when $x = 0$.

$$y = 3$$

$$y = -\frac{3}{2}(2) + 3$$

Solve for y when $x = 2$.

$$y = -3 + 3$$

$$y = 0$$

$$y = -\frac{3}{2}(-3) + 3$$

Solve for y when $x = -3$.

$$y = \frac{9}{2} + 3$$

$$y = \frac{9 + 6}{2}$$

$$y = \frac{15}{2} = 7\frac{1}{2}$$

It is acceptable to have a fractional value of y.

x	y
0	3
2	0
-3	$7\frac{1}{2}$

Make a table for the values of x and y.

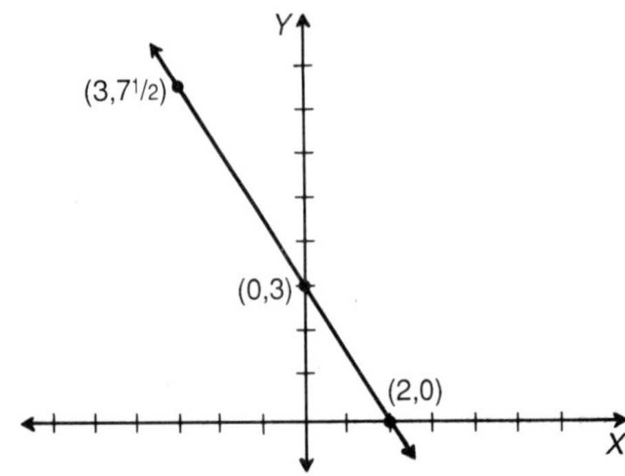

Graph these solutions, and draw a line through the points. If your points do not line up, an error has been made. Recheck your work.

Since two points are all that are necessary to make a line, we can make use of a quick method to graph a simple linear equation. This method is called the **intercept method.** To graph an equation by the intercept method, we do the following:

1. Let $x = 0$, and then solve for y. This gives one point, called the ***y* intercept**.
2. Let $y = 0$, and then solve for x. This gives the second point, called the ***x* intercept**.
3. You may want to let x equal to some different value and find the corresponding value of y. This will give you a check, since all three points must line up.

EXAMPLE 10.2.5 Graph the equation $2x - y = 3$ using the intercept method.

Solution

Comments

$2x - y = 3$

$2(0) - y = 3$

$-y = 3$

$y = -3$

Let $x = 0$, and then solve for y.

$2x - y = 3$
$2x - 0 = 3$
$2x = 3$

$x = \frac{3}{2}$

Let $y = 0$, and then solve for x.

x	y
0	-3
$\frac{3}{2}$	0

Make a table for the values of x and y.

$(0, -3), \left(\frac{3}{2}, 0\right)$

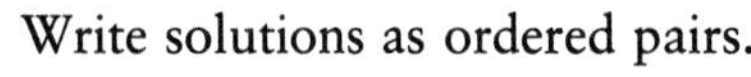

Write solutions as ordered pairs.

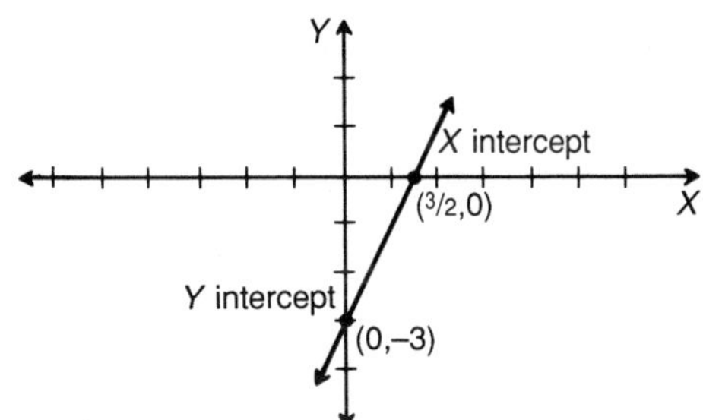

Check by finding a third point;

Graph the points.

You may encounter an equation that has its x intercept and y intercept both at the origin. Such an equation is

$$y = 3x$$

In this equation, since the x and y intercepts are the same, choose another convenient point for x, and find the corresponding value of y.

EXAMPLE 10.2.6 Graph $y = 3x$.

Solution

Comments

$y = 3(0)$
$y = 0$

Let $x = 0$, and solve for y.

$y = 3(2)$
$y = 6$

Let $x = 2$, and solve for y.

x	y
0	0
2	6

Make a table for the values of x and y.

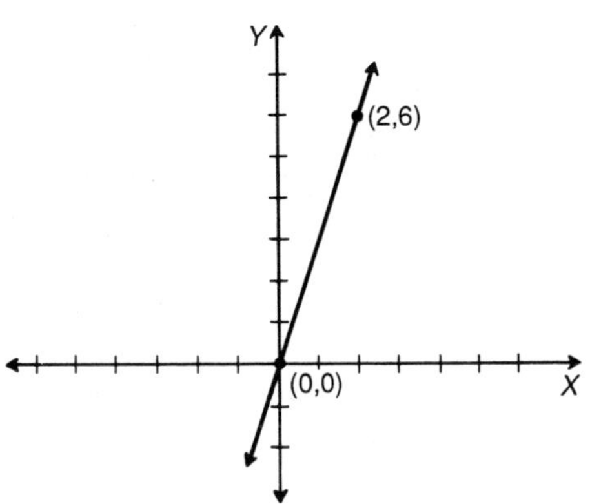

Graph the two ordered pairs [(0,0) and (2,6)]. You may use a third point as a check, if desired.

Sometimes a linear equation will have either the x term or y term missing, such as

$$x = 5 \quad (y \text{ not given})$$

or

$$y = -4 \quad (x \text{ not given}).$$

or, in general,

$$x = h$$

and

$$y = k$$

where h and k are constants.

To graph equations of this type, the variable not given in the equation may be any real number. The intercept method of graphing cannot be used to graph these types of equations since each equation yields only one intercept. The example that follows illustrates the method for graphing equations of this type.

EXAMPLE 10.2.7

Graph a. $x = 5$ b. $y = -4$.

Solution

a.

x	y
5	−1
5	2
5	4

b.

x	y
2	−4
−2	−4
0	−4

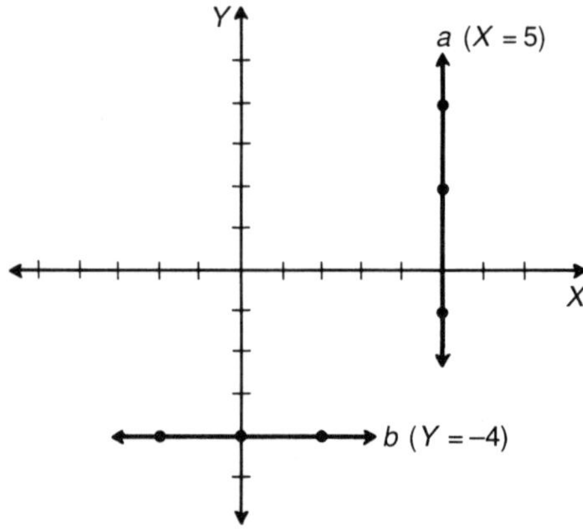

Comments

a. Make a table: x must equal to 5, but y can be any number. Choose small values, such as −1, 2, and 4.

b. Make a table: y must be −4, but x can be any number, such as 2, −2, and 0.

Plot both sets of points on one graph, and compare the resulting lines.

Equations in the form $x = h$ always result in vertical lines, and equations in the form $y = k$ always result in horizontal lines.

PROBLEM SET 1

Determine whether the point given is a solution of the equation.

1. $(4,1)$; $y = 2x + 1$
2. $(0,3)$; $y = -2x - 1$
3. $(-5,0)$; $y = 3x + 15$
4. $(-1,4)$; $2x + 3y = 6$
5. $(6,3)$; $x + 2y = 12$
6. $(1,1)$; $x = y$

Graph the following equation. Use at least three values of x, such as $x = -3, -2, -1, 0, 1, 2$, and so.

7. $y = 2x$
8. $y = -2x$
9. $y = -2x + 1$
10. $y = 2x + 1$
11. $y = \frac{3}{2}x$
12. $y = \frac{3}{2}x + 1$
13. $y = \frac{3}{2}x + 2$
14. $2x + 2y = -2$
15. $3x - 2y = -6$
16. $4x - 3y = 1$
17. $y = 2x + 5$
18. $-y = 2x + 5$
19. $y = \frac{1}{3}x + 3$
20. $y = \frac{1}{3}x - 3$
21. $x + 4y - 3 = 0$
22. $y = x$
23. $y = -x$

Graph using the intercept method. You may check by using a third point.

24. $y = x + 1$
25. $y = -x + 1$
26. $y = -x + 4$
27. $2y = -x + 4$
28. $3y = -x + 4$
29. $2y = -2x + 1$
30. $4x - 3y = 12$
31. $y = -\frac{1}{2}x + \frac{1}{3}$

Answers to odd-numbered problems appear on page 241.

10.3 GRAPHING DATA

A set of data, whether collected by experimentation, surveys, or other types of analyses, can be shown pictorally as a graph. Most graphs are in the first quadrant of the rectangular coordinate system, since most physical quantities are associated with positive numbers:

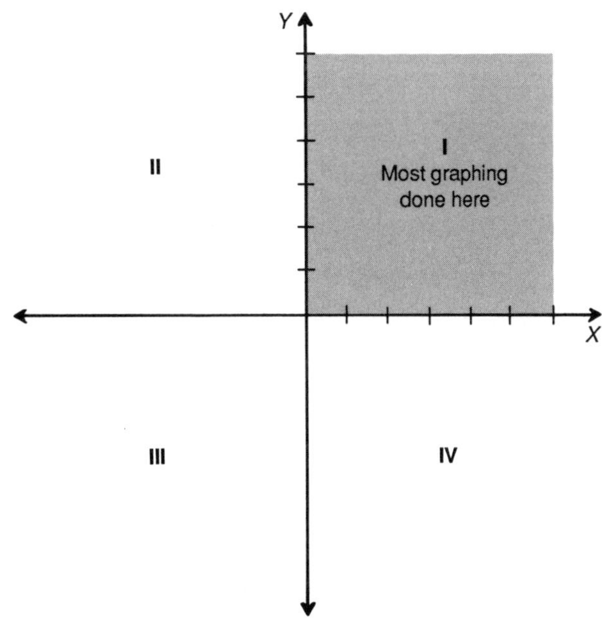

These are a few important points to remember when presenting data on a graph. Make use of them in your work.

Tips on Graphing Correctly

1. Use as much space for the graph as possible. Spread your units on the horizontal and vertical axes as much as possible.

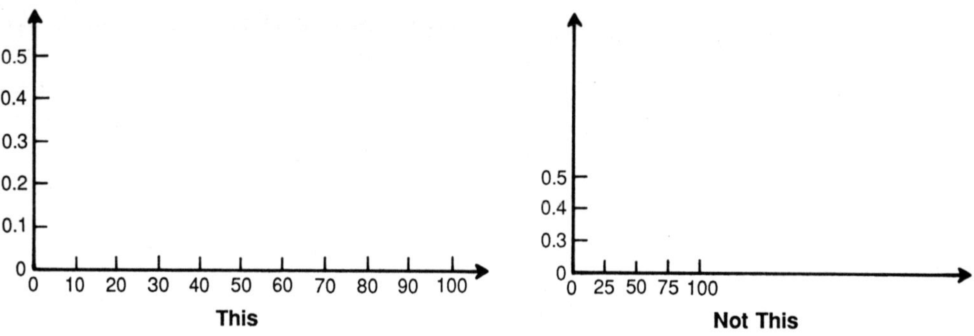

2. Make sure the units on each axis are of uniform width. The horizontal and vertical axes, however, do not have to be uniform with each other:

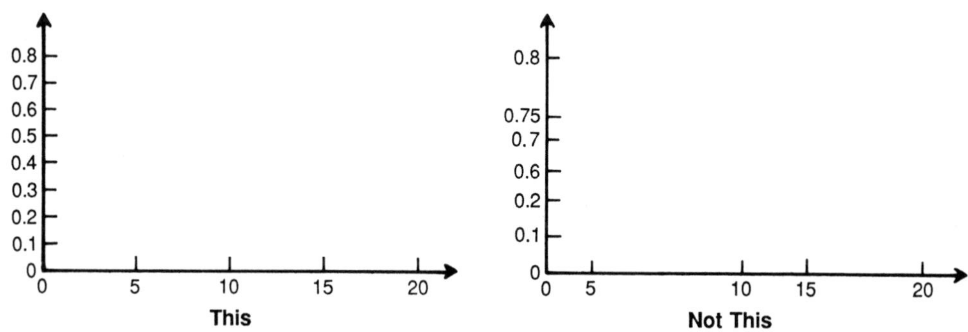

3. Label each axis as to what the axis represents:

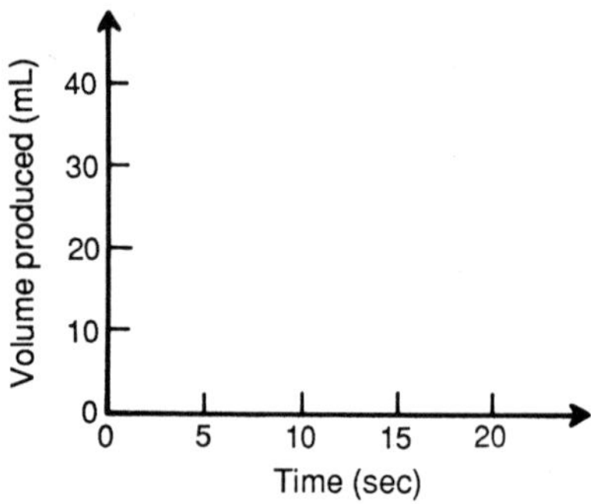

4. Place a title above the graph. The title should indicate what the graph represents:

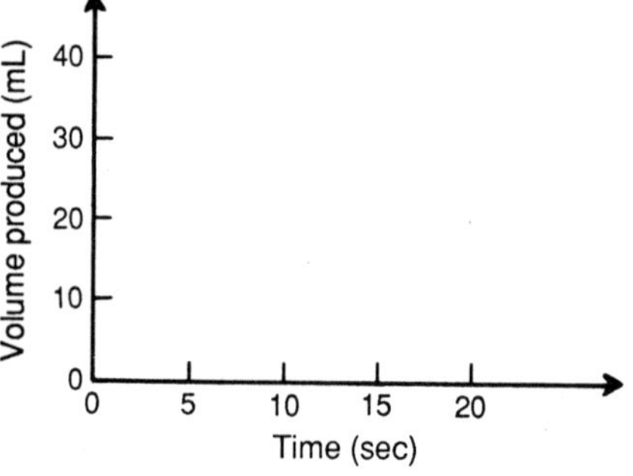

5. The **independent variable** is always placed on the horizontal axis. The independent variable is the quantity that is being changed or purposefully manipulated. The **dependent variable** is placed on the vertical axis. The dependent variable is the value that is altered by manipulation or by changing the independent variable.

   The figure below shows the relationship between distance traveled by a car and time spent traveling. Here, time is the independent variable and distance is the dependent variable.

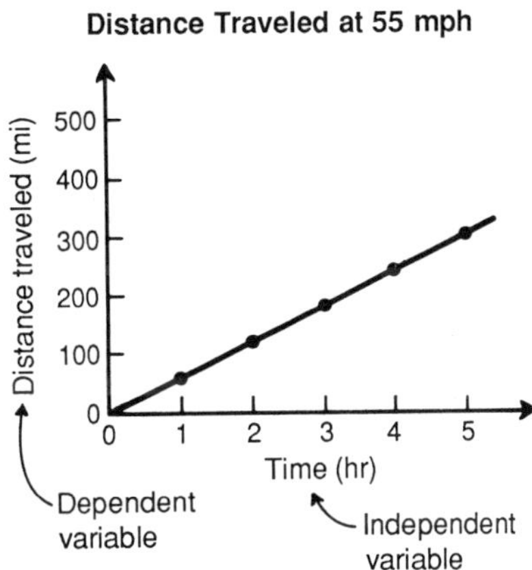

6. Try as best as possible not to *distort* the graph. Generally, begin each axis at zero if this is feasible. To aid in deciding how large each unit on each axis should be, determine the largest numerical value to be shown on the axis, then divide by the number of spaces available on that axis. This will give you the number to be represented by each space. (We will illustrate distortion in an example to follow.)

Continuous and Discrete Data

When data are as precise as is practical, they are said to be **continuous data.** If, however, the collected data contain items that are not numerical (such as the names of elements, companies, diseases, and so on) or that cannot be measured any more precisely (such as a count), then the data are said to be **discrete data.** Examples of each type are shown below.

Continuous data: Time, length, volume, and mass measurements. These can be made as precisely as our instruments allow.

Discrete data: Name of elements, compounds, diseases, automobiles, drugs, and so forth. A count, such as a number of people in a classroom, the number of times an event occurs, the number of births in a country, etc.

To summarize, continuous data are numerical values obtained by measurement, whereas, discrete data are numerical values obtained by a count.

When drawing graphs using continuous data, we usually join the points with a smooth curve. When drawing graphs of discrete data, we join the points with straight lines or use bar graphs.

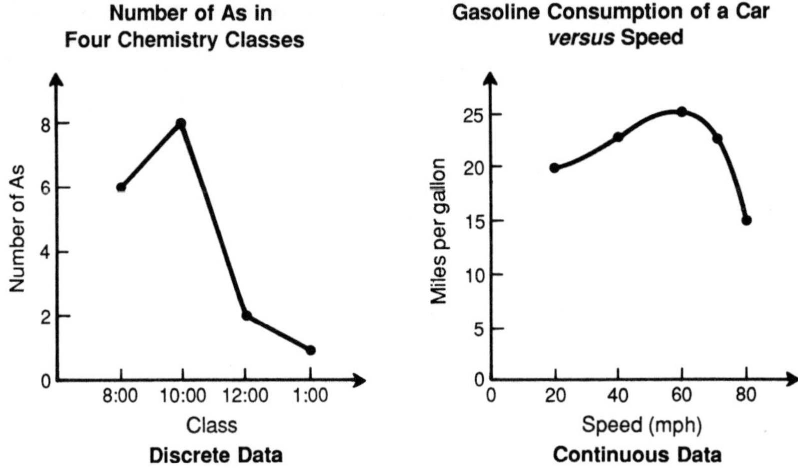

We now apply the material presented thus far to a number of examples.

EXAMPLE 10.3.1

The number of calories required daily by growing boys of various ages can be represented by the following table:

Age	Calories
8	1700
9	1900
10	2100
11	2100
12	2300
13	2500
14	2600
15	2700
16	2700
17	2800

Represent these data in a graph.

Solution

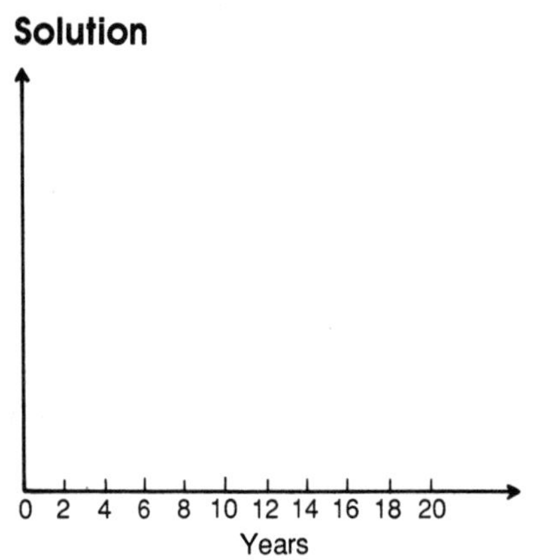

Comments

The horizontal axis represents age. Begin at 0, proceed in steps of 2 up to 20 years. Label that axis.

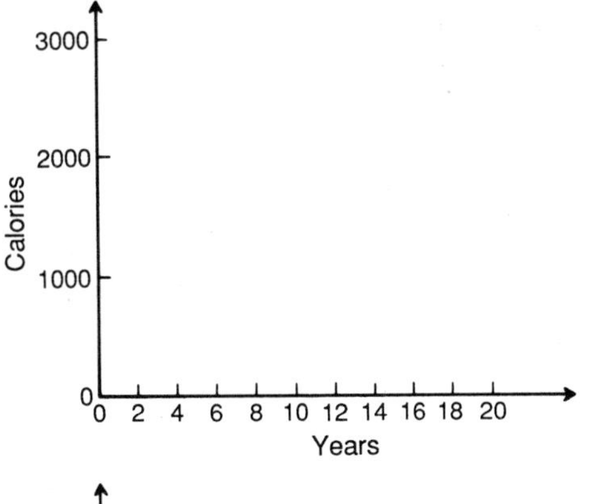

The vertical axis represents calories. Begin at 0 calories, and mark off uniform steps of 1000 until 3000 calories are at the top most part of the vertical axis.

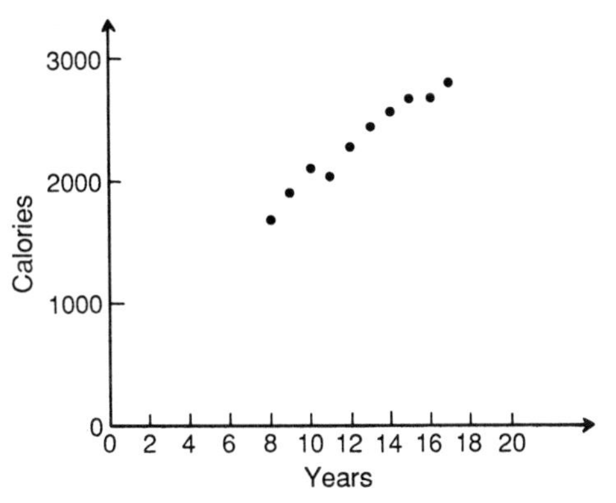

Plot the points from the table. The data are in the form of the ordered pair (age, calories).

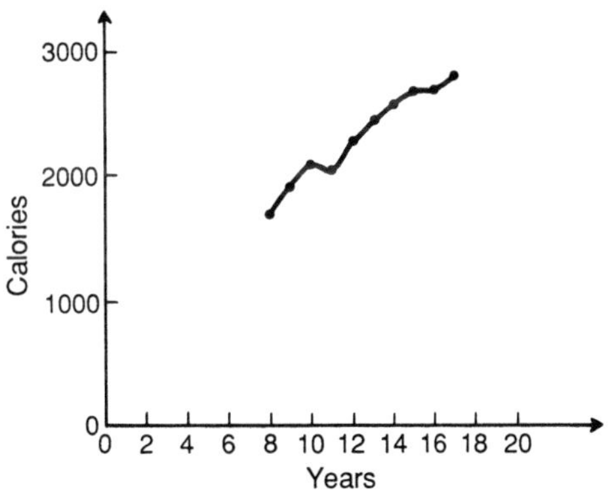

Draw a smooth curve through the points.

The graph in example 10.3.1 contains some empty space near the bottom. We could redraw the graph by beginning the horizontal axis at 5 years and by beginning the vertical axis at 1500 calories, and marking off uniform units to 2000 calories, as is shown below:

Daily Calories Required by Growing Boys *versus* Age

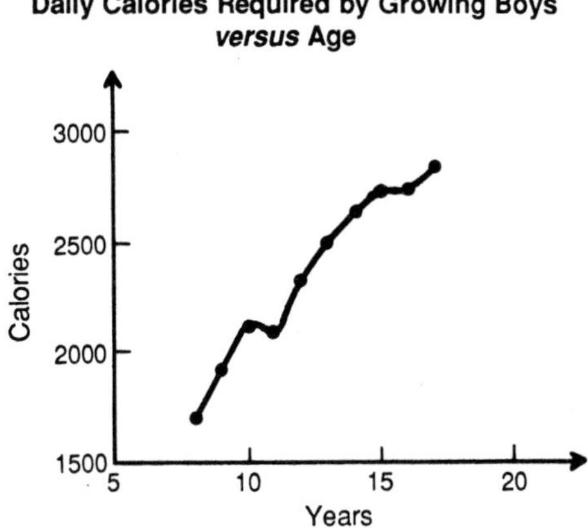

This type of graph can cause a distortion of the data, however. It looks as if the number of calories increases more dramatically than it actually does.

Where it is important to save space and eliminate blank spots, we can use interruption symbols, as is illustrated below:

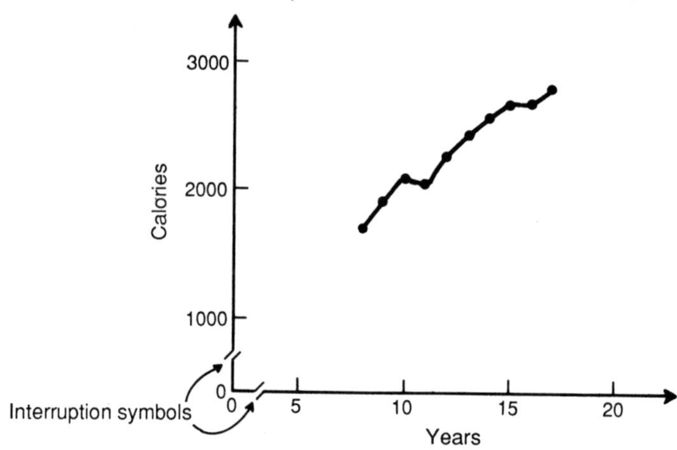

EXAMPLE 10.3.2

A patient ingests 100 g of glucose, and the blood sugar level is checked at 20-minute intervals for 2 hours. The table below summarizes the results. (Normal glucose levels range from 65 to 110 mg/dL.)

Minutes After Ingestion	Glucose Level (mg/dL)
0	110
20	125
40	200
60	240
80	255
100	250
120	240

Represent these data in a graph.

Solution

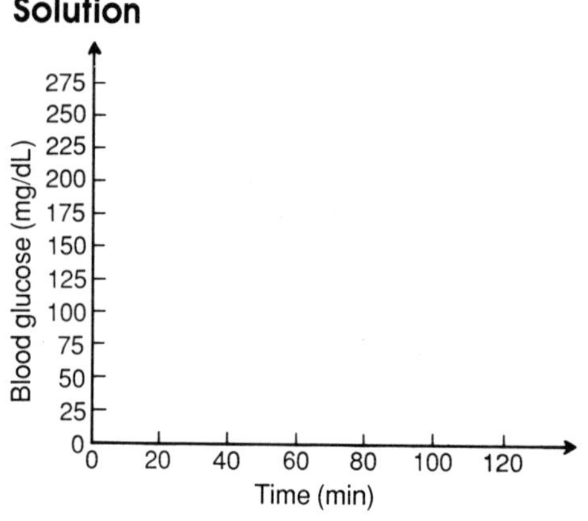

Comments

Time is placed on the horizontal axis—begin at 0 minutes and mark off to 120 in steps of 20 minutes.

The glucose level is placed on the vertical axis. Begin at 0 mg/dL, and mark off in steps of 25 up to at least 275 mg/dL.

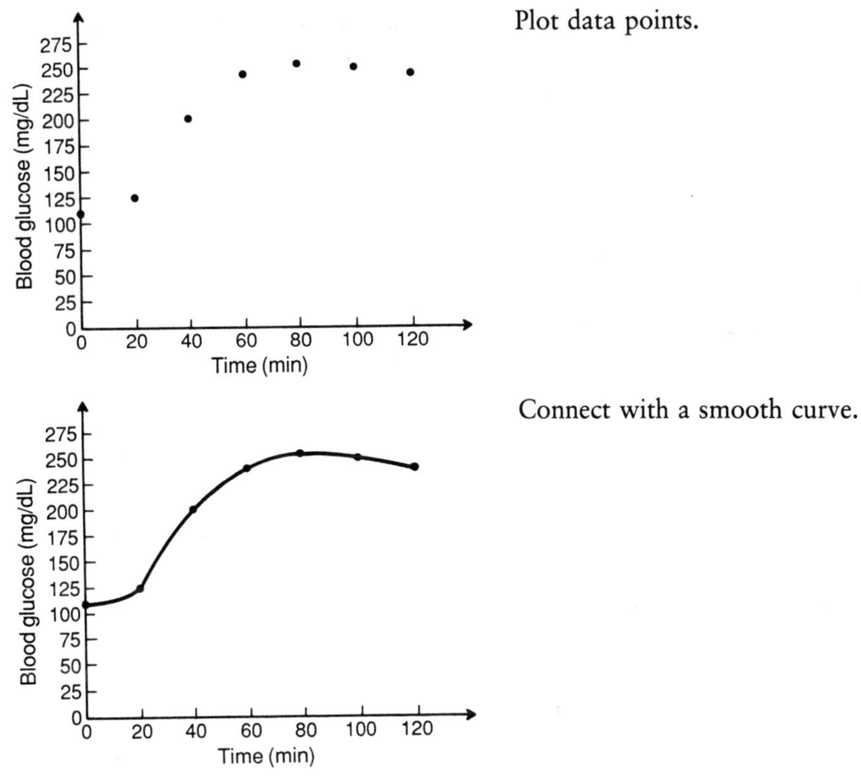

Plot data points.

Connect with a smooth curve.

A second patient was given 100 g of glucose, and had his blood glucose level tested every 20 minutes for 2 hours. The following data were obtained:

Time After Glucose (min)	Glucose Level (mg/dL)
0	80
20	135
40	125
60	98
80	96
100	90
120	85

Let us plot these points on the graph obtained from example 10.3.2:

Blood Glucose *versus* Time for Two Patients

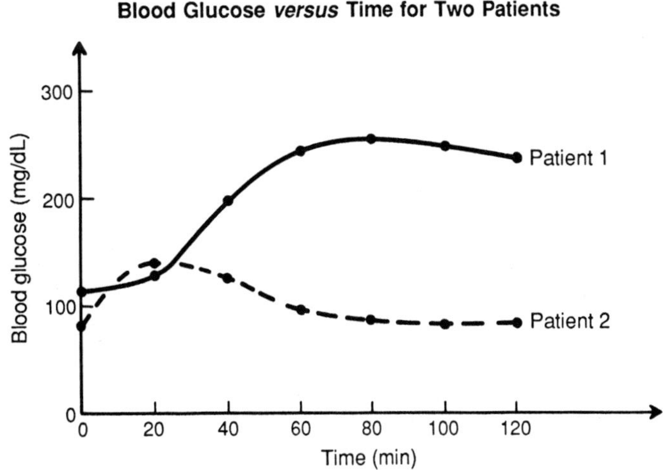

It is easy to make comparisons between the two sets of data by plotting them on the same graph. Be careful, however, to label plainly the two curves either by words or by varying the type of line drawn (solid line, dashes, dots, and so on).

The next example involves an application of spectrophotometry. The concentrations of **standard solutions** are known. If their absorbances are measured with a spectrophotometer and plotted on a graph, a **standard curve** results. Most solutions have absorbances that obey **Beer's law**, which means that, when plotted on a graph, a straight line can be drawn through them.

EXAMPLE 10.3.3 Draw a standard curve for a nickel solution given the following:

Concentration (mol/L)	Absorbance
0.0125	0.076
0.0250	0.145
0.0500	0.281
0.0750	0.419
0.100	0.550

Solution

Comments

Concentration is the independent variable. Place it on the horizontal axis. Place units as far apart as possible. Begin at 0, advance up to 0.1 in steps of 0.01. Label the axis.

Absorbance is placed on the vertical axis. Start at 0 and advance up to 0.6 in steps of 0.1. Label both axes.

Plots points (concentration, absorbence).

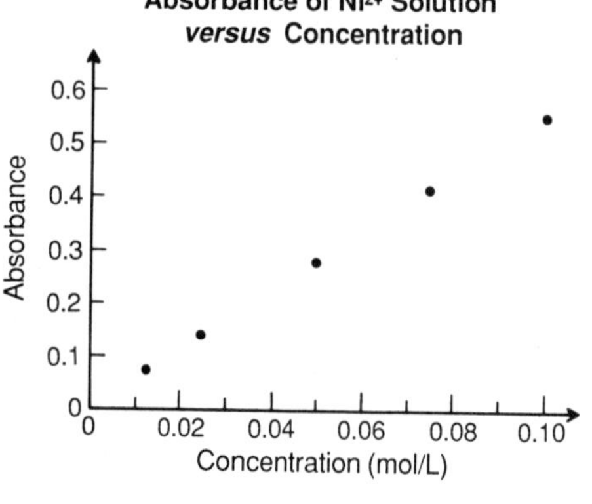

Absorbance of Ni^{2+} Solution *versus* Concentration

Absorbance: 0, 0.1, 0.2, 0.3, 0.4, 0.5, 0.6

0, 0.02, 0.04, 0.06, 0.08, 0.10

Concentration (mol/L)

If the points do not all lie in a straight line, draw a line of best fit. Some of the points should lie below the line, some on the lie, and some above the line. You may use the origin as a point.

EXAMPLE 10.3.4

Assume that a sample of the same solution as in example 10.3.3 with an unknown concentration is placed in the spectrophotometer, and the absorbance is found to be 0.387. Using the standard curve in example 10.3.3, find the concentration of the solution.

Solution

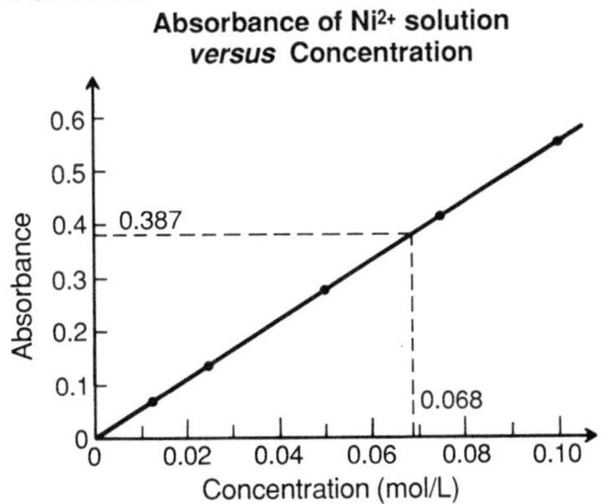

Comments

Using the previous graph, find the absorbance (0.387) along the vertical axis. Draw a dotted line at a right angle from the vertical axis at this point to the line. Drop a line perpendicular to the X axis. The intersection of this line and the X axis gives the concentration of the solution.

Concentration = 0.068 M.

Two Interesting Curves

If we graph the data obtained by manipulating the pressure of a gas and measuring resulting volume, an interesting curve results. This curve is described in the next example.

EXAMPLE 10.3.5

The volume of a sample of gas is related to its pressure by the formula $V = \frac{10 \text{ atm/L}}{P}$, where P = pressure in atm (atmospheres) and V = volume in liters. Complete the table below, and draw a graph of the data. Will the line ever touch the vertical axis? The horizontal axis?

P (atm)	*V* (L)
1.0	
2.0	
3.0	
4.0	
5.0	
8.0	
10.0	

Solution

$$V = \frac{10}{1.0} = 10 \text{ (L)}$$

$$V = \frac{1}{2.0} = 5 \text{ L}$$

$$V = \frac{10}{3.0} = 3.3 \text{ L}$$

$$V = \frac{10}{4.0} = 2.5 \text{ L}$$

$$V = \frac{10}{5.0} = 2.0 \text{ L}$$

$$V = \frac{10}{8.0} = 1.25 \text{ L}$$

$$V = \frac{10}{10} = 1.0 \text{ L}$$

P	V
1.0	10 L
2.0	5 L
3.0	3.3 L
4.0	2.5 L
5.0	2.0 L
8.0	1.25 L
10.0	1.0 L

Comments

First, complete the table by substituting P into the formula, and solving for V.

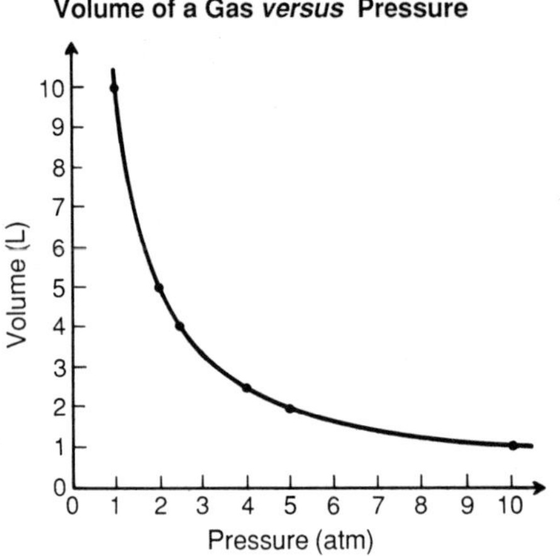

Use pressure as the independent variable and volume as the dependent variable.

Start pressure at 0 and advance to 10 atm. Start volume at 0, advance to 10 L.

Plot points (P,V).

Draw a smooth curve through the points.

The curve will never touch the vertical axis because P, which is in the denominator, can never be equal to zero. On the other hand, no matter how large pressure becomes, the volume will never completely become zero. Therefore, this curve, which is called a **hyperbola,** never touches either axis.

The next example illustrates another curve with many applications in the sciences, the **parabola.**

EXAMPLE 10.3.6

A beam of x-rays travels a distance of 10 cm and strikes a sheet of film. The area covered by the beam is measured to be 78.5 cm^2. The area covered by the x-ray beam is related to the distance traveled by the formula

$$A = kD^2$$

where $k = 0.785$. Find the area covered by the x-ray beam when the film distances (often called the film-focus distance) are 15, 20, 25, 30, 35, and 40 cm, respectively.

Solution

$A = kD^2$

$$\begin{aligned} A &= 0.785\ (15\ \text{cm})^2 \\ &= 0.785\ (225\ \text{cm}^2) \\ &= 177\ \text{cm}^2 \end{aligned}$$

$$\begin{aligned} A &= 0.785\ (20\ \text{cm})^2 \\ &= 0.785\ (400\ \text{cm}^2) \\ &= 314\ \text{cm}^2 \end{aligned}$$

$$\begin{aligned} A &= 0.785\ (25\ \text{cm})^2 \\ &= 0.785\ (625\ \text{cm}^2) \\ &= 491\ \text{cm}^2 \end{aligned}$$

$$\begin{aligned} A &= 0.785\ (30\ \text{cm})^2 \\ &= 0.785\ (900\ \text{cm}^2) \\ &= 706\ \text{cm}^2 \end{aligned}$$

$$\begin{aligned} A &= 0.785\ (35\ \text{cm})^2 \\ &= 0.785\ (1225\ \text{cm}^2) \\ &= 962\ \text{cm}^2 \end{aligned}$$

$$\begin{aligned} A &= 0.785\ (40\ \text{cm})^2 \\ &= 0.785\ (1600\ \text{cm}^2) \\ &= 1256\ \text{cm}^2 \end{aligned}$$

Comments

Determine the area associated with each distance, and then make a table of values.

D (cm)	A (cm^2)
10	78.5
15	177
20	314
25	491
30	706
35	962
40	1256

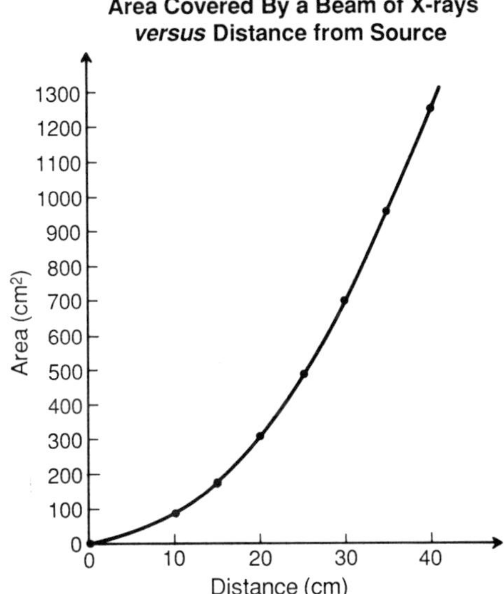

Set up the graph. Since the distances range from 10 to 40 cm, let the horizontal axis begin at 0 and continue to 40 cm.

The area ranges from 78.5 cm^2 to 1256 cm^2. Begin at 0 and continue up to 1300 cm^2.

Label each axis and title the graph.

Plot the data points.

This graph shows one half (one limb) of a parabola. If negative distances were plotted (not allowed in the real world), we would obtain a mirror image of the graph pictured. Both halves form the whole parabola.

PROBLEM SET 2

Draw graphs of the following data. Label each axis, arrange units to use as such room as is available, and be sure to title the graph.

1. Distance traveled versus time of a car at 50 mph.

Time (hr)	Distance (miles)
0.5	25
1.0	50
1.5	75
2.0	100
2.5	125
3.0	150

2. Minimum stopping distances: stopping distance of an automobile versus speed.

Speed (mph)	Total Stopping Distance (ft)
5	9.5
15	29.5
25	55.5
35	90.5
45	141.5
55	208.5
65	291.5

3. Reaction time to grasp a 18-inch ruler dropped through open fingers.

Distance Ruler Falls (inches)	Reaction Time (sec)
2	0.1
4	1.4
6	1.8
8	0.20
10	0.22
12	2.35
14	0.26
16	0.28
18	0.30

4. Blood alcohol level of 160-lb man 2 hours after eating versus number of 1-oz drinks (86 proof).

Number of Drinks	Blood Alcohol Level (%)
1	0.01
3	0.04
5	0.07
7	0.11
9	0.14
11	0.17
13	0.20

At what point would this man become legally drunk? (A person is legally drunk at .10%)

5. Vapor pressure of water versus temperature.

Temperature (°C)	Vapor Pressure (mm Hg)
0	4.58
10	9.21
20	17.54
30	31.82
40	55.3
50	92.5
60	149.4
70	233.7
80	355.1
90	525.8
100	760.0

a. At what temperature is the vapor pressure of water equal to the normal air pressure (760.0 mm Hg)?

b. What is the vapor pressure of water at 55°C?

6. Mass of radioactive strontium-90 (^{90}Sr) undecayed versus time.

Time (yr)	Mass of ^{90}Sr (g)
0	10.0
10	7.0
20	6.0
30	4.5
40	3.7
50	2.4
60	2.2
70	1.7
80	1.4
90	1.0
100	0.6

a. How long will it take for only half of the ^{90}Sr to remain (the half-life)?

b. How much ^{90}Sr remains after two half-lives?

7. Atmospheric CO_2 concentration as a function of time.

Time (yr)	Atmospheric CO_2 (ppm)
1870	290
1880	288
1895	290
1910	302
1917	301
1922	305
1933	310
1938	324
1946	314
1955	330

(*Hint:* This table is based on experimental data. You must draw a curve of best fit.)

a. Are the data best graphed by using a straight line or a smooth curve?

b. Can you predict what has happened to the level of CO_2 since 1955?

8. Average daily concentration of nitrogen dioxide (NO_2) over Los Angeles, California, on a day in July, 1965.

Time of Day	NO_2 (ppm)
Midnight	0.02
3:00	0.03
6:00	0.06
9:00	0.23
12:00 Noon	0.15
3:00	0.12
6:00	0.13
9:00	0.12
Midnight	0.06

9. Calibration curve for a drying oven. A drying oven used in a chemistry lab has a dial with settings from 0 to 8. To determine what temperature corresponds to each dial setting a thermometer was placed in the oven, and the following data was obtained.

Dial Setting	Temperature (°C)
55.0	3.2
65.0	3.6
75.0	4.0
88.0	4.4
102.0	5.0
118	5.6
127	6.0
140	6.4
154	7.0
168	7.6
180	8.0

a. What dial setting would be necessary to maintain a 135°C temperature inside the oven?

b. A lab assistant checks the drying oven and finds the dial set at 7.4. What is the temperature inside the oven?

10. Population of bacteria cells versus time.

Time (hr)	Number of Cells
0	2
2	11
4	50
6	120
8	240
10	340
12	400
14	429
16	450
18	447

a. What is the population of the bacteria cells after 15 hours?

b. What would you estimate the population to be after 24 hours?

(*Note:* This type of curve, which begins as an exponential growth curve and then levels off, is called a *sigmoid curve.* It is typical of many growth patterns where food is limited.)

Answer the following questions from the graphs provided.

11. Standard curve: Cholesterol in blood serum at 600 nm.

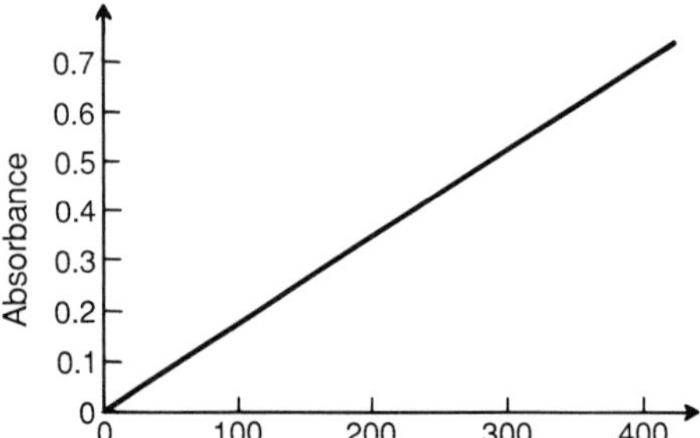

a. A blood serum sample when mixed with the proper reagents and placed in a spectrophotometer was found to have an absorbance of 0.38. What is the concentration of cholesterol in the bloodstream?

b. A patient was found to have a cholesterol level of 165 mg/dL. From the standard curve, what absorbance corresponds with this cholesterol level?

c. If normal cholesterol levels range from 150 to 300 mg/dL, determine the absorbance range that corresponds to these normal levels.

12. Pulmonary function: Liters of air expelled versus time (a test of the lung capacity of one of the authors).

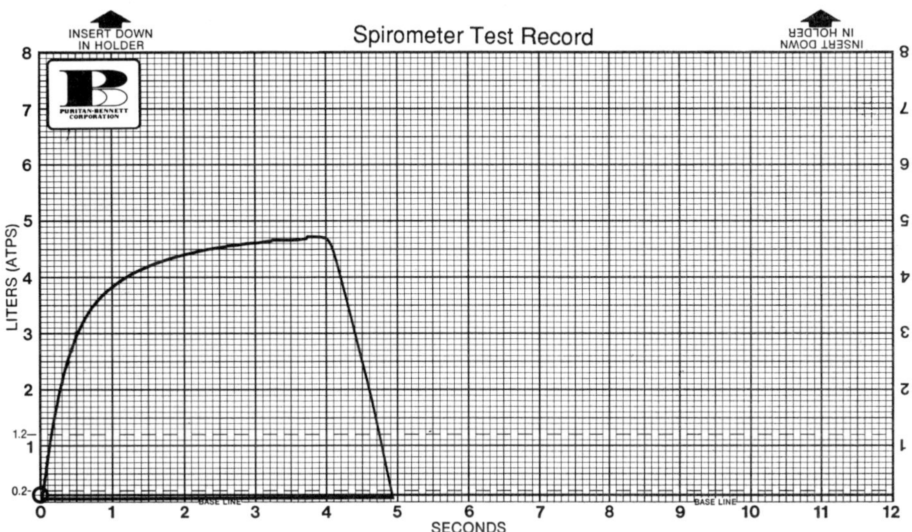

a. How long did the author expel air from his lungs?

b. How many liters of air were expelled?

c. What accounts for the straight line extending downward on the right?

d. It was predicted, for the author's age, that he would expel 5.46 L of air. What percent of the predicted value did the author score?

13. Solubility curve: Solubility of NaCl and KNO_3 versus temperature.

The Solubility of Two Common Ionic Solids

Solubility (NaCl/100 g H_2O)
100
90
80
70
60
50
40
30
20
10
0
KNO_3
NaCl
0 10 20 30 40 50 60 70 80 90 100
Temperature (°C)

a. What is the solubility of NaCl in grams per 100 g of water at 24°C?

b. What is the solubility of KNO_3 in grams per 100 g of water at 24°C?

c. Compare the solubilities of NaCl and KNO_3 at 45°C. What has happened to the solubilities of the two substances?

d. A student completely dissolved 48 g of KNO_3 in 100 g of water, and the solution was saturated. What was the temperature of the water?

e. How much more NaCl can be dissolved at 100°C than at 0°C?

g. Can you tell from the graph how much KNO_3 can be dissolved in 100 g of water at 100°C?

14. Daily variations in temperature and humidity.

Temperature versus time
Humidity (%) versus time

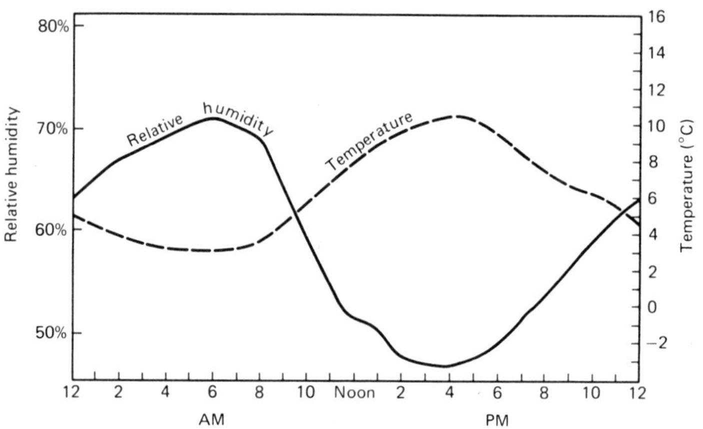

(From Lutgens, F. and Tarbuck, E. *The atmosphere* (2nd ed.). Englewood Cliffs, N.J.: Prentice-Hall, 1985).

[*Note:* The left side axis gives the relative humidity (%), and the right side axis gives the Temperature (°C).]

a. At what time does the maximum temperature occur? What is the maximum temperature?

b. At what time does the maximum humidity occur? What is the maximum humidity?

c. At what time does the minimum temperature occur? What is it?

d. At what time does the minimum humidity occur? What is it?

e. Is there an apparent relationship between temperature and humidity? State the relationship.

Answers to odd-numbered problems appear on page 245.

10.4 CIRCLE AND BAR GRAPHS

Circle Graphs

The circle graph is especially useful when comparing the relationship among the parts of a whole. The circle graph below compares the categories of expenses of a typical family.

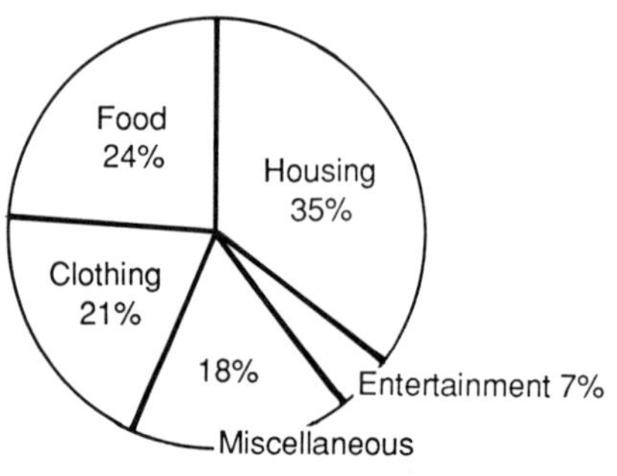

Expenses of a Typical Family of Four

It is obvious from the graph that housing makes up the largest share of the expenses, whereas money spent for entertainment is only a small portion. In any circle or "pie" graph, the percentages should always add up to 100. Each slice of the pie represents a component of the whole, with the component in greatest abundance represented by the largest slice. Consider the following example.

EXAMPLE 10.4.1

The following table gives the percent abundances of some of the elements naturally occurring in the earth's crust. Construct a circle graph from the data.

Element	Weight (%)
Oxygen	49.5
Silicon	25.7
Aluminum	7.5
Iron	4.7
All others	12.6

Solution	Comments
$\frac{\%}{100} = \frac{\text{Part}}{\text{Whole}}$	Since a circle contains 360°, find the number of degrees to be allotted to each component. Use the percent formula from Chapter 4: % = given; part = x; and whole = 360°.
$\frac{49.5}{100} = \frac{x}{360}$ $\frac{(360)(49.5)}{100} = x$ $178° = x$	Determine the number of degrees of the circle allotted for oxygen: % = 49.5; whole = 360°; and part allotted for oxygen = x.
$\frac{25.7}{100} = \frac{x}{360}$ $93° = x$	Determine the number of degrees allotted for silicon: % = 25.7; whole = 360°; and part allotted for silicon = x.
$\frac{7.5}{100} = \frac{x}{360}$ $27° = x$	Determine the number of degrees allotted for aluminum: % = 7.5; whole = 360°; and part allotted for aluminum = x.
$\frac{4.7}{100} = \frac{x}{360}$ $17° = x$	Determine the number of degrees allotted for iron: % = 4.7; whole = 360°; and part allotted for iron = x.
$\frac{12.6}{100} = \frac{x}{360}$ $45° = x$	Determine the number of degrees allotted for all other elements. % = 12.6; whole = 360°; part allotted for all other elements = x.
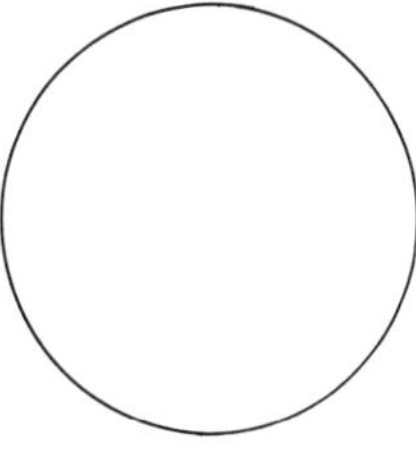	Draw a circle large enough to subdivide easily. Locate the center. Using a protractor, lay off sectors of the appropriate size for each component.

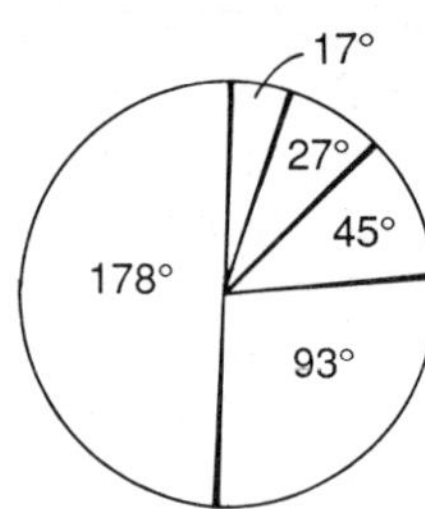

Oxygen	=	178°
Silicon	=	93°
Aluminum	=	27°
Iron	=	17°
All others	=	45°
Total	=	360°

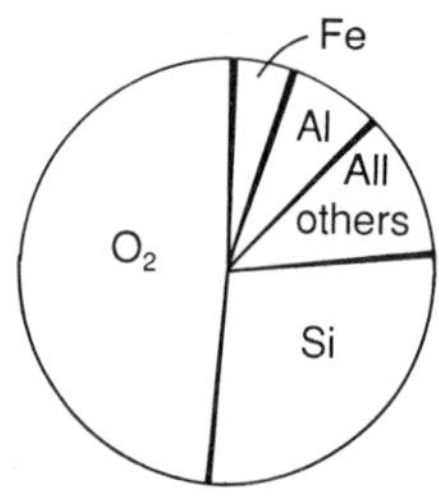

Now, label the "slices" with three proper elements.

You may be given a set of data where the percentages are not given, as in the next example. Using the percent formula, the percentages may be calculated, and the pie graph readily drawn.

EXAMPLE 10.4.2

The amount of water excreted by various organs of the body in one day is given in the table below. Construct a pie graph of the data.

	Output (mL/day)
Kidneys	1400
Lungs	350
Skin	440
Intestines	210

Solution

$$\text{Total} = 1400 \text{ mL} + 350 \text{ mL} + 440 \text{ mL} + 210 \text{ mL} = 2400 \text{ mL}$$

Comments

Determine the total output from all organs. This is the "whole" in the percent formula.

$$\frac{\%}{100} = \frac{\text{Part}}{\text{Whole}}$$

Determine the percent of the total excreted by each organ.

$$\% = \frac{1400 \text{ mL}}{2400 \text{ mL}} \cdot 100$$

$$\% = 58.3$$

First, determine the percent excreted by the kidneys: part = 1400 mL; and whole = 2400 mL.

$$\frac{58.3}{100} = \frac{x}{360°}$$

$$x = \frac{(58.3)(360°)}{100}$$

$$x = 2\bar{1}0°$$

Determine the size of the "slice" allotted to the kidneys: part = 58.3; and whole = 360°.

$$\% = \frac{350 \text{ mL}}{2400 \text{ mL}} \cdot 100$$

$$\% = 14.6$$

Determine the percent excreted by the lungs: part = 350 mL; and whole = 2400 mL.

$$\frac{14.6}{100} = \frac{x}{360°}$$

Determine the size of the slice allotted to the lungs: part = 14.6; and whole = 360°.

$$x = \frac{(14.6)(360°)}{100}$$

$$x = 52.6°$$

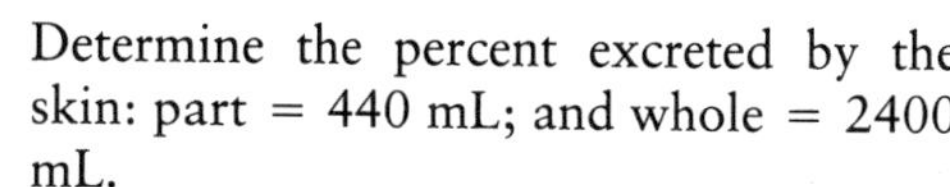

Determine the percent excreted by the skin: part = 440 mL; and whole = 2400 mL.

$$\% = \frac{440 \text{ mL}}{2400 \text{ mL}} \cdot 100$$

$$\% = 18.3$$

Determine the size of the slice allotted to the skin: part = 18.3; and whole = 360°.

$$\frac{18.3}{100} = \frac{x}{360°}$$

$$x = \frac{(18.3)(360°)}{100}$$

$$x = 65.9$$

Lastly, determine the percent excreted by the intestines: part = 210 mL; and whole = 2400 mL.

$$\% = \frac{210 \text{ mL}}{2400 \text{ mL}} \cdot 100$$

$$\% = 8.75$$

Determine the size of the slice allotted to the intestines: part = 8.75; whole = 360°.

$$\frac{8.75}{100} = \frac{x}{360°}$$

$$x = \frac{(8.75)(360°)}{100}$$

$$x = 31.5°$$

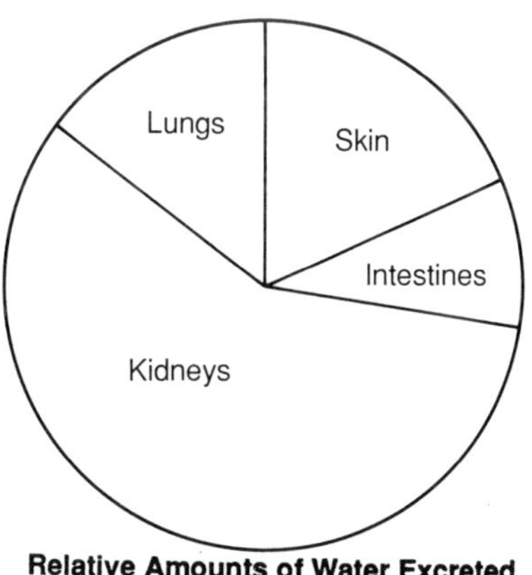

Relative Amounts of Water Excreted Daily by Various Organs

To summarize, the circle will be sliced up as follows:

Kidneys	210°
Lungs	52.6°
Skin	65.9°
Intestines	31.5°

Use a protractor to lay out the slices as illustrated in example 10.4.1.

Bar Graphs

When analyzing data of a discrete sort, we often resort to the **bar graph**.

EXAMPLE 10.4.3

Draw a bar graph of the following data:

Element	Average Intake (mg/day)
Iron (males)	10
Iron (females)	18
Zinc	15
Manganese	3.8
Fluorine	2.8
Copper	2.5
Molybdenum	0.3
Iodine	0.15

Solution

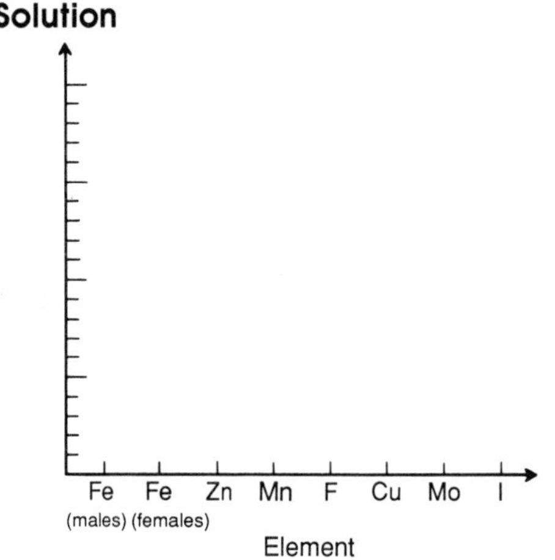

Comments

Use the horizontal axis to list the elements; use uniform spacing. Use element symbols to save space.

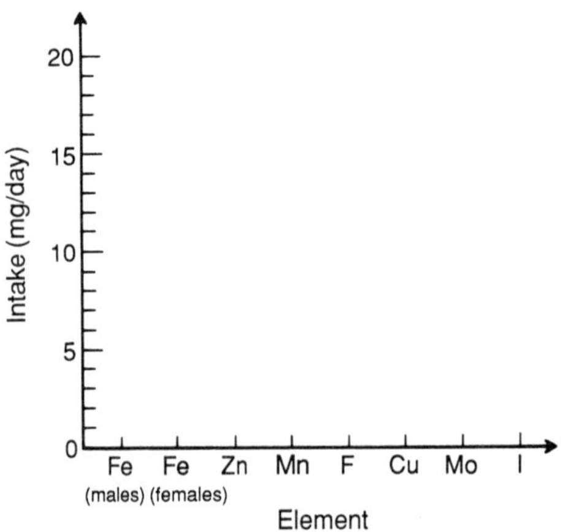

Use the vertical axis for the intake units. Begin at 0, and mark off the axis uniformly up to at least 18 mg/day.

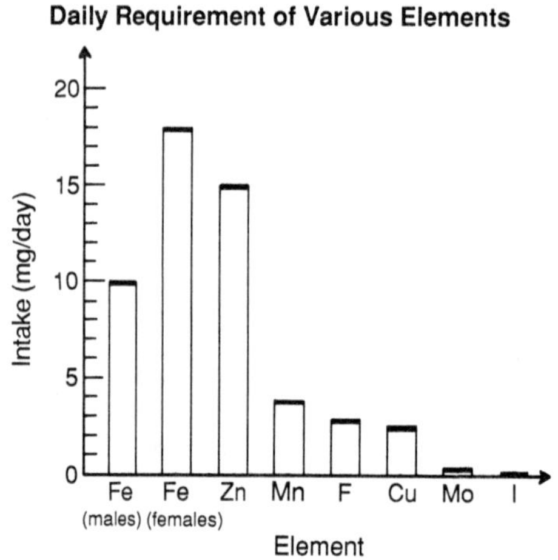

Use a bar to extend from zero up to the intake for the element in question. The bar should be centered over the element symbol. A space is left between bars.

The bar graph is excellent for comparison purposes. Several items can be compared at the same time, and trends spotted easily. The bar graph is often used in the fields of economics and business to show trends from month to month or year to year in sales, earnings, or production.

The bar graph can be presented in another form. Instead of drawing a bar, we graph single points at the top of each bar. The points can be joined by a series of straight lines (not a smooth curve). The following figure illustrates the data from example 10.4.3 presented in this type of bar graph.

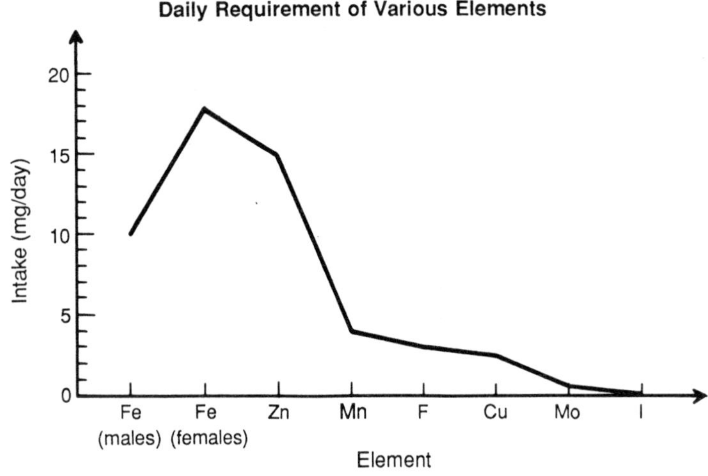

PROBLEM SET 3

Draw circle graphs for each set of data that follows.

1. Ethanol consists of the following three elements (by weight): carbon = 52.5%; hydrogen = 13.0%; and oxygen = 34.8%.

2. A family of three spends its monthly budget of $1800 in the following manner: food = 16.2%; clothing = 8.2%; shelter = 32.5%; entertainment = 12.4%; installment loans = 23.7%; and miscellaneous = 7%.

3. The approximate elemental analysis of the human body is as follows: oxygen = 65%; carbon = 18%; hydrogen = 10%; nitrogen = 3%; and all others = 4%.

4. There were 124 graduates at a small college, with the following number of students in each major: mathematics and science = 22; business = 43; languages and literature = 28; health and physical education = 12; and social sciences = 19.

   (*Hint:* First find the percent each major contributed to the whole before drawing the graph.)

Draw bar graphs for each of the following sets of data. Try to avoid distortion if possible.

5. Top six chemicals produced in 1984.

Chemical	Billions of Pounds Produced
Sulfuric acid	79.4
Ammonia	32.4
Lime	32.2
Oxygen	31.04
Nitrogen	43.4
Ethylene	32.2

6. Typhoid and related death rates in the United States, 1900–1935.

Year	Death Rate per 100,000 Population
1900	35
1905	28
1910	24
1915	12
1920	8
1925	8
1930	3
1935	2

Approximately how many deaths from typhoid were there in 1935 if the population was approximately 150 million?

7. pH values for certain common solutions

Solution	pH
Gastric fluid	1.5
Orange juice	3.7
Coffee	5.2
Milk	6.4
Pure water	7.0 (neutral)
Milk of Magnesia	9.0
Household ammonia	11.0
Lye	13.0

8. Normal values for various blood components.

Component	Normal Values (mg/dL)
Triglycerides	10–195
Glucose	65–110
BUN	10–20
Cholesterol	150–300
Calcium	8.6–10.7

(*Hint:* For each component, draw a bar from the lowest number of each range to the highest number of each range.)

9. Causes of death (1970).

Cause	Deaths per 100,000
Cardiovascular disease	340
Cancer	190
Cerebrovascular disease	120
Trauma	55
Pneumonias	43
Neonatal disease	35
Diabetes mellitus	32
Cirrhosis	30

Answers to odd-numbered problems appear on page 246.

CHAPTER REVIEW

(10.2)

1. Determine whether the given ordered pair is a solution to the equation.
   a. $(3,1);\ y = 3x - 5$
   b. $(0,2);\ x + 2y = 4$
   c. $(-5,3);\ y = \frac{1}{5}x + 4$

2. Graph the following equations using at least three points.
   a. $y = -2x + 3$
   b. $y = -\frac{2}{3}x + 5$
   c. $2x + y = -1$
   d. $4x + \frac{1}{2}y = 7$

(10.3)

Graph the following data. Be sure to label each axis and place a title above the graph.

3. Cooling curve: Cooling of a glass of hot tap water in a room at 24.5°C.

Elapsed Time (min)	Temperature (°C)
0	35.5
5	34.5
10	33.5
15	32.5
20	31.8
25	31.4
30	30.9

   a. What will the temperature of the water be after 17 minutes of cooling?
   b. Does the water cool at a constant rate? When does it begin leveling off?

4. Hemoglobin–oxygen dissociation curve: Percent saturation of hemoglobin versus the partial pressure of oxygen (Po_2) in the bloodstream (at 38°C).

Po_2 (mm Hg)	Saturation (%)
0	0
10	12
20	34
30	61
40	75
50	85
60	91
70	95
80	97
90	98
100	99

   a. What is the partial pressure of oxygen (Po_2) when the percent saturation of hemoglobin is 48%?

b. The normal P_{O_2} is 100 mm Hg. If it falls to 64 mm Hg, by how much would the percent saturation decline?

(10.4) 5. Draw a circle graph to represent these data.

FEDERAL BUDGET FUNDS ALLOTTED TO VARIOUS RESEARCH AND DEVELOPMENT DEPARTMENTS (1985)

Department	Funds (%)
Defense	66%
Health and Human Services	10%
Energy	9%
NASA	7%
National Science Foundation	3%
Other	5%

6. Draw a bar graph to represent the following data.

CASES OF HUMAN ANTHRAX IN THE US (1930–1979)

Year	Approximate Number of Cases
1930–1934	305
1935–1939	300
1940–1944	400
1945–1949	270
1950–1954	230
1955–1959	145
1960–1964	95
1965–1969	30
1970–1974	15
1975–1979	10

Answers to all problems appear on page 248.

Appendix A: Temperature Measurement and Conversions

A.1 THE TEMPERATURE SCALES

Temperature measurement, which is the measure of heat, is an important part of many laboratory procedures. In this section, we study the three major temperature measuring scales, and methods of converting from one scale to another.

Most laboratories use mercury thermometers to measure temperature. Thermometers may be calibrated with the **Fahrenheit** scale or the **Celsius** (also called centigrade) scale. Usually, these thermometers are read to the nearest tenth of a "degree." A comparison of the two scales is shown in the following figure:

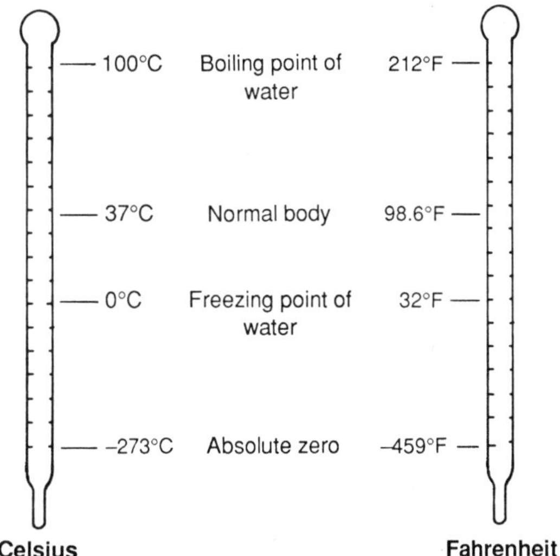

The Fahrenheit scale is used more frequently in our daily affairs, such as in weather reports and in cooking. The Celsius scale is the scale of choice for the sciences, and is considered to be the metric temperature scale.

A.2 TEMPERATURE CONVERSION

To convert from Fahrenheit temperature to Celsius temperature, we make use of the following formula:

$$°C = \frac{5}{9}(°F - 32)$$

where °F is the Fahrenheit temperature and °C is the Celsius temperature.

EXAMPLE A.2.1

Change 38°F to °C.

Solution	Comments
$°C = \frac{5}{9}(°F - 32)$	Write down the formula. Let °F = 38 and solve for °C.
$°C = \frac{5}{9}(38 - 32)$	Use the order of operations: simplify inside the parenthesis first.
$°C = \frac{5}{9}(6)$	Multiply by $\frac{5}{9}$.
$°C = \frac{30}{9}$	
$°C = 3.3$	38°F = 3.3°C.

A helpful fact to remember is that Fahrenheit temperature is always numerically larger than the equivalent Celsius temperature at temperatures above the freezing point of water.

To convert from Celsius temperature to Fahrenheit temperature, we make use of the following formula:

$$°F = \frac{9}{5}°C + 32$$

EXAMPLE A.2.2

Change 84.0°C to °F. (Recall that the corresponding Fahrenheit temperature will be numerically larger than the equivalent Celsius temperature.)

Solution	Comments
$°F = \frac{9}{5}°C + 32$	Write down the formula. Let °C = 84.0 and solve for °F.
$°F = \frac{9}{5}(84.0) + 32$	Following the order of operations we will multiply before adding.
$°F = \frac{756}{5} + 32$	
$°F = 151 + 32$	
$°F = 183$	183°F = 84.0°C.

You should memorize both formulas presented, and learn how to use them. Your instructor may show you some other variations of these two formulas.

A.3 ABSOLUTE TEMPERATURE MEASUREMENT

When using temperature as a variable in certain formulas, such as the gas laws, it must be expressed as a positive number; otherwise we may obtain an answer with a negative or undefined value. Both the Fahrenheit and Celsius scales have numerical values that are negative, and therefore cannot be used in such formulas. These two scales are called **relative temperature scales** because you can only tell relatively how much heat is present.

For example, if the high temperature yesterday was −10°F and the high temperature today is 0°F, we can say only that it has warmed up by 10 degrees, but not absolutely how much heat is present today or was present yesterday.

In order to avoid the problem of negative temperatures, scientists used the **absolute temperature scale.** On this scale, the temperature where no heat is present, absolute zero, is 0 **Kelvin.** The Kelvin scale is considered a **companion scale** to the Celsius scale because a 1° rise on the Celsius is equivalent to a 1° rise on the Kelvin scale. Since it is impossible to have a temperature colder than absolute zero, there is no need for negative temperature readings. The following figure illustrates the Celsius scale and the companion Kelvin scale:

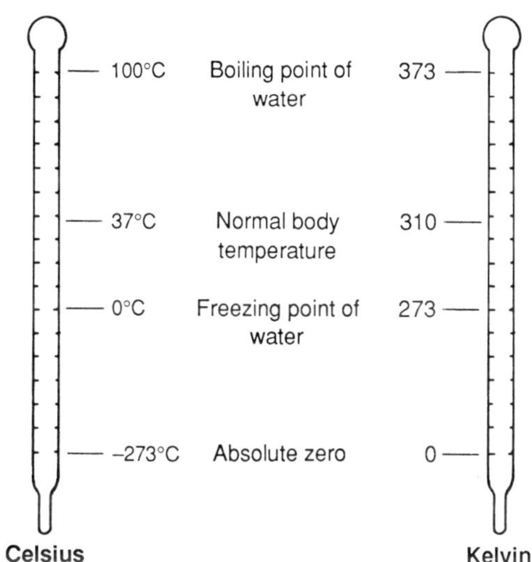

Any temperature recorded in the lab with a Fahrenheit or Celsius thermometer must be changed to the Kelvin scale before using it in a formula. This is easy to do, using the formula

$$K = °C + 273$$

where °C is the Celsius temperature and K is the Kelvin temperature.

EXAMPLE A.2.3

Mercury freezes at −39°C (mercury thermometers cannot be used at temperatures this low). What is the equivalent Kelvin temperature?

Solution	**Comments**
$K = °C + 273$ $K = -39 + 273$	Using the formula, let °C = −39 and solve for K. Be careful with the negative sign.
$K = 234$	234 K = −39°C

EXAMPLE A.2.4

Helium boils at 4.2 K. Find the equivalent Celsius temperature.

Solution	**Comments**
$K = °C + 273$ $K - 273 = °C$ $4.2 - 273 = °C$	Using the Kelvin conversion formula, let K = 4.2 and solve for °C by subtracting 273 from both sides of the equation.
$-269 = °C$	−269°C = 4.2 K.

PROBLEM SET 1

1. Change the following Celsius temperatures to °F:
   a. 45
   b. 20
   c. −40
   d. 121
   e. 448.2
   f. −236.4
2. Change the following Fahrenheit temperatures to °C:
   a. 113
   b. 68
   c. 5
   d. −40
   e. 167.6
   f. −273.2
3. Change the following Celsius temperatures to Kelvin temperatures:
   a. 100
   b. 273
   c. −273
   d. 412.2
   e. 1622
   f. 16,024
4. Normal body temperature is considered to be 98.6°F. What is this in °C? In K?
5. Nitrogen boils at 77 K. What is this in °C? In °F?
6. Physicians have recommended that children with a fever under 100°F not be given an antipyretic for the first 24 hours of the fever. What is this temperature in °C?
7. The temperature of the surface of a star was found to be 35,000 K. What is this temperature in °C?
8. A supersaturated glucose solution was prepared at 95.2°C. It was cooled to room temperature (20.0°C). By how much did the solution cool in °C? In K?

Answers to odd-numbered problems appear on page 250.

Appendix B: Radiographic Exposure Factors

B.1 THE BASIC EXPOSURE FACTORS

To make an acceptable radiograph (x-ray), several factors must be considered:

1. Current flowing through the X-ray tube, measured in milliamperes (mA)
2. Focus-film distance (D), measured in feet or inches
3. Time (T) of exposure, measured in seconds

Any change in one of these factors will necessitate a change in one of the others to produce radiographs of similar quality. We examine three relationships involving these factors, and the application of each, in this appendix:

1. The milliampere–time relation
2. The focus-film distance–time relation
3. The milliampere-second–distance relation

B.2 THE MILLIAMPERE–TIME RELATION

To obtain similar exposures, the milliamperage required is *inversely* proportional to the time of exposure. That is, a shorter exposure requires a higher milliamperage, and a longer time requires a lower milliamperage. This relationship may be written as the following inverse proportion:

$$\frac{\text{mA}_O}{\text{mA}_n} = \frac{T_n}{T_O}$$

where mA_O is the original milliamperage, T_O is the original time, mA_n is the new milliamperage, and T_n is the new time.

If we cross multiply in the above formula, we obtain a variation of the formula that is easier to remember:

$$\text{mA}_O T_O = \text{mA}_n T_n$$

The product of $\text{mA}_O T_O$ may be considered as a single factor that is a constant, as in $\text{mA}_n T_n$. This factor is called the "milliampere-second" factor, and we will make use of it in another section. The following example will clarify the use of the milliampere–time relation.

EXAMPLE B.2.1

A milliamperage of 25 and an exposure time of 0.375 seconds are needed to obtain a proper exposure. If we wish to decrease the exposure time to exactly 0.25 seconds, what milliamperage is necessary to obtain the proper exposure?

Solution	Comments
$mA_O T_O = mA_n T_n$ $(25)(0.375 \text{ scc}) = mA_n(0.25 \text{ sec})$ $\frac{(25)(0.375 \cancel{\text{sec}})}{(0.25 \cancel{\text{sec}})} = mA_n$	Write down the formula. Let $mA_O = 25$, $T_O = 0.375$ sec, $T_n = 0.25$ sec, and solve for mA_n.
$37.5 \text{ mA} = mA_n$	The new milliamperage is 37.5 mA.

EXAMPLE B.2.2

Proper radiographs have been made at 30.0 mA with an exposure time of exactly 1.5 seconds. If we wish to increase the exposure time to exactly 2 seconds, what milliamperage is required?

Solution	Comments
$mA_O T_O = mA_n T_n$ $(30)(1.5 \text{ sec}) = mA_n(2 \text{ sec})$ $\frac{(30)(1.5 \cancel{\text{sec}})}{2 \cancel{\text{sec}}} = mA_n$	Write down the formula. Let $mA_O = 30.0$ mA, $T_O = 1.5$ sec, $T_n = 2$ sec, and solve for mA_n.
$22.5 = mA_n$	The new milliamperage is 22.5 mA.

B.3 THE FOCUS-FILM DISTANCE–TIME RELATION

When the distance between the x-ray source and the film (the focus-film distance) is increased, the intensity of the x-ray beam per surface area is decreased; therefore in order to maintain an exposure of similar quality, the time of exposure must be increased. If the distance is decreased, then the time of exposure must be decreased to compensate for the increased intensity per surface area. In general, we may say that the time of exposure is *directly* related to the *square* of the distance between the x-ray source and the film. This relation is expressed algebraically as the direct ratio

$$\frac{T_n}{T_O} = \frac{D_n^2}{D_O^2}$$

where T_O is the original time, T_n is the new time, D_O is the old distance (in feet or inches), and D_n is the new distance.

The following two examples illustrate the utility of this proportion.

EXAMPLE B.3.1

Good quality radiographs may be made with an exposure time of 2.0 seconds where the distance is 35.0 inches. What time is required if the distance is shortened to 30.0 inches?

Solution	Comments
$\frac{T_n}{T_O} = \frac{D_n^2}{D_O^2}$ $\frac{T_n}{2 \text{ sec}} = \frac{(30.0 \text{ inches})^2}{(35.0 \text{ inches})^2}$ $\frac{T_n}{2.0 \text{ sec}} = \frac{90\bar{0} \cancel{\text{inches}^2}}{1225 \cancel{\text{inches}^2}}$ $T_n = \frac{(2.0 \text{ sec})(90\bar{0})}{1225}$	Write down the proportion. Let $T_O = 2.0$ sec, $D_O = 35.0$ inches, $D_n = 30.0$ inches and solve for T_n. Be sure to square the distances.
$T_n = 1.47 \text{ sec} \approx 1.5 \text{ sec}$	The new exposure time is 1.5 sec.

EXAMPLE B.3.2

The original exposure time for a radiograph was 1.0 second with a distance of 60.0 inches. If the exposure time needs to be reduced to 0.25 second, what distance will be required?

Solution	Comments
$\frac{T_n}{T_O} = \frac{D_n^2}{D_O^2}$	Write down the proportion. Let $T_n = 0.25$ sec, $T_O = 1.0$ sec, $D_O = 60.0$ inches, and solve for D_n.
$\frac{(0.25 \text{ sec})}{1.0 \text{ sec}} = \frac{D_n^2}{(60.0 \text{ inches})^2}$	
$\frac{(0.25 \not{\text{sec}})(60.0 \text{ inches}^2)^2}{1.0 \not{\text{sec}}} = D_n^2$	
$\frac{(0.25 \not{\text{sec}})(36\bar{0}0 \text{ inches}^2)}{1.0 \not{\text{sec}}} = D_n^2$	
$9\bar{0}0 \text{ inches}^2 = D_n^2$	
$\sqrt{900 \text{ inches}^2} = D_n$	Take the square root of both sides of the equation.
$3\bar{0} \text{ inches} = D_n$	The new distance is $3\bar{0}$ inches.

B.4 THE MILLIAMPERE-SECOND–DISTANCE RELATION

When the milliampere–time ($mA_O T_O = mA_n T_n$) and time–distance $\left(\frac{T_n}{T_O} = \frac{D_n^2}{D_O^2}\right)$ relations are combined into one equation, we obtain the milliampere-second–distance equation:

$$\frac{mA_n T_n}{mA_O T_O} = \frac{D_n^2}{D_O^2}$$

The variables "$mA_n T_n$" and "$mA_O T_O$" are called the "milliampere-second" values. This equation is used in the following two examples.

EXAMPLE B.4.1

If a 100.0-milliampere-second (mA-sec) exposure is required at a distance of $6\bar{0}$ inches, what distance is required for a 20.0-mA-sec exposure?

Solution	Comments
$\frac{mA_n T_n}{mA_O T_O} = \frac{D_n^2}{D_O^2}$	Write down the equation. Let $mA_n T_n$ = 20.0 mA-sec, mA_O-T_O = 100.0 mA-sec, $D_O = 6\bar{0}$ inches, and solve for D_n.
$\frac{20.0 \text{ mA-sec}}{100.0 \text{ mA-sec}} = \frac{D_n^2}{(6\bar{0} \text{ inches})^2}$	
$\frac{(20.0 \text{ mA-sec})(6\bar{0} \text{ inches})^2}{100.0 \text{ mA-sec}} = D_n^2$	
$\frac{(20.0 \not{\text{mA-sec}})(3600 \text{ inches}^2)}{100.0 \not{\text{mA-sec}}} = D_n^2$	
$\frac{72{,}000 \text{ inches}^2}{100.0} = D_n^2$	
$720 \text{ inches}^2 = D_n^2$	Take the square root of both sides of the equation.
$\sqrt{720 \text{ inches}^2} = D_n$	
$26.8 \text{ inches} = D_n$	
$27 \text{ inches} \approx D_n$	The new distance is 27 inches

EXAMPLE B.4.2

The usual factors for a radiograph of the hip require a distance of 45.0 inches and a milliampere-second value of 75.0. Certain limitations of the patient permit a distance of only 35.0 inches. What new milliampere-second value is required?

Solution	**Comments**
$\frac{mA_nT_n}{mA_OT_O} = \frac{D_n^2}{D_O^2}$	Write down the formula. Let mA_OT_O = 75.0 mA-sec, D_O = 45.0 inches, D_n = 35.0 inches, and solve for mA_nT_n. (Consider mA_nT_n as a single value.)
$\frac{mA_nT_n}{75.0 \text{ mA-sec}} = \frac{(35.0 \text{ inches})^2}{(45.0 \text{ inches})^2}$	
$mA_nT_n = \frac{(75.0 \text{ mA-sec})(35.0 \text{ inches})^2}{(45.0 \text{ inches})^2}$	
$mA_nT_n = \frac{(75.0 \text{ mA-sec})(1225 \text{ inches}^2)}{2025 \text{ inches}^2}$	
$mA_nT_n = 45.4$ mA-sec	The new milliampere-second value is 45.4 mA-sec.

In actual practice, there are several commercially prepared tables available relating the exposure factors discussed in this appendix. It is important, however, that the student understand the origin of these tables, and how these factors are related to proper exposures of radiographs.

PROBLEM SET 1

1. A milliamperage of $3\bar{0}$ mA and an exposure time of 0.5 second are required for the proper exposure of an x-ray. If we wish to decrease the time to 0.1 second, what milliamperage will be required to maintain the same exposure?
2. An x-ray requires a time of 2.0 seconds, with a milliamperage of 45 mA. What time will be required for a milliamperage of $10\bar{0}$ mA?
3. Good quality radiographs may be made with an exposure time of 1.5 seconds where the distance is 45.0 inches. What time is required if the distance is shortened to 25.0 inches?
4. A radiograph requires a time of 2.5 seconds at a distance of 50.0 inches. If the exposure time is reduced to 1.0 second, what distance will be required?
5. A 125 milliampere-second exposure is required with a distance of 72 inches. What distance is required for a $10\bar{0}$ milliampere-second exposure?
6. A special technique requires a distance of 3.0 feet at 175 mA-sec. If the mA-sec value is lowered to 80.0, what distance is then required?
7. To obtain proper exposure, these values are required: mA = $8\bar{0}$; T = 1.5 sec; D = 2.0 feet. What distance is required if mA = $12\bar{0}$ amd T = 0.5 sec? Hint: milliampere-seconds = mA × T.

Answers to odd-numbered problems appear on page 250.

Appendix C: Logarithm Tables

LOGARITHMS OF NUMBERS

N	0	1	2	3	4	5	6	7	8	9
1.0	.0000	.0043	.0086	.0128	.0170	.0212	.0253	.0294	.0334	.0374
1.1	.0414	.0453	.0492	.0531	.0569	.0607	.0645	.0682	.0719	.0755
1.2	.0792	.0828	.0864	.0899	.0934	.0969	.1004	.1038	.1072	.1106
1.3	.1139	.1173	.1206	.1239	.1271	.1303	.1335	.1367	.1399	.1430
1.4	.1461	.1492	.1523	.1553	.1584	.1614	.1644	.1673	.1703	.1732
1.5	.1761	.1790	.1818	.1847	.1875	.1903	.1931	.1959	.1987	.2014
1.6	.2041	.2068	.2095	.2122	.2148	.2175	.2201	.2227	.2253	.2279
1.7	.2304	.2330	.2355	.2380	.2405	.2430	.2455	.2480	.2504	.2529
1.8	.2553	.2577	.2601	.2625	.2648	.2672	.2695	.2718	.2742	.2765
1.9	.2788	.2810	.2833	.2856	.2878	.2900	.2923	.2945	.2967	.2989
2.0	.3010	.3032	.3054	.3075	.3096	.3118	.3139	.3160	.3181	.3201
2.1	.3222	.3243	.3263	.3284	.3304	.3324	.3345	.3365	.3385	.3404
2.2	.3424	.3444	.3464	.3483	.3502	.3522	.3541	.3560	.3579	.3598
2.3	.3617	.3636	.3655	.3674	.3692	.3711	.3729	.3747	.3766	.3784
2.4	.3802	.3820	.3838	.3856	.3874	.3892	.3909	.3927	.3945	.3962
2.5	.3979	.3997	.4014	.4031	.4048	.4065	.4082	.4099	.4116	.4133
2.6	.4150	.4166	.4183	.4200	.4216	.4232	.4249	.4265	.4281	.4298
2.7	.4314	.4330	.4346	.4362	.4378	.4393	.4409	.4425	.4440	.4456
2.8	.4472	.4487	.4502	.4518	.4533	.4548	.4564	.4579	.4594	.4609
2.9	.4624	.4639	.4654	.4669	.4683	.4698	.4713	.4728	.4742	.4757
3.0	.4771	.4786	.4800	.4814	.4829	.4843	.4857	.4871	.4886	.4900
3.1	.4914	.4928	.4942	.4955	.4969	.4983	.4997	.5011	.5024	.5038
3.2	.5051	.5065	.5079	.5092	.5105	.5119	.5132	.5145	.5159	.5172
3.3	.5185	.5198	.5211	.5224	.5237	.5250	.5263	.5276	.5289	.5302
3.4	.5315	.5328	.5340	.5353	.5366	.5378	.5391	.5403	.5416	.5428
3.5	.5441	.5453	.5465	.5478	.5490	.5502	.5514	.5527	.5539	.5551
3.6	.5563	.5575	.5587	.5599	.5611	.5623	.5635	.5647	.5658	.5670
3.7	.5682	.5694	.5705	.5717	.5729	.5740	.5752	.5763	.5775	.5786
3.8	.5798	.5809	.5821	.5832	.5843	.5855	.5866	.5877	.5888	.5899
3.9	.5911	.5922	.5933	.5944	.5955	.5966	.5977	.5988	.5999	.6010
4.0	.6021	.6031	.6042	.6053	.6064	.6075	.6085	.6096	.6107	.6117
4.1	.6128	.6138	.6149	.6160	.6170	.6180	.6191	.6201	.6212	.6222
4.2	.6232	.6243	.6253	.6263	.6274	.6284	.6294	.6304	.6314	.6325

LOGARITHMS OF NUMBERS (*Continued*)

N	0	1	2	3	4	5	6	7	8	9
4.3	.6335	.6345	.6355	.6365	.6375	.6385	.6395	.6405	.6415	.6425
4.4	.6435	.6444	.6454	.6464	.6474	.6484	.6493	.6503	.6513	.6522
4.5	.6532	.6542	.6551	.6561	.6571	.6580	.6590	.6599	.6609	.6618
4.6	.6628	.6637	.6646	.6656	.6665	.6675	.6684	.6693	.6702	.6712
4.7	.6721	.6730	.6739	.6749	.6758	.6767	.6776	.6785	.6794	.6803
4.8	.6812	.6821	.6830	.6839	.6848	.6857	.6866	.6875	.6884	.6893
4.9	.6902	.6911	.6920	.6928	.6937	.6946	.6955	.6964	.6972	.6981
5.0	.6990	.6998	.7007	.7016	.7024	.7033	.7042	.7050	.7059	.7067
5.1	.7076	.7084	.7093	.7101	.7110	.7118	.7126	.7135	.7143	.7152
5.2	.7160	.7168	.7177	.7185	.7193	.7202	.7210	.7218	.7226	.7235
5.3	.7243	.7251	.7259	.7267	.7275	.7284	.7292	.7300	.7308	.7316
5.4	.7324	.7332	.7340	.7348	.7356	.7364	.7372	.7380	.7388	.7396
5.5	.7404	.7412	.7419	.7427	.7435	.7443	.7451	.7459	.7466	.7474
5.6	.7482	.7490	.7497	.7505	.7513	.7520	.7528	.7536	.7543	.7551
5.7	.7559	.7566	.7574	.7582	.7589	.7597	.7604	.7612	.7619	.7627
5.8	.7634	.7642	.7649	.7657	.7664	.7672	.7679	.7686	.7694	.7701
5.9	.7709	.7716	.7723	.7731	.7738	.7745	.7752	.7760	.7767	.7774
6.0	.7782	.7789	.7796	.7803	.7810	.7818	.7825	.7832	.7839	.7846
6.1	.7853	.7860	.7868	.7875	.7882	.7889	.7896	.7903	.7910	.7917
6.2	.7924	.7931	.7938	.7945	.7952	.7959	.7966	.7973	.7980	.7987
6.3	.7993	.8000	.8007	.8014	.8021	.8028	.8035	.8041	.8048	.8055
6.4	.8062	.8069	.8075	.8082	.8089	.8096	.8102	.8109	.8116	.8122
6.5	.8129	.8136	.8142	.8149	.8156	.8162	.8169	.8176	.8182	.8189
6.6	.8195	.8202	.8209	.8215	.8222	.8228	.8235	.8241	.8248	.8254
6.7	.8261	.8267	.8274	.8280	.8287	.8293	.8299	.8306	.8312	.8319
6.8	.8325	.8331	.8338	.8344	.8351	.8357	.8363	.8370	.8376	.8382
6.9	.8388	.8395	.8401	.8407	.8414	.8420	.8426	.8432	.8439	.8445
7.0	.8451	.8457	.8463	.8470	.8476	.8483	.8488	.8494	.8500	.8506
7.1	.8513	.8519	.8525	.8531	.8537	.8543	.8549	.8555	.8561	.8567
7.2	.8573	.8579	.8585	.8591	.8597	.8603	.8609	.8615	.8621	.8627
7.3	.8633	.8639	.8645	.8651	.8657	.8663	.8669	.8675	.8681	.8686
7.4	.8692	.8698	.8704	.8710	.8716	.8722	.8727	.8733	.8739	.8745
7.5	.8751	.8756	.8762	.8768	.8774	.8779	.8785	.8791	.8797	.8802
7.6	.8808	.8814	.8820	.8825	.8831	.8837	.8842	.8848	.8854	.8859
7.7	.8865	.8871	.8876	.8882	.8887	.8893	.8899	.8904	.8910	.8915
7.8	.8921	.8927	.8932	.8938	.8943	.8949	.8954	.8960	.8965	.8971
7.9	.8976	.8982	.8987	.8993	.8998	.9004	.9009	.9015	.9020	.9025
8.0	.9031	.9036	.9042	.9047	.9053	.9058	.9063	.9069	.9074	.9079
8.1	.9085	.9090	.9096	.9101	.9106	.9112	.9117	.9122	.9128	.9133
8.2	.9138	.9143	.9149	.9154	.9159	.9165	.9170	.9175	.9180	.9186
8.3	.9191	.9196	.9201	.9206	.9212	.9217	.9222	.9227	.9232	.9238
8.4	.9243	.9248	.9253	.9258	.9263	.9269	.9274	.9279	.9284	.9289
8.5	.9294	.9299	.9304	.9309	.9315	.9320	.9325	.9330	.9335	.9340
8.6	.9345	.9350	.9355	.9360	.9365	.9370	.9375	.9380	.9385	.9390
8.7	.9395	.9400	.9405	.9410	.9415	.9420	.9425	.9430	.9435	.9440
8.8	.9445	.9450	.9455	.9460	.9465	.9469	.9474	.9479	.9484	.9489
8.9	.9494	.9499	.9504	.9509	.9513	.9518	.9523	.9528	.9533	.9538
9.0	.9542	.9547	.9552	.9557	.9562	.9566	.9571	.9576	.9581	.9586
9.1	.9590	.9595	.9600	.9605	.9609	.9614	.9619	.9624	.9628	.9633
9.2	.9638	.9643	.9647	.9652	.9657	.9661	.9666	.9671	.9675	.9680
9.3	.9685	.9689	.9694	.9699	.9703	.9708	.9713	.9717	.9722	.9727
9.4	.9731	.9736	.9741	.9745	.9750	.9754	.9759	.9763	.9768	.9773

LOGARITHMS OF NUMBERS (*Continued*)

N	0	1	2	3	4	5	6	7	8	9
9.5	.9777	.9782	.9786	.9791	.9795	.9800	.9805	.9809	.9814	.9818
9.6	.9823	.9827	.9832	.9836	.9841	.9845	.9850	.9854	.9859	.9863
9.7	.9868	.9872	.9877	.9881	.9886	.9890	.9894	.9899	.9903	.9908
9.8	.9912	.9917	.9921	.9926	.9930	.9934	.9939	.9943	.9948	.9952
9.9	.9956	.9961	.9965	.9969	.9974	.9978	.9983	.9987	.9991	.9996

(From Seese, W., Daub, G. *In preparation for college chemistry.* Englewood Cliffs, N.J.: Prentice-Hall, 1980.)

Appendix D: Table of Atomic Weights

TABLE OF ATOMIC WEIGHTS (BASED ON CARBON-12)

Element	Symbol	Atomic Number	Atomic Weight	Element	Symbol	Atomic Number	Atomic Weight
Actinium	Ac	89	[227]*	Iridium	Ir	77	192.2
Aluminum	Al	13	26.9815	Iron	Fe	26	55.847
Americium	Am	95	[243]	Krypton	Kr	36	83.80
Antimony	Sb	51	121.75	Lanthanum	La	57	138.91
Argon	Ar	18	39.948	Lawrencium	Lw	103	[257]
Arsenic	As	33	74.9216	Lead	Pb	82	207.19
Astatine	At	85	[210]	Lithium	Li	3	6.939
Barium	Ba	56	137.34	Lutetium	Lu	71	174.97
Berkelium	Bk	97	[247]	Magnesium	Mg	12	24.312
Beryllium	Be	4	9.0122	Manganese	Mn	25	54.9380
Bismuth	Bi	83	208.980	Mendelevium	Md	101	[256]
Boron	B	5	10.811	Mercury	Hg	80	200.59
Bromine	Br	35	79.909	Molybdenum	Mo	42	95.94
Cadmium	Cd	48	112.40	Neodymium	Nd	60	144.24
Calcium	Ca	20	40.08	Neon	Ne	10	20.183
Californium	Cf	98	[249]	Neptunium	Np	93	[237]
Carbon	C	6	12.01115	Nickel	Ni	28	58.71
Cerium	Ce	58	140.12	Niobium	Nb	41	92.906
Cesium	Cs	55	132.905	Nitrogen	N	7	14.0067
Chlorine	Cl	17	35.453	Nobelium	No	102	[253]
Chromium	Cr	24	51.996	Osmium	Os	76	190.2
Cobalt	Co	27	58.9332	Oxygen	O	8	15.9994
Copper	Cu	29	63.546	Palladium	Pd	46	106.4
Curium	Cm	96	[247]	Phosphorus	P	15	30.9738
Dysprosium	Dy	66	162.50	Platinum	Pt	78	195.09
Einsteinium	Es	99	254	Plutonium	Pu	94	[212]
Erbium	Er	68	167.26	Polonium	Po	81	[210]
Europium	Eu	63	151.96	Potassium	K	19	39.102
Fermium	Fm	100	[253]	Praseodymium	Pr	59	140.907
Fluorine	F	9	18.9984	Promethium	Pm	61	[145]
Francium	Fr	87	[223]	Protactinium	Pa	91	[231]
Gadolinium	Gd	64	157.25	Radium	Ra	88	[226]
Gallium	Ga	31	69.72	Radon	Rn	86	[222]
Germanium	Ge	32	72.59	Rhenium	Re	75	186.2
Gold	Au	79	196.967	Rhodium	Rh	45	102.905
Hafnium	Hf	72	178.49	Rubidium	Rb	37	85.47
Helium	He	2	4.0026	Ruthenium	Ru	44	101.07
Holmium	Ho	67	164.930	Samarium	Sm	62	150.35
Hydrogen	H	1	1.00797	Scandium	Sc	21	44.956
Indium	In	49	114.82	Selenium	Se	34	78.96
Iodine	I	53	126.9044	Silicon	Si	14	28.086

TABLE OF ATOMIC WEIGHTS (BASED ON CARBON-12) (*Continued*)

Element	Symbol	Atomic Number	Atomic Weight	Element	Symbol	Atomic Number	Atomic Weight
Silver	Ag	47	107.870	Tin	Sn	50	118.69
Sodium	Na	11	22.9898	Titanium	Ti	22	47.90
Strontium	Sr	38	87.62	Tungsten	W	74	183.85
Sulfur	S	16	32.064	Uranium	U	92	238.03
Tantalum	Ta	73	180.948	Vanadium	V	23	50.942
Technetium	Tc	43	[99]	Xenon	Xe	54	131.30
Tellurium	Te	52	127.60	Ytterbium	Yb	70	173.04
Terbium	Tb	65	158.924	Yttrium	Y	39	88.905
Thallium	Tl	81	204.37	Zinc	Zn	30	65.37
Thorium	Th	90	232.038	Zirconium	Zr	40	91.22
Thulium	Tm	69	168.934				

* A value given in brackets denotes the mass number of the longest-lived or best-known isotope.

(From Nelson, J. H., Kemp, K. C. *Laboratory experiments for Brown and LeMay chemistry*, Englewood Cliffs, N.J.: Prentice-Hall, 1977.)

Appendix E: Periodic Table of Elements

PERIODIC TABLE OF THE ELEMENTS

GROUPS

PERIODS	IA	IIA	IIIB	IVB	VB	VIB	VIIB	VIII			IB	IIB	IIIA	IVA	VA	VIA	VIIA	0
1	1.008 H 1																	4.003 He 2
2	6.941 Li 3	9.012 Be 4											10.81 B 5	12.011 C 6	14.007 N 7	15.999 O 8	18.998 F 9	20.179 Ne 10
3	22.990 Na 11	24.305 Mg 12	TRANSITION ELEMENTS										26.982 Al 13	28.086 Si 14	30.9738 P 15	32.06 S 16	35.453 Cl 17	39.948 Ar 18
4	39.102 K 19	40.08 Ca 20	44.956 Sc 21	47.90 Ti 22	50.941 V 23	51.996 Cr 24	54.938 Mn 25	55.847 Fe 26	58.933 Co 27	58.71 Ni 28	63.546 Cu 29	65.37 Zn 30	69.72 Ga 31	72.59 Ge 32	74.922 As 33	78.96 Se 34	79.904 Br 35	83.80 Kr 36
5	85.468 Rb 37	87.62 Sr 38	88.906 Y 39	91.22 Zr 40	92.9064 Nb 41	95.94 Mo 42	98.906 Tc 43	101.07 Ru 44	102.906 Rh 45	106.4 Pd 46	107.868 Ag 47	112.40 Cd 48	114.82 In 49	118.69 Sn 50	121.75 Sb 51	127.60 Te 52	126.904 I 53	131.30 Xe 54
6	132.906 Cs 55	137.34 Ba 56	138.906 *La 57	178.49 Hf 72	180.948 Ta 73	183.85 W 74	186.2 Re 75	190.2 Os 76	192.22 Ir 77	195.09 Pt 78	196.967 Au 79	200.59 Hg 80	204.37 Tl 81	207.2 Pb 82	208.981 Bi 83	(209) Po 84	(210) At 85	(222) Rn 86
7	(223) Fr 87	226.025 Ra 88	(227) **Ac 89	[(261) Rf 104]	[(260) Ha 105]	[(263) 106]												

***Lanthanides**	140.12 Ce 58	140.908 Pr 59	144.24 Nd 60	(145) Pm 61	150.4 Sm 62	151.96 Eu 63	157.25 Gd 64	158.925 Tb 65	162.50 Dy 66	164.930 Ho 67	167.26 Er 68	168.934 Tm 69	173.04 Yb 70	174.97 Lu 71
****Actinides**	232.038 Th 90	231.031 Pa 91	238.029 U 92	237.048 Np 93	(244) Pu 94	(243) Am 95	(247) Cm 96	(247) Bk 97	(251) Cf 98	(254) Es 99	(253) Fm 100	(256) Md 101	(253) No 102	(257) Lr 103

Numbers below the symbol of the element indicate the atomic numbers. Atomic masses, above the symbol of the element, are based on the assigned relative atomic mass of ^{12}C — exactly 12; ( ) indicates the mass number of the isotope with the longest half-life. [ ] indicates not officially approved or named.

(From Seese, W., Daub, G. *In preparation for college chemistry.* Englewood Cliffs, N.J.: Prentice-Hall, 1980.)

Appendix F: Answers to Odd-Numbered Problems and to All Reviews

CHAPTER 1

Problem Set 1

1. 3
3. 2
5. −35.7
7. −271.26
9. 0.6
11. 1002.5
13. 18.48
15. −16
17. −2423.925
19. −394.5
21. $-\frac{29}{42}$
23. −4.8
25. −16
27. 8
29. 1.1
31. 2
33. 125

Problem Set 2

1. 27
3. 48
5. 51.84
7. 6.25
9. $\frac{1}{125}$
11. 144
13. −51.2
15. 576
17. $-\frac{1}{4}$
19. 72

Problem Set 3

1. 21
3. 45
5. −2
7. −14
9. 123
11. 44
13. 0
15. 141
17. 46
19. 46

Chapter Review

1. real; rational; integer
2. real; rational
3. real; rational; integer; whole; natural
4. real; rational
5. real; irrational
6. 8
7. −7
8. −1
9. 297
10. −150
11. 9.75
12. 9
13. 6
14. 48
15. −38
16. 12
17. −16.5
18. 4.2
19. 0
20. 81
21. −32
22. −1
23. $-\frac{8}{27}$
24. $6\frac{4}{39}$
25. −3
26. 31
27. 128
28. 17
29. 84
30. $-\frac{19}{4}$

CHAPTER 2

Problem Set 1

1. a. 2401

   c. 16

   e. 2.25

   g. 128

   i. −16
3. 150.72 m^2
5. −17
7. $2.61\overline{6}$ in^3
9. 32.1536 m^3

Problem Set 2

1. $2^9 = 512$
3. $2^6 = 64$
5. x^{12}
7. x^5y^5
9. $8x^7y^4$
11. $\frac{x^8}{16y^4}$
13. $\frac{x^7y}{2}$
15. 1
17. $\frac{x}{2z^2y}$

Problem Set 3

1. 4.2
3. $5x$
5. 7.4
7. 9
9. $\frac{1}{5}$
11. $2^{1/2}xy^{3/2}$
13. $4y^{1/3}z^{4/3}$
15. $2y^{4/5}z^{2/5}$
17. $144x^2\sqrt{y}$
19. $\sqrt[4]{2x^2y}$
21. $9\sqrt[6]{x^8y^3}$

Problem Set 4

1. no
3. no
5. yes
7. $9y$
9. $29xy - 22yz + 6xz$
11. $prs^2 - 19pr^2s + 16p^2rs$
13. $9qz^2 + 14qzt - 4qzt^2$
15. $18ab^3 - 91a^3b - 10a^3b^3 + 17ab$

Chapter Review

1. a. 3^4
   b. x^5
   c. $8y^3$
2. 288 ft
3. 18.1 ft^2
4. a. $8x^6$
   b. $15y^3$
   c. $\frac{16z^{12}}{y^4}$
   d. $324x^8y^6z^{12}$
   e. $8x^5y^{11}$
5. a. 5
   b. 1
   c. $\frac{108}{y^7}$
   d. 81
   e. $\frac{16}{9x^4y^6}$
   f. $\frac{y^3}{2}$
   g. 1
   h. $\frac{3z^3}{xy^4}$
   i. $3xy$
   j. $\frac{x^2y^{21}}{72z^2}$
6. a. 10.4
   b. 56.0
   c. 1.7
   d. -9
7. 9.2
8. a. $3\sqrt[3]{x}$
   b. $\sqrt[3]{3x}$
   c. $\sqrt[5]{4y^3z}$
   d. $4\sqrt[3]{x^2y}$
   e. $7\sqrt[4]{y^3z}$
9. a. $2^{1/4}x^{1/4}y^{3/4}$ or $(2xy^3)^{1/4}$
   b. $\left(\frac{1}{g}\right)^{1/2}$
   c. $3xy^{1/2}$
   d. $5^{1/3}x^{2/3}y^{4/3}$ or $(5x^2y^4)^{1/3}$
   e. $\left(\frac{3}{4}\right)^{1/3}v^{2/3}$
10. a. 16
    b. 1331
    c. 216
    d. $\frac{1}{9}$
    e. $\frac{1}{81}$
11. a. $25.5x^2 - 5x^2y - 2.5xy^2$
    b. $9x^2yz - 4xyz^2 - 100xy^2z$
    c. $-\frac{1}{4}pr^2 + \frac{17}{24}p^2r + \frac{1}{3}p^2r^2$
    d. $-2y^2z - 6.5yz^2 - 3yz$
    e. $-6x^2z^2q - 9xz^2q^2 + 20x^2zq^2$

CHAPTER 3

Problem Set 1

1. 3
3. 1
5. 4
7. 1

9. 4
11. infinite
13. 3
15. 4
17. 1
19. 5

Problem Set 2

1. 39 cm
3. 7.7 m
5. $1\bar{0}0$ mL
7. 0.37 cg
9. 5.0 g
11. 1.9 mm
13. 1.0 a.m.u.
15. 12.0 a.m.u.
17. 39.1 a.m.u.
19. 24.3 a.m.u.
21. 14.0 a.m.u.
23. 63.5 a.m.u.

Problem Set 3

1. 16.9
3. 50
5. 0.000063
7. 633.1
9. 2000
11. 22.23
13. $50\bar{0}$
15. ≈ 2
17. 167

Problem Set 4

1. $5.0 \cdot 10^7$
3. $3.909 \cdot 10^{10}$
5. $4.6 \cdot 10^1$
7. $5.09 \cdot 10^9$
9. 10^8
11. $2.7 \cdot 10^{-7}$
13. $2.0 \cdot 10^1$
15. $3.48 \cdot 10^4$
17. $2 \cdot 10^1$
19. $7.06 \cdot 10^7$
21. $8.34 \cdot 10^5$
23. $2.1 \cdot 10^{-3}$
25. $3.08 \cdot 10^{-2}$
27. $7.922 \cdot 10^4$
29. $6 \cdot 10^8$ problems
31. $1.80 \cdot 10^{10}$ m
33. $1.0 \cdot 10^4$ mg

Chapter Review

1. 3
2. 2
3. 4
4. 3
5. 3
6. 1
7. 4.84 cL
8. 864 m
9. 2.01 dg
10. 1,290,000 mi
11. $1.00 \cdot 10^5$ hm
12. 16.0 a.m.u.
13. 2.65
14. 32,000
15. $14\bar{0}$
16. 1.0
17. $3.2014 \cdot 10^2$
18. $8.01 \cdot 10^{-1}$
19. $1.821 \cdot 10^8$
20. $2.22 \cdot 10^{-4}$
21. $4.60 \cdot 10^5$
22. $2.99 \cdot 10^{22}$
23. 1
24. $1.35 \cdot 10^6$
25. $2.1 \cdot 10^{-3}$
26. $8.70 \cdot 10^{-10}$ m

CHAPTER 4

Problem Set 1

1. 2600
3. 0.04
5. 100,000
7. 20
9. 4,330,000
11. 0.0084
13. 0.02999
15. 10,000
17. 1,000,000
19. 1
21. 2070
23. 0.0002384
25. 1,000,000
27. 0.003267

Problem Set 2

1. 14.7 mL
3. 120,000 cc
5. measure out 520 mL of water
7. about 70 g

Problem Set 3

1. 165 lb
3. 3.2 kg
5. 91.4 m
7. 188 cm
9. 60.0 mi/hr
11. answers vary
13. 120 mL
15. 28.8 m^2
17. $\approx$ 6100 mL
19. 5.7 L
21. 800 g

Chapter Review

1. 23.5 mm
2. 19,200 g
3. 0.039 dL
4. 2 dag
5. 2.1 mL
6. 803,000 dL
7. 14,200 mg
8. 0.0000000024 L
9. 780 dg
10. 0.0963 km
11. $\approx 5\bar{0}$ g
12. $\approx$ 25.2 g
13. $\approx$ 76,000 kg
14. $\approx$ 170 lb
15. 4.0 kg
16. $25\overline{00}$ mL
17. 2.4 L
18. 270 gtt
19. 4600 mg

CHAPTER 5

Problem Set 1

1. Identity Rule for Multiplication
3. Inverse Rule for Addition
5. Associative Rule for Addition
7. Identity Rule for Addition
9. Distributive Property

Problem Set 2

1. -1
3. -8
5. 307
7. 2
9. -121
11. -7
13. $\frac{10}{9}$
15. $-\frac{13}{7}$
17. 6
19. $-\frac{9}{4}$
21. $-\frac{1}{6}$
23. $-\frac{10}{3}$
25. $+\frac{31}{4}$
27. $\frac{32}{13}$
29. $+\frac{123}{11}$

Problem Set 3

1. 68
3. $\frac{7}{3}$
5. $\frac{3}{4}$
7. $\frac{33}{136}$
9. $\frac{20}{7}$
11. $-\frac{1}{48}$
13. 3
15. $\frac{504}{11}$
17. $-\frac{4}{3}$
19. $\frac{17}{71}$

Problem Set 4

1. P_1/P_2
3. TR/k
5. $C/2\pi$
7. E/c^2
9. $2E/V^2$
11. $P - P_1 - P_2$
13. $7 - 16b/5$
15. $4R + 6/3$
17. $\frac{5}{9}(F - 32)$
19. $28 - 2M/M$
21. $fv/v - f$
23. $6 - 3x/x + 2$

Problem Set 5

1. 35
3. $\frac{432}{13}$
5. 2
7. 4
9. $\frac{25}{18}$
11. $1\frac{1}{4}$ inches
13. 0.0004%
15. $94.\overline{4}$%
17. 3.875 g
19. 14
21. 0.00003%
23. Caustic Chemical Co. $\approx$ \$.58/oz

Problem Set 6

1. $V = kR$
3. $W = k/L$
5. $X = kN/L$
7. $D = kr\sqrt{t}/4e$
9. $W = 2/L$
11. $D = 8r\sqrt{t}/4e$
13. 9 cc
15. Area is doubled.
17. Hydrogen is 4 times faster.
19. It would be $\frac{1}{16}$ as much.

Chapter Review

1. Inverse Rule for Multiplication
2. Distributive Rule
3. Associative and Commutative Rules for Multiplication
4. 17
5. -5
6. $\frac{24}{7}$
7. $\frac{20}{3}$
8. -3
9. $\frac{34}{3}$
10. $2A/h$
11. PV/nT
12. $P_2V_2T_1/P_1V_1$
13. $\frac{3tq}{2t-q}$
14. $2tR/R + 3t$
15. 3
16. 5
17. 1000
18. $\frac{3}{7}$
19. 2.625 mi
20. Company A, about 46¢/oz.
21. 512 mi
22. 9
23. $W = kx$
24. $Z = k/Y$
25. $Q = kPRS/T$
26. $W = 3x$
27. $Z = 2/Y$
28. $Q = 0.5PRS/T$
29. $G = 100ht^2/q$
30. 1000

CHAPTER 6

Problem Set 1

1. 1.0%
3. 15.7%
5. 5.00%
7. Use $6\overline{0}$ g benzalkonium chloride.
9. ≈ 1100 mL
11. 2.50%
13. 80 mL
15. Use 34.0 g $FeSO_4$; add 816 g H_2O.
17. 1.20 mg %
19. 0.05 mg % to 0.18 mg %

Problem Set 2

1. 0.0018%
3. 0.0020%
5. 820 ppb < 1.2 ppm
7. 0.02%
9. 74% N_2O; 25% O_2; 1% halothane
11. Left for the student to prove.
13. 0.02%
15. 750 mL

Problem Set 3

1. a. 200.6 g
   c. 106.8 g
   e. 159.8 g
   g. 80.0 g
   i. 84.0 g
   k. 46.0 g
2. a. 0.444 mol
   c. 0.953 mol
   e. 0.000035 mol
   g. 4.5 mol
   i. 17 mol
   k. 0.5906 mol
3. 4.9 *M*
5. 4.0 *M*
7. 2.35 *M*
9. 0.338 *M*
11. $6\overline{0}$ g NaOH needed
13. 22.5 g
15. Need 0.800 mol; have 0.685 mol
17. 0.636 *M*

Problem Set 4

1. a. 32.7 g
   c. 37.0 g
   e. 20.0 g
   g. 41.0 g
2. a. $1\overline{0}0$ mEq
   c. 505 mEq
   e. $15\overline{0}$ mEq
   g. 350 mEq
3. a. 9.59 Eq
   c. 0.262 Eq
   e. 0.307 Eq
   g. 0.45 Eq
4. a. 1.46 *N*
   c. 0.893 *N*
   e. 10.5 *N*
5. 74 mL
7. $8\overline{0}$ Eq
9. 36.2 *N*

Problem Set 5

1. Use 42 mL 12.0 *M* HCl.
3. $3\overline{0}$%
5. Add 600 mL H_2O.
7. Use $28\overline{0}$ mL of 9.00 *N* H_2SO_4.
9. Dilute 15 mL of 12 *M* HCl up to 900 mL.
11. Beaker # 1 = 0.20%
    Beaker #2 = $2.0 \cdot 10^{-3}$%
    Beaker #3 = $2.0 \cdot 10^{-5}$%
    Beaker #4 = $2.0 \cdot 10^{-7}$%

Chapter Review

1. 7.28%
2. 0.011%
3. 215 mL
4. Use 65 g of $KMnO_4$.
5. 939 mg
6. $1.3 \cdot 10^{-2}$ g
7. $2.0 \cdot 10^{4}$ ppm
8. 360 g
9. 0.28*M*
10. 0.377 N
11. a. 61.5 mEq
    b. 197 mEq
12. Use 236 mL of 95% alcohol solution.
13. 5000 mL
14. Beaker #1 = 0.300 *M*
    Beaker #2 = 0.0150 *M*
    Beaker #3 = 0.00075 *M*

CHAPTER 7

Problem Set 1

1. 0.659
3. −1.133
5. −2.405
7. 3.9518
9. 5.990783
11. −0.04503
13. 1.5901
15. 3.8319
17. −2.3169
19. 0.01870
21. 4 log(2.3)
23. log(2.3) + log(4.2) − log(1.5)

Problem Set 2

1. 50.80
3. 3240
5. 0.0001000
7. 0.0938
9. 0.005370
11. 5.492
13. $5.994 \cdot 10^{6}$
15. 158.0
17. 21.30
19. $9.9 \cdot 10^{-3}$

Problem Set 3

1. 11.8
3. 2.39
5. 1.42
7. $6.67 \cdot 10^{3}$
9. $5.98 \cdot 10^{-3}$
11. 3.28
13. 0.3776
15. $2.4 \cdot 10^{7}$
17. 0.2143
19. $3.2 \cdot 10^{-12}$

Problem Set 4

1. a. 2
   b. 4.28
   c. 4.10
   d. 12.1
   e. 6.59
2. a. $1.7 \cdot 10^{-7}$ mol/L
   c. $6.2 \cdot 10^{-4}$ mol/L
   e. $6.0 \cdot 10^{-14}$ mol/L
3. $9.8 \cdot 10^{-10}$ mol/L
5. pH = 2.6
7. 4.06
9. 0.418
11. 0 = 100%T
    4 = 0.01%T

Chapter Review

1. a. 1.450
   b. 2.1544
   c. −2.107
   d. 3.1072
2. a. 498.0
   b. 2563
   c. 0.01093
   d. $1.535 \cdot 10^{-4}$
3. a. 13.5
   b. 1.71
   c. 11.16
   d. 0.258
4. a. 5.291
   b. 2.515
5. a. $3.9 \cdot 10^{-9}$ mol/L
   b. $5 \cdot 10^{-3}$ mol/L
6. 3.65
7. 1.6%

CHAPTER 8

Problem Set 1

1. $\overline{MN}$, $\overline{NO}$, $\overline{OP}$, $\overline{PM}$
3. $\overline{MN}$, $\overline{NO}$
5. a. *DCFE* b. *ABCD*, *ADEH* c. $\overline{BC}$, $\overline{FG}$, $\overline{EH}$
7. $\angle FGE$ and $\angle AGF$; $\angle BGC$ and $\angle CGD$
9.
11. $\angle a$—acute
    $\angle b$—acute
    $\angle c$—right
    $\angle d$—acute
    $\angle e$—obtuse

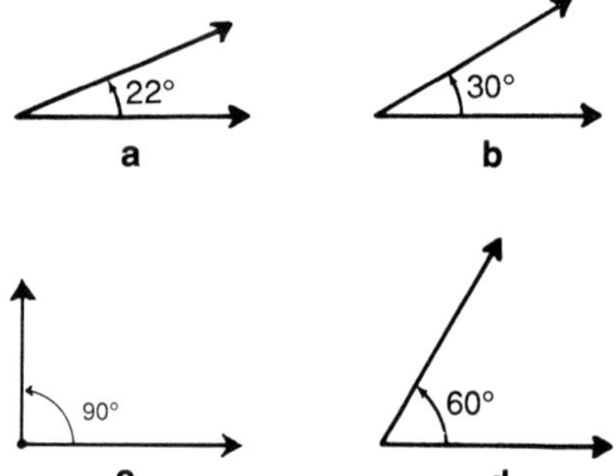

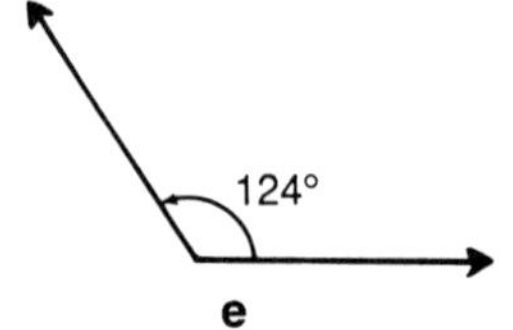

Problem Set 2

1. **a.** right triangle; **b.** rhombus; **c.** isoceles triangle; **d.** square;
   e. rectangle; **f.** parallelogram; **g.** scalene triangle.
3. **a.** 16 cm^2; **b.** 2000 yd^2;
   c. 12.6 cm^2, round to 13 cm^2; **d.** 94.5 m^2;
   e. 357 km^2 + 59.5 km^2 = 416.5 km^2; round to $4.2 \cdot 10^2$ km^2;
   f. 253.12 m^2; round to $2.5 \cdot 10^2$ m^2;
   g. 175.5 ft^2; round to $1.8 \cdot 10^2$ ft^2;
   h. 240.3 cm^2; round to $2.40 \cdot 10^2$ cm^2;
   i. 615.44 cm^2; round to $6.2 \cdot 10^2$ cm^2;
   j. 5460.1146 mm^2; round to $5.46 \cdot 10^3$ mm^2;
   k. 113.04 cm^2; round to $1 \cdot 10^2$ cm^2.
5. 1155 lb
7. 3612.5 ft^2
9. 56.5 cm^2
11. **a.** 864 mm^2
    b. $\approx$ 43 mm

Problem Set 3

1. a. 624.24 m^2; round to $6.24 \cdot 10^2$ m^2
   b. 369.92 mm^2; round to $3.7 \cdot 10^2$ mm^2
   c. 1256 m^2; round to $1.26 \cdot 10^3$ m^2
   d. 1153.153 in^2; round to $1.15 \cdot 10^3$ m^2
   e. 6847.2096 ft^2; round to $6.85 \cdot 10^3$ ft^2
3. $59.40\overline{6}$ m^3; round to $5.9 \cdot 10$ in^3
5. 6.28 in^3; round to 6.3 in^3
7. $5 \cdot 10^{-7}$ cm^3
9. $9.4 \cdot 10^3$ lb
11. a. 206.58766 cm^3; round to $2.1 \cdot 10^2$ cm^3
    b. 344.27509 cm^3; round to $3.4 \cdot 10^2$ cm^3
    c. 25,120 mm^3; round to $2.5 \cdot 10^4$ mm^3
    d. 712,152 mm^3; round to $7.1 \cdot 10^5$ mm^3
    e. 86.23225 mm^3; round to $8.6 \cdot 10$ mm^3
13. 13.6 kg
15. 8694 g; round to $8.7 \cdot 10^3$ g
17. $6.35 \cdot 10^2$ m

Chapter Review

1. a. $\overleftrightarrow{AB}$, $\overleftrightarrow{DC}$; b. $\angle HGI$, $\angle GIH$, $\angle IHG$
   c. $\angle HIG$ and $\angle FIG$; $\angle FIG$ and $\angle FID$; $\angle FID$ and $\angle DIH$; $\angle DIH$ and $\angle HIG$; $\angle EHG$ and $\angle GHI$; $\angle GHI$ and $\angle AHI$; $\angle AHI$ and $\angle AHE$; $\angle AHE$ and $\angle EHG$; $\angle HGI$ and $\angle CGH$; $\angle CGH$ and $\angle CGB$; $\angle CGB$ and $\angle BGI$; $\angle BGI$ and $\angle HGI$.
   d. $\angle GHI$, $\angle EHG$, $\angle EHA$, $\angle AHI$.
   e. $\overline{CG}$, $\overline{CI}$, $\overline{CD}$, $\overline{GI}$, $\overline{GD}$, $\overline{ID}$; end points may be reversed, i.e., $\overline{CG}$ and $\overline{GC}$ are the same segment.
   f. no
2. a. 40° b. 125°
3. 45° is an acute angle; 135° is an obtuse angle; 390° coincides with an acute angle of 30°.

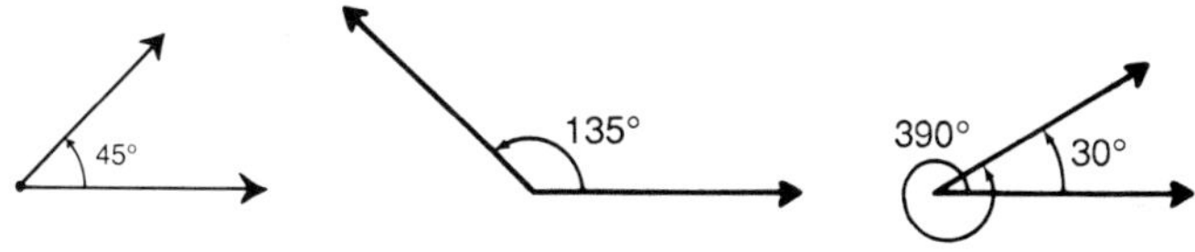

4. 113.9 ft^2; round to $1.1 \cdot 10^2$ ft^2
5. 196 cm^2
6. about 71.7 cm
7. 1439 cm^2; round to $1.44 \cdot 10^3$ cm^2
8. 244.4 ft^2; round to $2.4 \cdot 10^2$ ft^2
9. 19

10. **a.** $2.7 \cdot 10^{13}$ dm^3; **b.** $3.35 \cdot 10^4$ cm^3; **c.** $3.34 \cdot 10^6$ mm^3; **d.** $1.33 \cdot 10^2$ cm^3
11. **a.** $5.4 \cdot 10^9$ dm^2; **b.** $5.02 \cdot 10^3$ cm^2; **c.** $1.24 \cdot 10^5$ mm^2
12. $1.81 \cdot 10^3$ g
13. $5 \cdot 10^{-10}$ g
14. $6 \cdot 10^6$ atoms

CHAPTER 9

Problem Set 1

1. $\bar{x}$ = \$40.83
   $\tilde{x}$ = \$40.00
   mode = \$40.00
3. $\bar{x}$ = 63.4 inches
   $\tilde{x}$ = 63 inches
   bimodal
5. $\bar{x}$ = 3.82
   $\tilde{x}$ = 4.05
   mode = 4.5
7. Yes, examples will vary.
   2,3,4
   $\bar{x} = 3$
   $\tilde{x} = 3$
   mean = median

   2,3,3,3,4
   $\bar{x} = 3$
   mode = 3

   3,3,3
   $\bar{x} = 3$
   $\tilde{x} = 3$
   mode = 3

Problem Set 2

1. $s \approx \$6.15$
5. $s \approx 3.7$ inches
3. $s \approx 0.67$ kg
7. $z_1 = \dfrac{70 - 60}{10} = 1$

   $z_2 = \dfrac{75 - 66}{2} = 4.5$

   75 is more deviant.

Problem Set 3

1.

Entry	*Frequency*
32	1
38	1
40	2
45	1
50	1

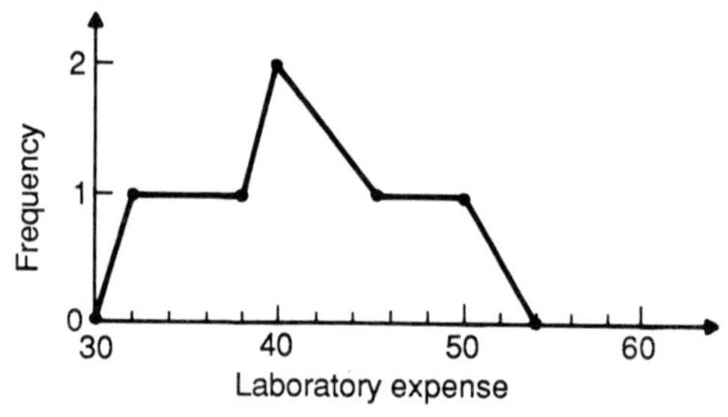

3.

Entry	*Frequency*
58	1
60	2
62	1
63	2
64	1
66	1
68	1
70	1

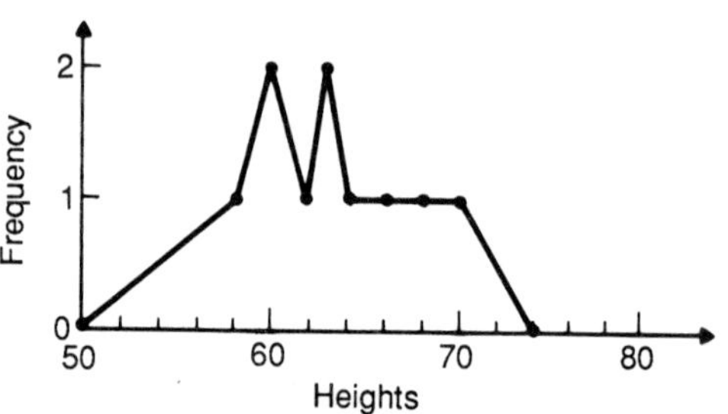

5.

Entry	*Frequency*
2.4	1
3.1	1
3.2	1
3.5	2
4.0	1
4.1	1
4.2	1
4.3	1
4.5	3

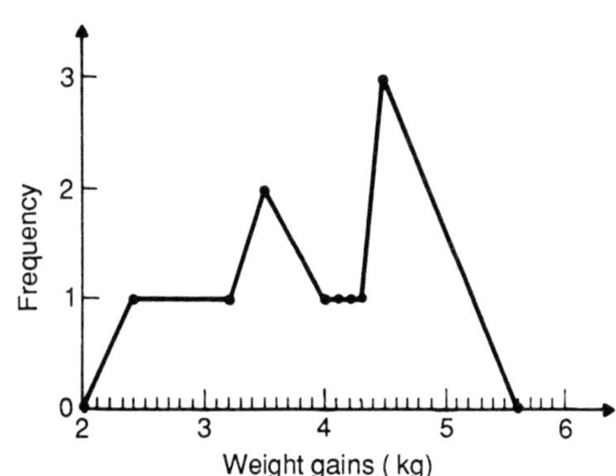

7. a. $\bar{x} = 24.9$ days
$\tilde{x} = 24.5$ days
mode = 24
$s \approx 3.0$

b. $\bar{x} = 296.9$ mg/dL
$\tilde{x} = 282$ mg/dL
mode = 282 mg/dL
$s \approx 41.2$ mg/dL

Problem Set 4

1. a. Answers may vary. The following is one possibility.

x	f	X	Xf	X^2	X^2f
60–66	4	63	252	3969	15876
67–73	3	70	210	4900	14700
74–80	10	77	770	5929	59290
81–87	2	84	168	7056	14112
88–94	5	91	455	8281	41405
95–101	3	98	294	9604	28812
102–108	3	105	315	11025	33075

$$\Sigma f = 30$$
$$\Sigma X = 588$$
$$\Sigma Xf = 2464$$
$$\Sigma X^2 = 50764$$
$$\Sigma X^2 f = 207{,}270$$

b. $\bar{x} = 82.1$

c. $\tilde{x} = 76$

d. $R = 44$

e. $s \approx 13$

Problem Set 5

1.

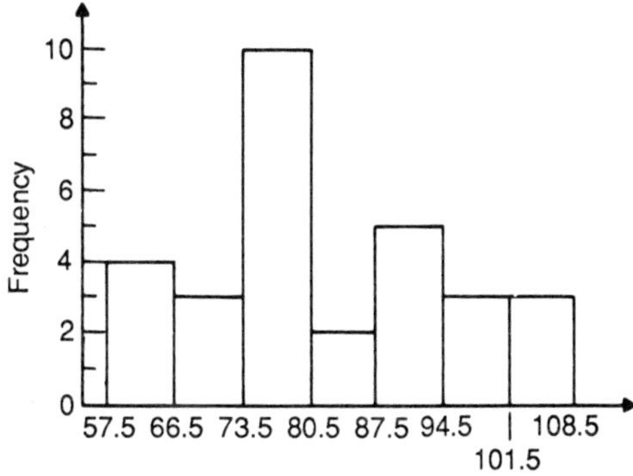

Chapter Review

1. a. $\bar{x} = 4.8$

   b. $\tilde{x} = 4.5$

   c. mode = 6

   d. $s \approx 2.6$

   e.

Entry	*Frequency*
1	3
2	4
3	4
4	4
5	2
6	5
7	3
8	1
9	3
10	1

   f.

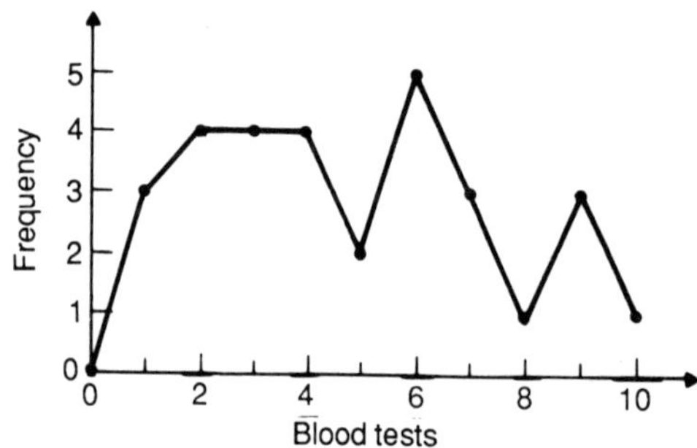

2. a. $\bar{x} = 25.2$

   b. $\tilde{x} = 26$

   c. mode = 26

   d. $s \approx 3.3$

   e.

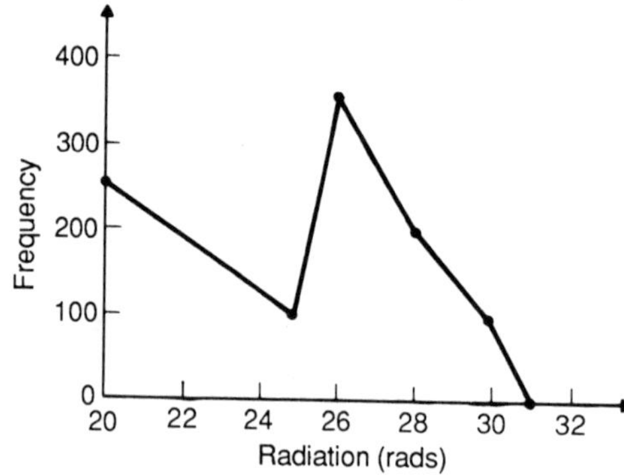

3. a. $\bar{x} = 250$

   b. $\tilde{x} = 250$

   c. mode = 250

   d. $s \approx 63.1$

4. The patient with reading of 150 is only 1 standard deviation above the mean in the group, whereas the patient with a reading of 146 is 2.3 standard deviations above

the mean in that group. Therefore the patient with a reading of 150 has lower relative blood pressure.

5. Answers will vary. The following is one possibility.

x	f	X	Xf	X^2	X^2f
45–59	12	52	624	2704	32,448
60–74	18	67	1206	4489	80,802
75–89	16	82	1312	6724	107,584
90–104	4	97	388	9409	37,636

$\Sigma f = 50$
$\Sigma X = 298$
$\Sigma Xf = 3530$
$\Sigma X^2 = 23326$
$\Sigma X^2 f = 258{,}470$

6. a. $\bar{x} = 70.6$

b. $\tilde{x} = 70$

c. mode $= 68$

d. $R = 49$

e. $s \approx 13.7$

7. 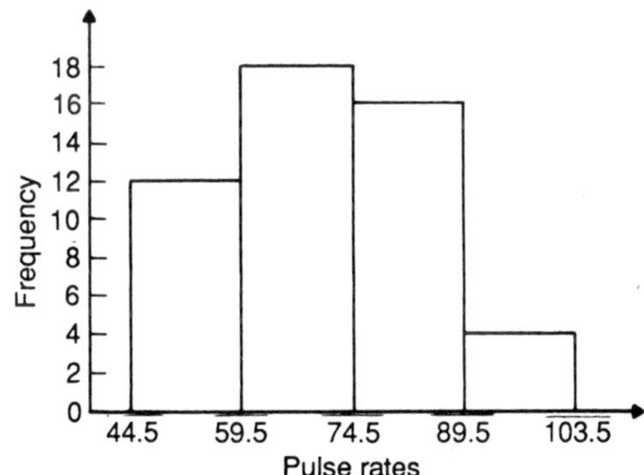

CHAPTER 10

Problem Set 1

1. no 3. yes 5. yes

7. 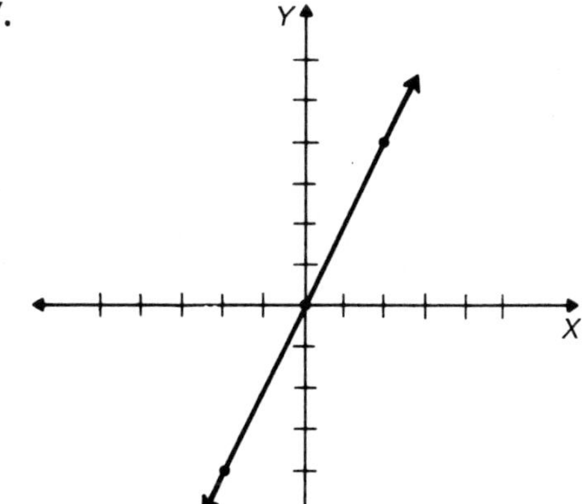

x	y
0	0
−2	−4
2	4

9.

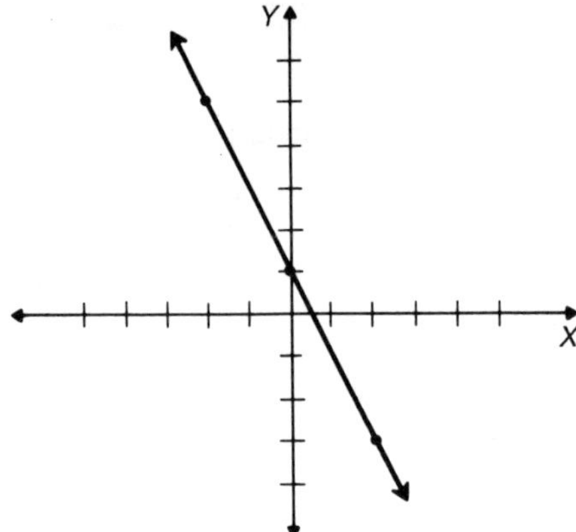

x	y
0	1
2	−3
−2	5

11.

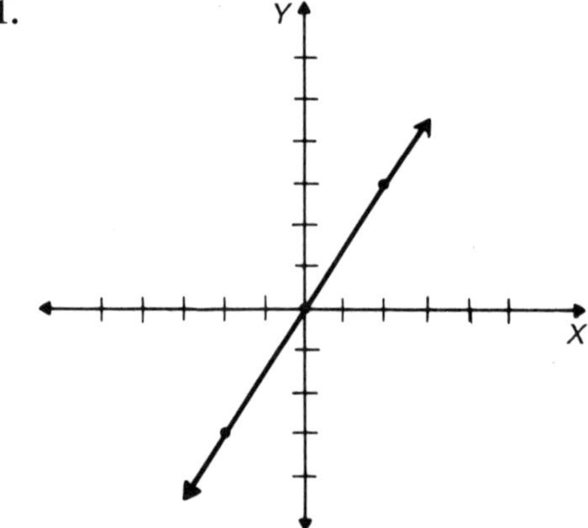

x	y
2	3
0	0
−2	−3

13.

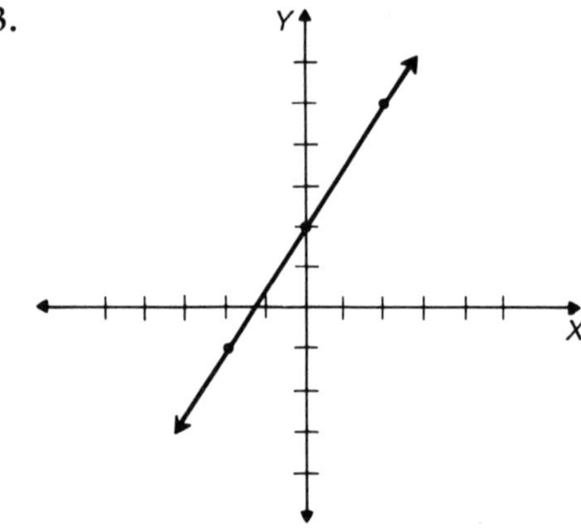

x	y
0	2
2	5
−2	−1

15.

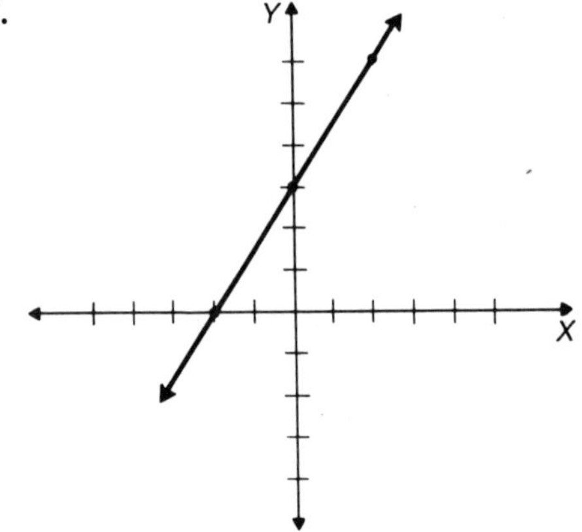

x	y
0	3
2	6
−2	0

17.

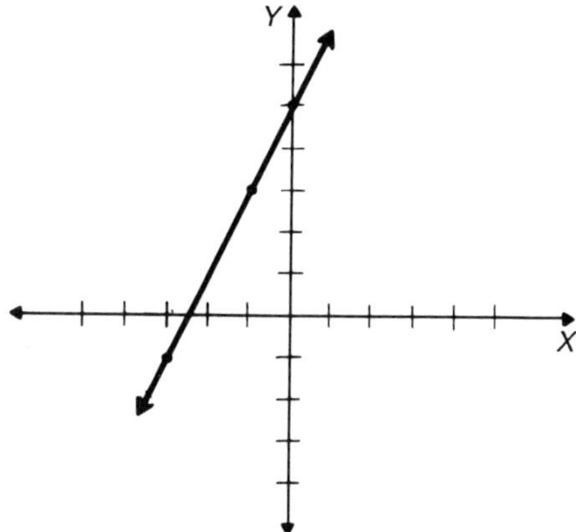

x	y
0	5
−3	−1
−1	3

19.

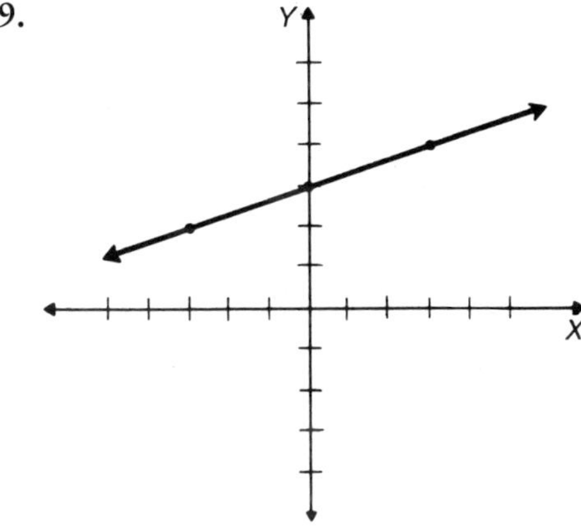

x	y
0	3
3	4
−3	2

21.

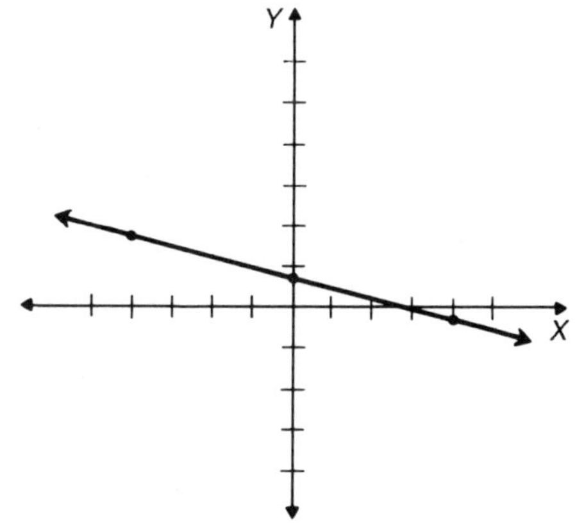

x	y
0	$\frac{3}{4}$
4	$-\frac{1}{4}$
−4	$1\frac{3}{4}$

23.

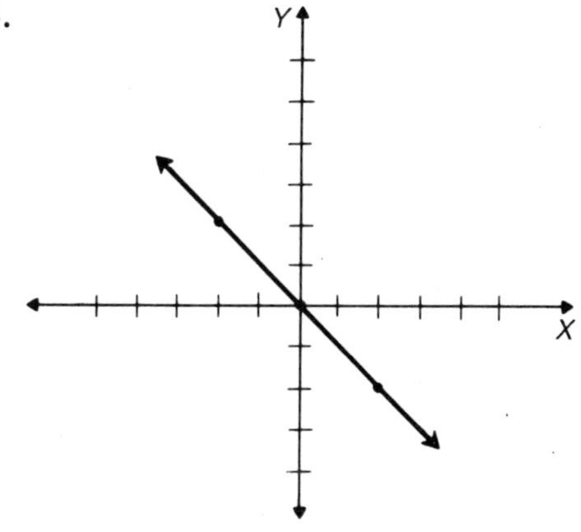

x	y
0	0
−2	2
2	−2

25.

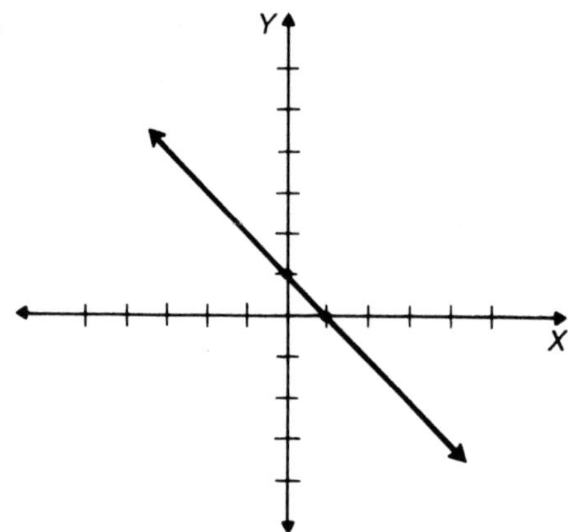

x	y
0	1
1	0

27.

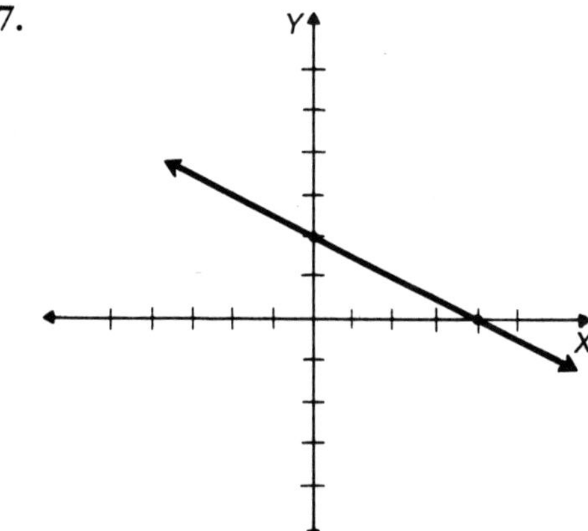

x	y
0	2
4	0

29.

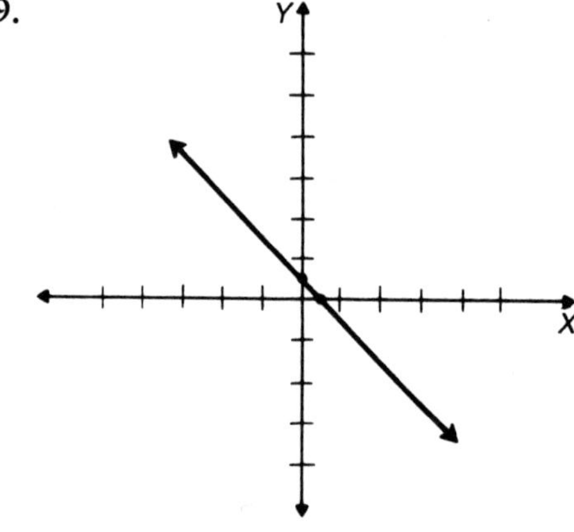

x	y
$\frac{1}{2}$	0
0	$\frac{1}{2}$

31.

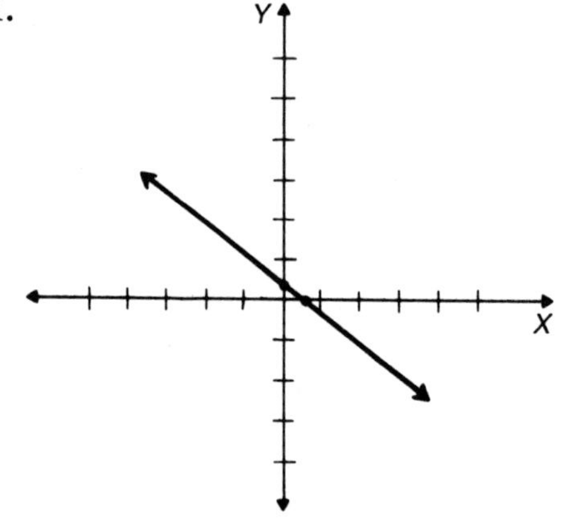

x	y
0	$\frac{1}{3}$
$\frac{2}{3}$	0

Problem Set 2

1. 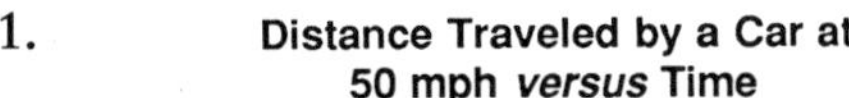

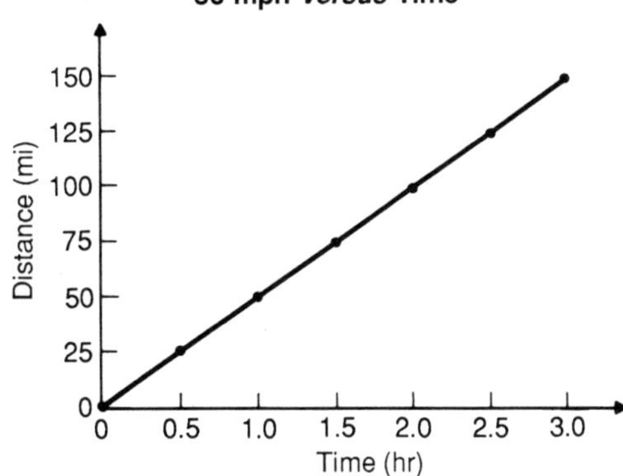

3. **Distance Ruler Falls *versus* Time to Grasp Between Thumb and Forefinger**

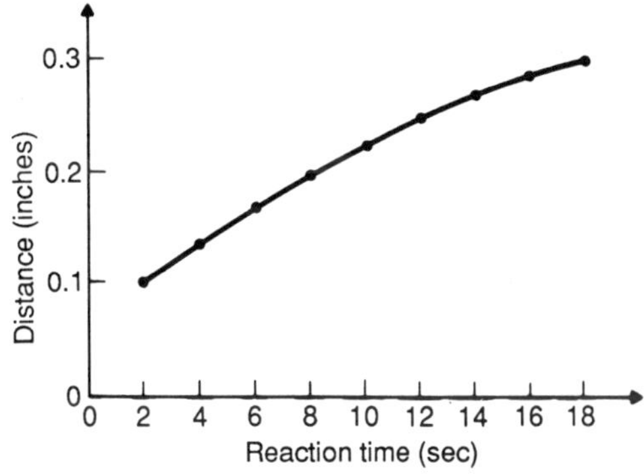

5. **Vapor Pressure of Water *versus* Temperature**

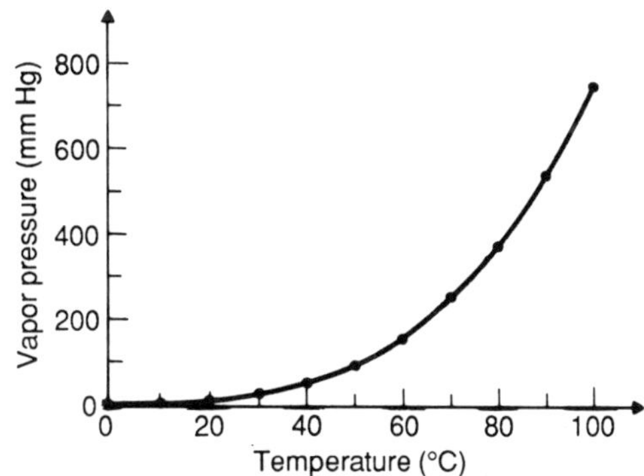

a. 100°C

b. approximately 118 mg Hg

7. 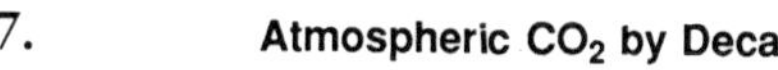

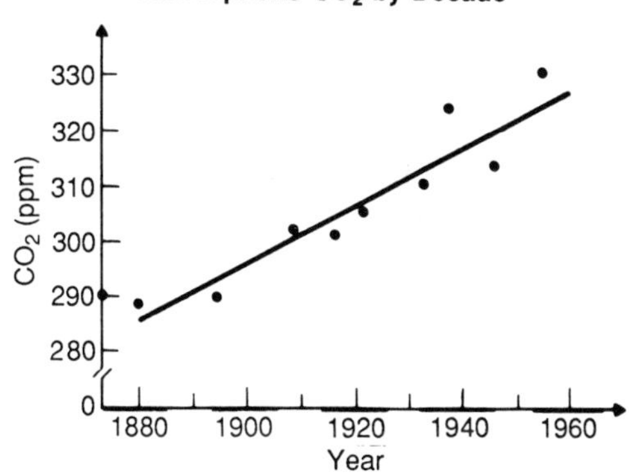

a. Straight line

b. It probably has continued to increase.

9.

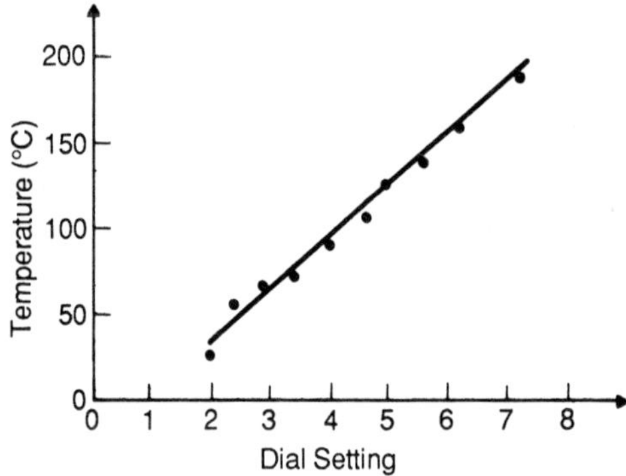

a. About 6.0

b. 161–162°C

11. a. Approximately 220 mg/dL

b. Approximately 0.28–0.29

c. Approximately 0.25–0.52

13. a. Approximately 36 g

b. Approximately 36 g

c. NaCl: approximately 38 g
KNO_3: approximately 85 g
The solubility of KNO_3 has more than doubled. The solubility of NaCl has barely changed.

d. Approximately 35°C

e. About 8 grams

f. No

Problem Set 3

1. **Percentage by Weight of Carbon, Hydrogen, and Oxygen in Ethanol**

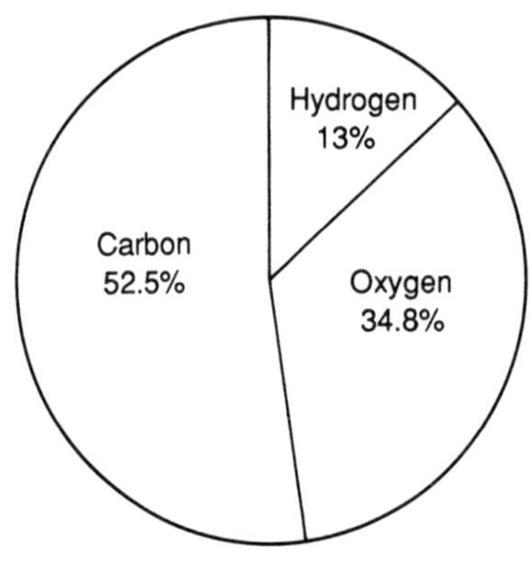

3. **Elemental Analysis of the Human Body**

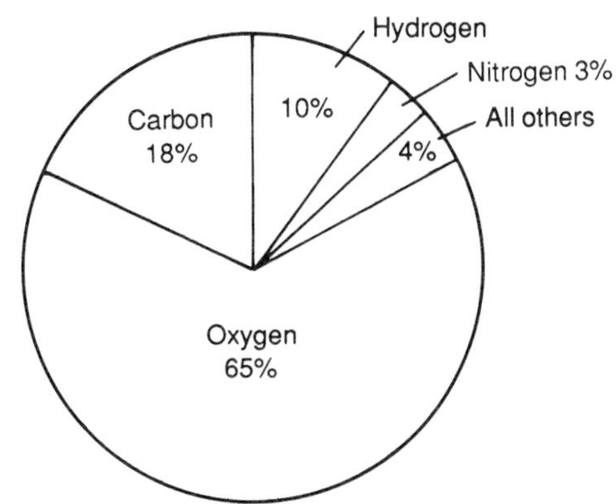

5. **Chemicals Produced in Greatest Quantities in 1984**

Billions of pounds produced

80
60
40
20
0

Sulfuric acid
Ammonia
Lime
Oxygen
Nitrogen
Ethylene

Chemicals

7. **pH Values For Some Common Solutions**

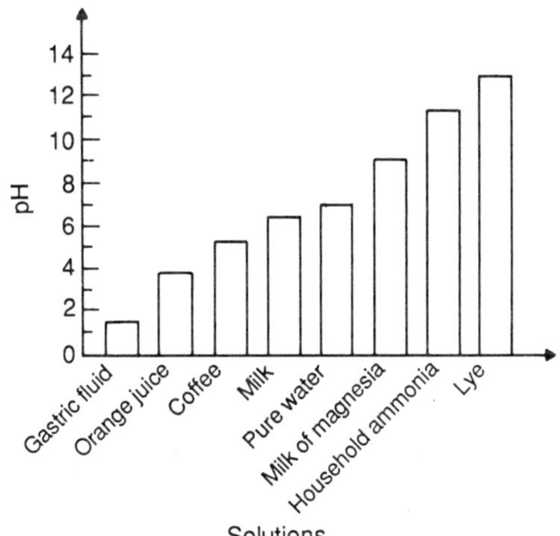

9.

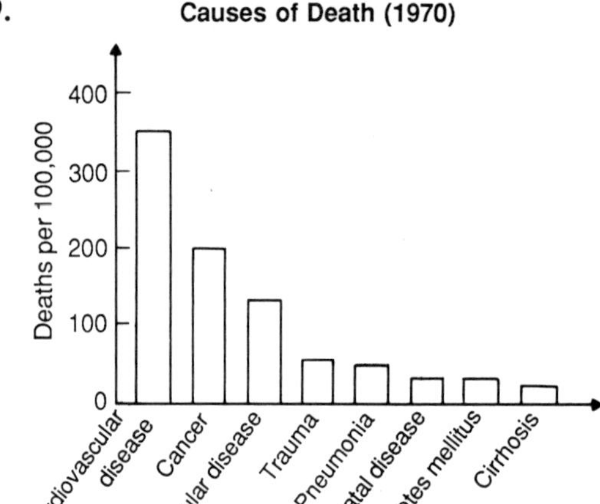

x	y
0	3
1	1
−1	5

Chapter Review

1. a. no b. yes c. yes

2. a.

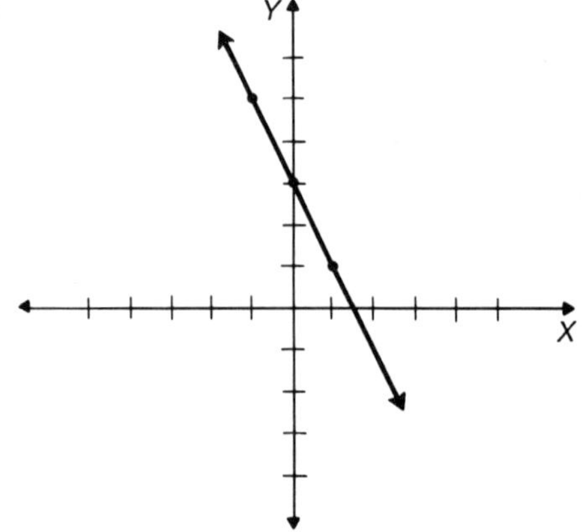

x	y
0	5
3	3
−3	7

b.

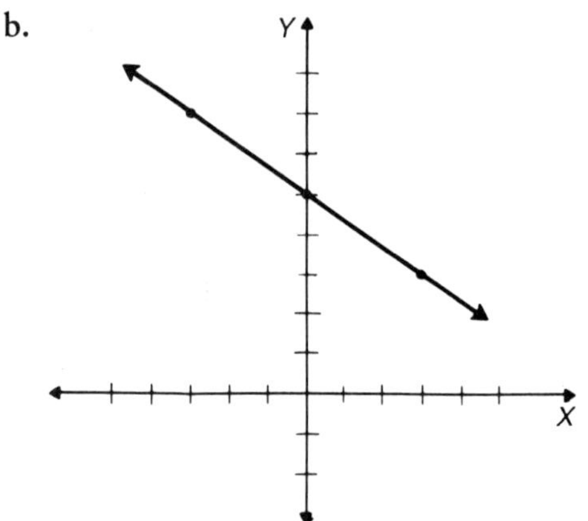

x	y
0	−1
$-\frac{1}{2}$	0
2	−5

c.

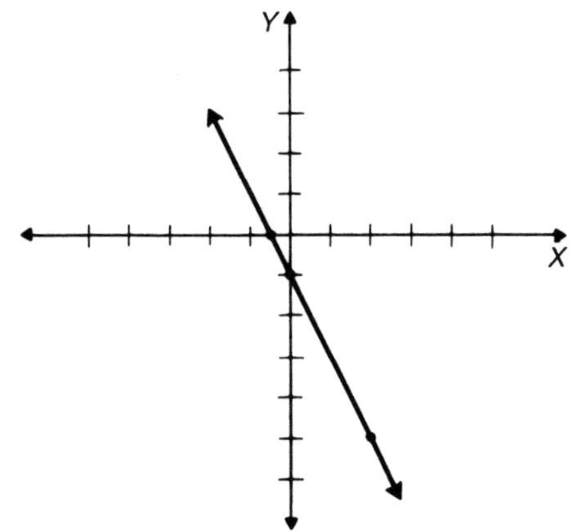

x	y
$1\frac{1}{2}$	2
1	6
2	−2

d.

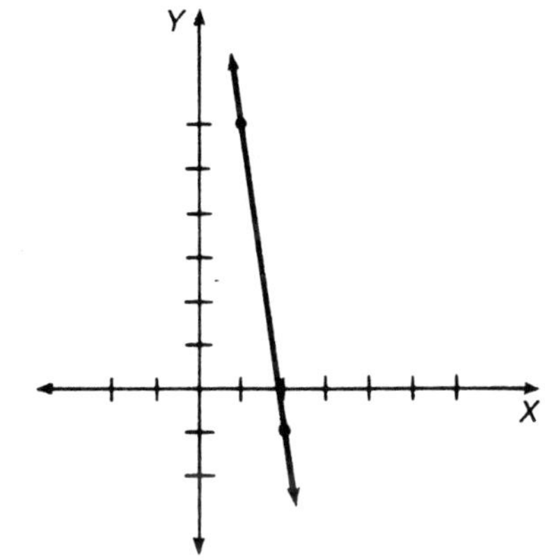

3. **Temperature of a Glass of Water *versus* Time**

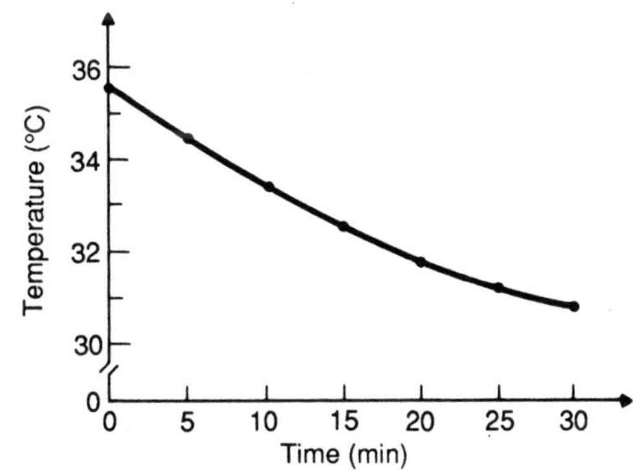

a. Approximately 33.8–33.9°C

b. No; after about 20 minutes

4. **Hemoglobin-Oxygen Dissociation Curve**

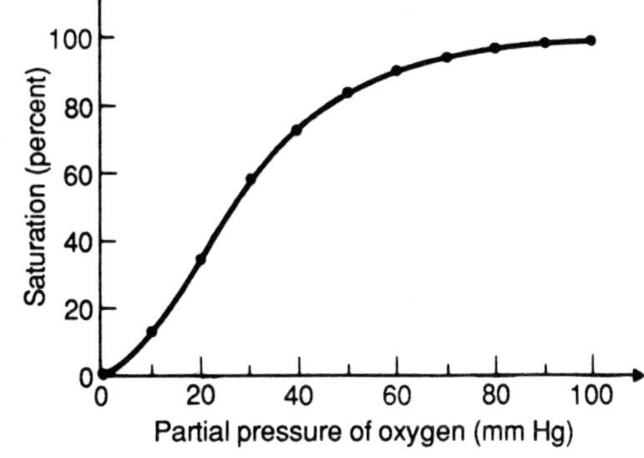

a. 24 mm Hg

b. About 6%

5. **Federal Budget Funds Allotted to Various Research and Development Departments (1985)**

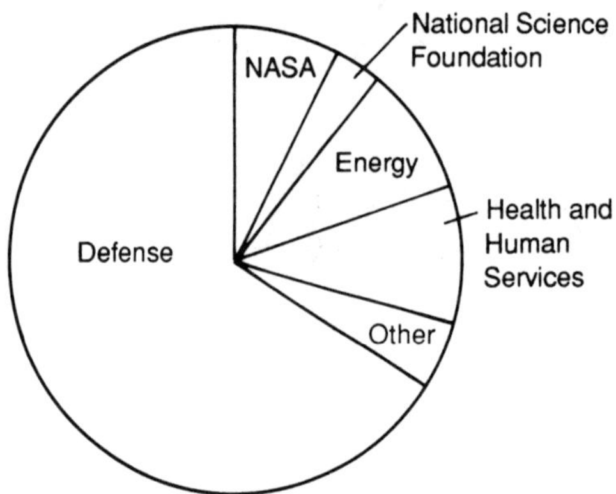

6. **Cases of Human Anthrax in the United States (1930-1979)**

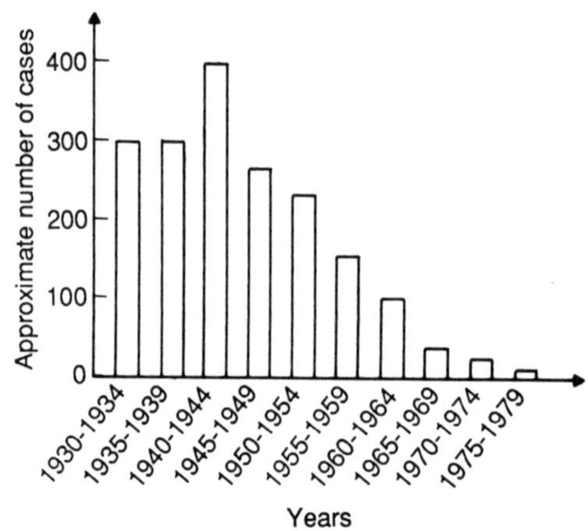

APPENDIX A

1. a. 113°F
   c. −40°F
   e. 838.8°F
2. a. 45°C
   c. −15°C
   e. 75.3°C
3. a. 373 K
   c. 0 K
   e. 1895 K
5. −196°C; −320.8°F
7. 34,727°C

APPENDIX B

1. 150 mA
3. 0.46 sec
5. 64 inches
7. 1.4 ft

Glossary

Abscissa. The horizontal axis (x axis) in the Cartesian Coordinate System

Absolute temperature. Temperature measurement beginning with zero degrees Kelvin at the point where no heat is present

Absolute value. The distance of a number from zero on a number line, regardless of direction

Absorbance. A measure of how much light is retained by a solution; the common logarithm of the inverse of the transmittance

Acid. Classically, a compound that yields hydrogen ions in a water solution

Accuracy. Closeness of a measurement to a standard or a true value

Acute angle. An angle which measures less than 90 degrees

Acute triangle. A triangle which has only acute angles

Altitude. Perpendicular distance between a vertex of a triangle and the opposite side; in a solid figure, the perpendicular distance between two faces

Angle. Two rays joined at a common endpoint

Antilogarithm. *See* Inverse logarithm

Apex. Point where the edges of the sides of a pyramid intersect

Area. Number of square units necessary to completely cover the interior of a plane figure

Atomic weight. The mass of one atom of an element; measured in atomic mass units

Bar graph. In statistics, a rectangular display of the frequencies of each class of a grouped frequency distribution

Base. Classically, a compound that yields hydroxide ions in a water solution *or* a number raised to a power; in 3^2, 3 is the base

Beer's law. An equation relating solution concentration to absorbance; usually results in a straight line when graphed

Bimodal distribution. A set of data containing two values which occur with equal frequency that is greater than that of all other values

Cartesian Coordinate System. A system of graphing which is based on two number lines at right angles; points are located by ordered pairs; also called the Rectangular Coordinate System

Center (of a circle). Point equidistant from all points on the circle

Circle. The set of all points in a plane equidistant from a given point called the center

Circumference. The perimeter of a circle; equal to pi times the diameter of the circle

Class boundaries. The number or limits obtained by extending class limits by one half of a unit

Class limits. The largest and smallest numbers of each interval in a grouped frequency distribution

Class mark. The number which represents all numbers in a class of a grouped frequency distribution; it is the mean of the class limits

Class width. The difference between the lower class limits of two adjoining classes in a grouped frequency distribution

Coefficient. The numerical part of an algebraic term

Colorimeter. An instrument used to measure the amount of light of a predetermined frequency passing through a solution

Companion scales. Different measuring scales with increments of the same width, as with Celsius and Kelvin temperature scales

Complementary angles. Two angles whose sum is 90 degrees

Conjugate base. The negative portion of an acid molecule after the hydrogen ion dissociates

Constant. A symbol which always represents the same numerical value

Continuous data. Values that can be measured as precisely as is practical, such as time, mass, volume, etc.

Conversion factor. An equivalence written as a fraction and multiplied by some other value in order to obtain a desired answer

Counting numbers. Natural numbers; 1, 2, 3, 4 . . .

Cube. The quantity that results when a number is raised to the third power *or* a box with all edges of equal length

Data. Numerical information collected from statistical samples

Decimal system. Any numerical system based on powers of 10

Dependent variable. A quantity that is changed because a related quantity (the independent variable) is changed

Diameter. A line segment passing through the center of a circle whose endpoints are on the circle

Dilution. The act of adding more solvent to a solution in order to lower the ratio of solute to solution; making a solution weaker

Dimensional analysis. A method of problem solving whereby units are used to aid in setting up a problem

Direct variation. An equation relating two variables in the form $y = kx$; as one variable increases, the other increases

Discrete data. Values that cannot be measured more precisely, such as a count of items

Edge. In a solid figure, the intersection of two faces (planes)

Equation. A statement that two quantities are equal

Equilateral triangle. A triangle with all sides of equal length

Equivalent. The amount of substance that will yield one mole of hydrogen ions or hydroxide ions, or one mole of charge

Exponent. The power to which a base is raised; as in 3^2, 2 is the exponent; the number of times a base is used as a factor

Exponential notation. Numbers written as powers of a base, commonly with a base of 10

Face. One side of a polyhedron

Focus-film distance. The distance, usually measured in inches, from the x-ray source to the x-ray film

Formula. An equation involving more than one variable, each representing actual measured quantities

Formula weight. The sum of the masses of all of the elements in a compound; measured in atomic mass units

Frequency histogram. *See* Bar graph

Frequency polygon. Pictoral display of the frequency of each class in a grouped frequency distribution, where each class is represented by the class mark

Frequency table. The listing of each individual piece of data together with the number of times it occurs

Gram. A unit of mass in the metric system; the mass of exactly one cubic centimeter of pure water at 4.5°C

Gram atomic weight. The atomic weight of an element expressed in grams rather than atomic mass units; equal to one mole of the element

Gram formula weight. The formula weight of a compound expressed in grams rather than atomic mass units; equal to one mole of the compound

Grouped frequency distribution. A set of data organized into intervals of equal width

Hypotenuse. The side opposite the right angle in a right triangle; the longest side of a right triangle

Independent variable. A quantity that is intentionally manipulated, which in turn affects another variable (the dependent variable)

Index. A number which appears outside and to the above left of a radical symbol, indicating which root is being taken

Integers. $\ldots -4, -3, -2, -1, 0, 1, 2, 3, 4 \ldots$

Intercept. The point where a line crosses either the x axis or the y axis

Intersecting lines. Lines which have one and only one point in common

Inverse logarithm. The result of raising a base to a known power

Inverse operations. Operations which undo each other

Inverse variation. An equation relating two variables in the form $y = k/x$; as one variable increases, the other decreases

Ionization constant. A number that indicates the degree of ionization of a weak acid (k_a) or a weak base (k_b)

Ion-product constant. For a water solution, the product of the concentrations of hydrogen ions and hydroxide ions; equal to 1×10^{-14}

Irrational number. Any number which cannot be expressed exactly as the ratio of two integers

Isoceles triangle. A triangle in which exactly two sides are equal in length

Joint variation. An equation relating several variables in the form $y = kxyz \ldots$

Line segment. The portion of a line between two points

Linear equation. An equation in the form $ax + by = c$; the solutions lie on a straight line

Liter. A unit of volume in the metric system; 1000 cubic centimeters

Literal equation. An equation involving more than one variable

Logarithm. Exponent placed on one quantity (called a base) to obtain another given quantity

Lowest common denominator. The smallest number or quantity divisible by every denominator in a group of fractions

Mass. The amount of matter contained in an object

Mean. The sum of a set of scores divided by the nuumber of scores; given by the formula $\bar{x} = \Sigma x/n$

Median. The middle number of a set of data with an odd number of entries; the mean of the two middle numbers of a set of data with an even number of entries

Meter. The base unit of length in the metric system

Milliampere. A measure of current; 1/1000 of an ampere

Mode. The single most frequently occurring value in a set of data

Molarity. A measurement of solution concentration; moles of solute divided by liters of solution

Mole. That amount of substance that contains the same number of particles as exactly 12 grams of carbon-12; an amount equal to the gram atomic weight of an element or the gram formula weight of a compound

Multimodal distribution. A set of data containing three or more values with equal frequency that is greater than that of all the other values

Natural numbers. *See* Counting numbers

Normal distribution. The set of data with approximately 68% of the values within one standard deviation of the mean; approximately 95% of the values within two standard deviations of the mean; and approximately 99.7% of the values within three standard deviations of the mean

Normality. A measure of concentration, used with ionic substances; equivalents of solute divided by liters of solution

Obtuse angle. An angle which measures more than 90 degrees but less than 180 degrees

Obtuse triangle. A triangle which has exactly one obtuse angle

Ordered pair. Two numbers that locate a point on the Cartesian Coordinate System; the first gives the distance from the y axis and the second, the distance from the x axis

Ordinate. The vertical (y axis) in the Cartesian Coordinate System.

Parallel. Lines which are in the same plane and never intersect

Parallelogram. A four-sided figure whose opposite sides are equal and parallel

Percent. A part of 100

Perimeter. The sum of the measures of the sides of a figure

Perpendicular. Lines which intersect at a right angle

pH. The negative of the logarithm of the hydrogen ion concentration of a water solution; a measure of acidity and alkalinity

Plane. Two-dimensional surface determined by three points not on the same line

Polyhedra. Solid figures with flat surfaces

Polyhedron. Singular of polyhedra

Power. The number of times a base is used as a repeated factor; *see also* Exponent

Precision. The level of care taken in making a measurement as reflected in the smallest place value reported in the measurement

Principal root. The positive result of placing a quantity under a radical with an even index; the only result of placing a quantity under a radical with an odd index

Prism. A polyhedron with two congruent sides in parallel planes, with the remaining sides in the shape of a parallelogram

Proportion. A statement that two ratios are equal

Proportionality constant. A numerical value which indicates exactly how two quantities are related

Protractor. An instrument used to measure and draw angles

Pyramid. A solid figure with a number of triangular side faces corresponding to the number of sides of its base

Pythagorean theorem. The sum of the squares of the legs of a right triangle is equal to the square of the hypotenuse

Radical. The symbol indicating that a root of a number is being taken

Radicand. The quantity appearing under a radical

Radiograph. An x-ray photograph

Radius. A line segment whose endpoints are the center of a circle and a point on the circle

Range. The difference between the largest and smallest values in a set of data

Ratio. A comparison of two quantities, usually in fractional form

Rational number. Any number which can be expressed exactly as the ratio of two integers, with the divisor not equal to zero

Ray. A portion of a line beginning with a given point and extending infinitely in only one direction

Rectangle. A parallelogram containing one right angle

Rectangular box. A prism with all faces in the shape of a rectangle

Relative temperature. A measurement of heat using both positive and negative numbers, usually in the Fahrenheit and Celsius scales

Rhombus. A parallelogram with all four sides equal

Right angle. An angle which measures 90 degrees

Right circular cone. A solid figure having a circular base with line segments connecting all points on the circumference of the base to a point directly above the center of the base

Right circular cylinder. A solid figure formed by enclosing the space between two circles in parallel planes with perpendicular lines

Right triangle. A triangle that contains a right angle

Root. The result of placing a quantity under a radical

Saturated solution. A solution where the solvent holds all of the solute possible at a given temperature

Scalene triangle. A triangle with no two sides equal

Scientific notation. Numbers written in exponential notation with the significant digit portion having a value between 1 and 10

Significant digits. Numbers that are the result of a measurement; measured digits

Significant digit portion. The factor that contains the significant digits of a measurement and is multiplied by an exponential factor

Solute. That part of a solution that is dissolved, or is present in the lesser quantity

Solution concentration. A measure of the relative proportions of solute and total solution; a measure of the strength of a solution

Solvent. That part of a solution that does the dissolving, or is present in the greater quantity

Spectrophotometer. *See* Colorimeter

Sphere. The set of all points in space equidistant from a given point called the center

Square. A parallelogram which contains four equal sides and one right angle *or* of a number, the quantity that results when the number is raised to the second power

Standard curve. A graph of the absorbance of a solution versus the corresponding concentrations; may be used to determine the strength of a solution of unknown concentration

Standard deviation. A numerical indicator of how widely data are dispersed about the mean

Standard position. The position of the decimal point that makes the significant digit portion of scientific notation a value between 1 and 10

Standard score. *See* z-score.

Standard solution. A solution whose concentration has been precisely determined

Statistics. Organization and interpretation of numerical information

Supplementary angles. Two angles whose sum is 180 degrees

Surface area. The number of square units covering the outside of a three dimensional figure

Système International (SI). The official version of the metric system, with these fundamental units: meter (length), cubic meter (volume), and kilogram (mass); health occupations use a slightly different version of this system

Temperature. A measure of heat energy

Term. An expression involving only multiplication and/or division of variables and/or constants.

Transmittance. A measure of the transparency of a solution; the ratio of initial light intensity to final light intensity.

Triangle. A three-sided figure formed by three line segments

Uncertain digit. The last digit reported in a measurement, usually approximated

Variable. A symbol, usually a letter, which can represent different numerical values

Variance. The square of the standard deviation of a set of individual scores or a grouped frequency distribution

Vertex. The point where parts of a figure are joined

Volume. The amount of space occupied by an object

Whole numbers. 0, 1, 2, 3, 4 . . .

z-score. The number of standard deviations a value is above or below the mean

Index